Cardiology

'Medical teachers know that half of what they teach
is untrue − the trouble is that they don't know which half.'

Attributed to Dr. C. S. Burwell
(formerly Dean, Harvard Medical School)

Fifth Edition

Cardiology

Desmond G. Julian MA, MD, FRCP, FRCP(E), FRACP, FACC

Emeritus Professor of Cardiology,
University of Newcastle upon Tyne;
Consultant Medical Director,
British Heart Foundation

Baillière Tindall   London·Philadelphia
Toronto·Sydney·Tokyo

| Baillière Tindall | 24—28 Oval Road |
| W.B. Saunders | London NW1 7DX |

West Washington Square
Philadelphia, PA 19105, USA

1 Goldthorne Avenue
Toronto, Ontario M8Z 5T9, Canada

ABP Australia Ltd
44—50 Waterloo Road
North Ryde, NSW 2113, Australia

Harcourt Brace Jovanovich Japan Inc
Ichibancho Central Building, 22—1 Ichibancho
Chiyoda-ku, Tokyo 102, Japan

First published 1970
Fourth edition 1983
Fifth edition 1988

Typeset by Setrite Typesetters Ltd., HK.
Printed in Great Britain by The Alden Press, Oxford

British Library Cataloguing in Publication Data

Julian, Desmond G.
  Cardiology.—5th ed.
  1. Heart—Diseases
  I. Title
  616.1'2   RC681

ISBN 0—7020—1259—9

Contents

Preface

The primary purpose of this book is to describe and explain cardiac disease in a way that is comprehensible to the student embarking on clinical medicine. It is also intended as a handbook for physicians, general practitioners, and nurses. In a book as short as this, oversimplification and dogmatism are inevitable, and those who wish to go more deeply into a specific subject are advised to consult the references provided at the end of each chapter as well as one of the several large textbooks available.

Cardiology has progressed rapidly since the publication of the fourth edition of this book in 1983, and it has therefore been very substantially rewritten. Much has been learned about the mechanisms involved in myocardial infarction and angina, which has led to important changes in management. Thrombolytic therapy, the more rational use of antianginal agents, and more experience of angioplasty have had a considerable impact on the care of patients with ischaemic heart disease. Non-invasive techniques, especially in ultrasound, continue to erode the role of cardiac catheterization in diagnosis, while the newer methods for the non-surgical relief of congenital and valvar heart disease (such as balloon pulmonary valvotomy) are increasing the role of the physician. There have been major improvements in the understanding of heart failure, and treatment has become more effective, particularly with the introduction of angiotensin converting enzyme inhibitors. Finally, large trials in hypertension have helped to clarify the indications for treatment of this disorder.

I am again indebted to Dr J.I. Hall and to Mr D.P. Hammersley for providing the illustrations, and to Drs S. Hunter and R.J.C. Hall for the ultrasound records.

In preparing this new edition, I have been helped by the comments and criticisms of many colleagues and friends, to whom I express my gratitude.

January 1988   D.G. Julian

Introduction

Diseases of the cardiovascular system are the main causes of death in the richer countries of the world and are of increasing importance in underdeveloped areas. In most Western countries, cardiovascular disease is responsible for approximately 50% of deaths, of which about half are due to ischaemic (coronary) heart disease. After increasing in nearly all countries, deaths due to coronary disease have diminished during the last decade in the United States, Australia and some European countries but continue to rise in others. Hypertension is the other main cardiovascular cause of death, and predominates in some countries, especially Japan. Rheumatic heart disease is responsible for perhaps 2% of all deaths but is the most important cardiac cause of disability and death in many parts of Asia, Africa and South America. Pulmonary heart disease is commonest in communities which have a heavy consumption of cigarettes and which are exposed to severe atmospheric pollution.

Because congenital and rheumatic heart diseases and hypertension are compatible with a long life span the relative prevalence of these conditions in the community differs from their incidence as causes of death.

The importance of the different types of heart disease varies considerably with age. Under the age of 15, heart disease is most commonly congenital, whereas between the age of 20 and 35 rheumatic heart disease is the major problem in those countries in which it is prevalent. Over this age cardiac disease is most likely to be due to coronary disease or hypertension (or a combination of the two). Pulmonary heart disease is largely confined to men over 45.

The epidemiology of each of these types of heart disease is discussed in the relevant chapter.

Myocardial Function: Heart Failure

Normal myocardial function

The primary function of the heart is to provide the tissues and organs of the body with a flow of oxygenated blood sufficient for their metabolic needs. In order to do this, it must pump a cardiac output (in the adult) of about 5 litres per minute at rest, and be able to increase this to 15 litres per minute or more on exercise. It must also adjust to great variations in peripheral resistance and venous return without substantially altering arterial, venous or intracardiac pressures. This ability both to maintain an adequate flow and to keep intracardiac and vascular pressures within a limited range is lost when cardiac failure develops.

The ways in which the ventricles as a whole respond to changing demands can be, to a considerable extent, explained by the structure and function of the sarcomere, the fundamental unit of cardiac contraction.

The structure and function of the sarcomere

Each muscle cell contains, amongst other structures, a nucleus, numerous mitochondria, and a number of parallel fibrils. Each fibril is made up of functional sub-units or sarcomeres. The sarcomere is composed of parallel actin and myosin filaments, arranged with the thin actin filaments attached to its limiting membrane (or Z line) and interdigitating with the thicker myosin filaments which are placed centrally (Fig. 2.1).

The myosin filaments are lined with a series of 'heads', which can flex, thus bringing them into contact with the actin filaments, and causing them to be drawn towards the centre of the sarcomere. The actin filaments contain the protein actin, together with the two regulatory proteins, troponin and tropomyosin (Fig. 2.1). The thread-like tropomyosin molecules lie in the trough between the two twisting strands of actin molecules. Troponin molecules are attached to the tropomyosin molecules at regular intervals. In the resting state, when the calcium level is low, troponin binds with actin and prevents cross-bridging with myosin. When activation causes a rise in calcium level, calcium ions bind with troponin;

Fig. 2.1 (A) Diagram of actin filament, showing relationships of actin, tropomyosin and troponin. (B, C, D) Relationships of actin (thin horizontal lines) and myosin (thick horizontal bars) in the sarcomere. In (B) the actin filaments are overriding each other. In (C) all bridges (vertical lines) are available for binding. In (D) the sarcomere is overextended; some sites are not engaged. Contraction is maximal when the greatest number of sites are available for interaction as in (C).

contraction can then occur as the inhibitory effect of troponin on cross-bridging is abolished.

The number of cross-bridges that develop is dependent upon

the number of calcium molecules available; the more bridges there are for interaction, the more forceful will be the resulting contraction.

The law of the heart, as enunciated by Starling, states that the more myocardial fibres are stretched (or the greater the diastolic volume of the heart) within physiological limits, the greater the energy of the ensuing contraction. Beyond these limits, the energy of contraction falls off. As the diastolic volume of the heart is directly related to sarcomere length, it is reasonable to explain Starling's law in terms of the ultrastructure of the myocardial cell. As the sarcomere is progressively stretched to its optimal length, and the diastolic fibre lengthens proportionately, the force of contraction progressively increases. If the sarcomere (or heart muscle) is stretched excessively, less force is generated.

The mechanics of the myocardium

Two important characteristics of heart muscle are the force with which it contracts, and the velocity with which it shortens, for these determine the volume of blood expelled during systole. Three major factors are responsible for the force and velocity of cardiac contraction: (1) the extent to which the muscle is stretched prior to contraction ('preload'), (2) the load that the ventricle faces during contraction ('afterload'), and (3) the contractile state of the myocardium.

Preload

If other factors are held constant, the force with which the heart contracts depends on the extent to which it has been stretched prior to contraction. This is a restatement of Starling's law. In effect, the preload is the volume of the ventricle at the end of diastole, i.e. the *end-diastolic volume*. The end-diastolic volume is largely determined by the venous return, which is, in turn, dependent upon a number of influences including the blood volume and venous tone. Another important factor affecting venous return is the distensibility (compliance) of the ventricle. Atrial contraction contributes appreciably to ventricular end-diastolic volume as it occurs immediately before ventricular systole. This atrial component of ventricular filling assumes importance when the ventricle is hypertrophied because passive filling is then impeded by the indistensibility (lack of compliance) of the ventricle.

Afterload

The ventricle has to develop sufficient tension during systole to expel blood into the aorta in the face of the resistance (or, more correctly, impedance) imposed by the aorta and peripheral arterial vessels. A further factor which becomes of importance in the dilated ventricle is the end-diastolic volume (see p. 11).

The contractile state of the myocardium

If the end-diastolic volume and the aortic impedance are held constant, the force and velocity of contraction of the myocardium depend upon its contractile state. For a given end-diastolic volume, therefore, changes in contractility can alter the performance of the ventricle (see Fig. 2.2). Myocardial contractility is largely dependent upon the activity of the cardiac sympathetic nerves, but it can also be increased by circulating catecholamines, tachycardia, cardiac glycosides and isoprenaline. Myocardial contractility is depressed by hypoxia, quinidine and procainamide.

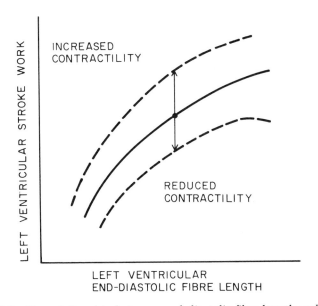

Fig. 2.2 The relationship between end-diastolic fibre length and the left ventricular stroke work. For any given end-diastolic fibre length, increased contractility, such as is produced by sympathetic action, produces more stroke work. Reduced contractility, as occurs in cardiac failure, produces less work. Similarly, if the arrows were drawn horizontally instead of vertically, it would be seen that for any given amount of work, increased contractility enables this to be performed at a smaller end-diastolic fibre length. In cardiac failure, a given amount of stroke work can only be achieved with a greater end-diastolic fibre length.

Mechanisms which lead to an increased ventricular perform-ance, such as an enlarged end-diastolic volume or sympathetic stimulation, also involve an increase in myocardial oxygen consumption. The greater ventricular performance does not neces-sarily, therefore, mean an increase in cardiac efficiency. Indeed, the increase in myocardial oxygen consumption is dispropor-tionately great in relation to the increase in work performed.

Impaired diastolic function

Disorders of relaxation of the ventricle are common, particularly in ischaemic heart disease. Ischaemia leads to increased stiffness in the myocardium and, therefore, to a raised end-diastolic pressure.

The effect of exercise

Cardiovascular changes take place as soon as exercise is antici-pated — as a result of vagal inhibition and a generalized sympa-thetic discharge. Both heart rate and myocardial contractility increase. The resistance vessels in the muscles dilate whilst those supplying the kidneys, abdominal viscera and skin constrict. The overall effect is to increase cardiac output and, specifically, the blood supply to the muscles.

With the onset of exercise, further dilatation of muscular arter-ioles and capillaries occurs and venous return is augmented by the pumping action of the muscles. The systolic blood pressure rises, the increase roughly corresponding to the severity of the exercise. Diastolic pressure changes little.

The energy supply of the myocardial cell

Energy is produced in the heart by the process of oxidative phosphorylation. This results from the conversion of the energy produced by the oxidation of substrates such as glucose, lactate and fatty acids into the energy of adenosine triphosphate (ATP) and creatine phosphate (CP). These substances provide the energy source for muscular contraction. Normally, free fatty acids are the main substrate, but in ischaemia the glycolytic pathway is stimulated.

Excitation–contraction coupling

The electrical excitation of the cell leads to a series of events which results in contraction of the heart muscle. This process, which is not as yet fully understood, involves transverse channels ('T' tubules) formed by invagination of the sarcolemma enshea-thing the cell, and the sarcoplasmic reticulum, a network of membrane-lined channels which run longitudinally in contact with the individual sarcomeres (Fig. 2.3). It has been postulated that the electrical stimulus traverses the transverse channels and then proceeds along the longitudinal channels releasing calcium. The calcium is then transferred into the fibril and causes contraction by activating adenosine triphosphatase (ATPase). Repolarization is associated with a reversal of the process and the active pumping of calcium back into the sarcoplasmic tubules.

The pressure and volume changes in the heart and great vessels during the cardiac cycle (Figs. 2.4 and 2.5)

With the onset of left ventricular systole, the mitral valve closes and the pressure in the ventricle rises rapidly. Until the aortic valve opens, the volume of the ventricle remains unchanged, this being the period of isovolumetric contraction. As soon as the aortic valve opens, blood is rapidly ejected from the ventricle into the aorta. This phase is followed by one of relatively slow ejection. Shortly after ejection ceases, the aortic valve closes. As the ventricle relaxes, the pressure within it falls rapidly, but until it has fallen to the level present in the left atrium, the volume in the ventricle remains unchanged, this being the period of isovolumetric relaxation. When the pressure in the ventricle falls below that in the atrium, the mitral valve opens and a period of rapid ventricular filling ensues. This is followed by a slow phase, or diastasis, during which the pressure rises slowly. This continues until atrial contraction propels more blood through the mitral valve and causes a small increase in left ventricular volume and pressure prior to the onset of the next ventricular systole.

Fig. 2.3 Note the relationship between the longitudinal tubules of the sarcoplasmic reticulum and the sarcomere, and between the lateral sac of the sarcoplasmic reticulum and the transverse channel ('T' tubule).

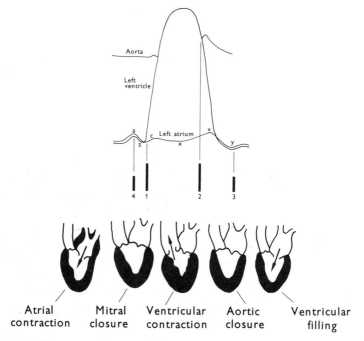

Fig. 2.4   Pressure pulses in the left atrium, left ventricle and aorta (see text).

In the left atrium, there are three waves in the cardiac cycle, the crests being designated 'a', 'c' and 'v', and the troughs 'x', 'y' and 'z'. The 'a' wave is due to atrial contraction, which is followed by a 'z' trough associated with atrial relaxation. After this, there is a 'c' wave as a result of upward movement of the mitral valve cusps, with a subsequent 'x' descent as the mitral valve ring descends as the ventricle contracts. During the latter portion of ventricular systole, with the mitral valve closed, there is a build up of pressure in the atrium with increasing pulmonary venous return. This rising pressure is terminated when the mitral valve opens. At this point, the peak of the 'v' wave is produced. The 'y' descent follows as blood flows into the ventricle during ventricular diastole. (From the opening of the mitral valve to its closure at the onset of ventricular systole, the pressures in the atrium and the ventricle are almost identical.) Events on the right side of the heart mirror those on the left but they take place slightly later so that tricuspid valve closure occurs shortly after mitral valve closure, and closure of the pulmonary valve follows that of the aortic valve. The timing of pulmonary valve closure varies with respiration. The increased negative pressure in the thorax during inspiration results in an augmented venous return to the right side of the heart. As a consequence of this transient increase in blood flow, ejection of blood in the right side of the heart is delayed and pulmonary valve closure occurs relatively later during inspiration than it does during expiration.

Heart failure

Failure in anything implies expectations unfulfilled, and one's definition of heart failure depends upon what one expects of the heart. No single definition suffices because the clinical and physiological criteria necessarily differ.

The clinician regards his patient as having heart failure when there are symptoms or physical signs attributable to inadequate cardiac performance. The physiologist regards the heart as failing when the contractility of the ventricles or the cardiac output falls outside the statistically defined normal range. There is no clear distinction between normality and abnormality; values in the 'abnormal' range may be found in normal hearts in the face of extreme demand, and 'normal' values may be encountered in diseased hearts when the demands are slight. Nonetheless, if one is aware of the shortcomings, some definitions of heart failure may be accepted.

To Sir Thomas Lewis, heart failure was 'an inability of the heart to discharge its contents adequately'; to Paul Wood it was 'a state in which the heart fails to maintain an adequate circulation for the needs of the body despite a satisfactory venous filling pressure' (thereby excluding from consideration inadequate cardiac output due to insufficient venous return).

Cardiac failure, as it is understood in clinical practice, denotes the presence of one of the complexes of symptoms and signs associated with the 'congestion' of tissues and organs or attributable to the inadequate perfusion of tissues and organs. Pulmonary venous congestion results from disordered function of the left ventricle or left atrium.

Systemic venous congestion is similarly due to disorders of the right ventricle and atrium, but is often the end-result of left-sided heart failure. The clinical features derive, in the main, from engorgement of the systemic veins and capillaries.

The heart has also failed when it cannot maintain an adequate blood pressure in spite of a peripheral vascular resistance that is normal or high but, by convention, this type of cardiac failure is referred to as acute circulatory failure or cardiogenic shock rather than heart failure.

Fig.2.5   Relationships between left ventricular pressure and left ventricular volume in the normal heart, in aortic stenosis and in mitral regurgitation. In the normal heart, following the closure of the mitral valve (M_1), there is a rapid rise in pressure without any change in volume until the aortic valve opens. Pressure then rises more slowly as the left ventricle ejects blood; in later systole, there is a fall-off in pressure, though ejection continues until the aortic valve closes (A_2). The phase of isovolumetric relaxation then occurs followed by diastolic filling with little change in pressure. The salient feature of aortic stenosis is the pressure load; mitral regurgitation is associated with a volume load leading to an increase in ventricular volume at the end of both systole and diastole.

The causes of heart failure

The heart fails either because it is subjected to an overwhelming load, or because the heart muscle is disordered, or as a result of a combination of the two.

An increased work load (Fig. 2.5) can be of two different types — a volume load (preload) and a pressure load (afterload). A volume load is imposed by disorders which demand that the ventricle expels more blood per minute than is normal. Examples include thyrotoxicosis and anaemia, in which the total cardiac output is increased; and mitral regurgitation and aortic regurgitation, in which the left ventricle has to expel not only the normal forward flow into the aorta but also the large volume of regurgitated blood as well.

Pressure loads are imposed by disorders which increase resistance to outflow from the ventricles (typified by systemic hypertension due to increased impedance of the peripheral arterioles, and by aortic stenosis in which there is narrowing of the outflow orifice of the left ventricle.)

Disorders of myocardial function result not only from diminished contractility but also from loss of contractile tissue, as occurs in myocardial infarction. An additional factor in this condition is a paradoxical movement of infarcted muscle which further increases the work of the remaining myocardium.

In rheumatic heart disease, the different mechanisms of heart failure are often combined, with myocardial damage, valve narrowing and valvar regurgitation all participating in its production.

Cardiac and circulatory responses in heart failure

The heart at first responds to pressure and volume overloads in much the same way as it does to normal increases in demand, such as those imposed by exercise. As the disorder progresses, more cardiac and circulatory adjustments take place which for a time, may maintain an adequate circulation but many of the so-called 'compensatory' mechanisms are inappropriate. As Harris has pointed out, during evolution the circulatory system has had to evolve methods of combating blood loss and trauma rather than, for example, myocardial infarction, and the responses invoked are relevant to the former stresses rather than the latter. Indeed, the clinical manifestations of heart failure are largely the effects of 'compensatory' mechanisms which eventually embarrass the circulation.

Dilatation of the heart — increase in end-diastolic volume

In response to a volume load, the heart dilates, i.e. the ventricular volume is increased. Up to a point, dilatation is a normal and efficient response but it is abnormal when it cannot be wholly ascribed to the volume load. Pathological dilatation of this kind occurs when there is myocardial disease, when, because of decreased contractility, the ventricle must be stretched to a greater extent for a given stroke volume. Even in those cases in which dilatation may at first be regarded as a physiological response, it eventually becomes disadvantageous because, as the ventricle increases in size, greater tension is required in the myocardium to expel a given volume of blood. This is in accordance with the law of Laplace which indicates that the tension in the myocardium (T) is proportional to the intraventricular pressure (P) multiplied by the radius (R) of the ventricular chamber ($T \propto PR$). The greater tension results in increased oxygen requirements and eventually leads to hypertrophy.

Hypertrophy of the heart

When the ventricle has to face a chronic increase of pressure load, such as that imposed by arterial hypertension, aortic stenosis or pulmonary hypertension, the myocardium hypertrophies, i.e. it increases in weight as a result of an enlargement of individual muscle fibres. The process affects only those chambers upon which there are increased demands. The mechanism responsible for the development of cardiac hypertrophy is uncertain but it seems likely that it is a response to increased stretching or tension in muscle fibres which result from a raised diastolic volume or pressure. Hypertrophy may be regarded as a normal compensatory mechanism which permits the heart to cope with the increased demands, but becomes self-defeating when it is excessive. The thickening of the fibres increases the distance which oxygen has to diffuse from the capillaries; eventually this leads to impaired oxygenation of the centre of the fibre. It is probable that this hypoxia is an important factor in the fibrosis which frequently develops in hypertrophied muscle.

Impaired myocardial contractility

In many types of heart disease, the major defect lies in the myocardium itself. This is the case in ischaemic heart disease, myocarditis and cardiomyopathy, and myocardial involvement is often considerable in rheumatic heart disease. Even when the primary disturbance is that of a volume or pressure overload, intrinsic myocardial function may be eventually affected adversely by dilatation and hypertrophy. Why the impaired myocardial contractility develops is uncertain, but it has been attributed by some to overstretching of the sarcomeres (see p. 4). There may be a slowing up in the conversion of chemical energy into muscular work as a result of depression in the activity of ATPase, the enzyme responsible for the release of energy from ATP. There may also be a defect in excitation—contraction coupling in heart failure because it has been noted that the cardiac glycosides which improve myocardial function in heart failure appear to enhance the release of calcium by the sarcoplasmic reticulum (see p. 6). A further factor which may reduce myocardial contractility is a depletion of noradrenaline (norepinephrine) stores in the myocardium.

The cardiac output in heart failure

By definition cardiac failure is present when the cardiac output is insufficient for the needs of the body, but some patients with an output in the normal range manifest the clinical features of cardiac failure, whereas other patients with low outputs are free of symptoms and signs. However, in cardiac failure, even if the cardiac output is normal at rest it usually responds inadequately to exercise. In conditions, such as beri-beri and thyrotoxicosis, in which the cardiac output is abnormally high, it is still insufficient for the exceptional metabolic demands.

Neuroendocrine response to heart failure

Cardiac failure activates several components of the neuroendocrine system, which play an important intermediary role in its clinical manifestations (Fig. 2.6).

Sympathetic nervous system. Activation of the sympathetic nervous system results in an increase in myocardial contractility, heart rate, and vasoconstriction of arteries and veins. Although this may be beneficial in maintaining blood pressure, it is adverse insofar as it increases preload, afterload, and myocardial oxygen requirement. There is also an increased plasma noradrenaline, but myocardial catecholamines are reduced.

Renin—angiotensin—aldosterone systems. Both the fall in cardiac output itself and the increase in sympathetic tone reduce effective blood flow to the kidney and consequently, increase renin secretion. Salt restriction and diuretic therapy also augment this. As a result, there is a rise in angiotensin II levels, which leads

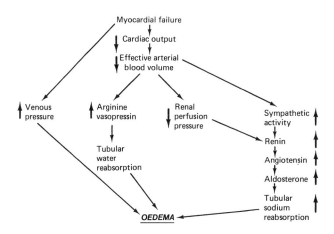

Fig. 2.6 Some of the neuroendocrine and renal responses to cardiac failure.

directly to vasoconstriction and indirectly, by stimulating aldosterone secretion, to sodium retention and the expansion of blood
volume. This is advantageous insofar as increasing preload helps
to maintain stroke volume by the Starling mechanism, but it does
so at the expense of circulatory congestion.

Arginine vasopressin (antidiuretic hormone). The reduced effective blood volume of heart failure stimulates the release of arginine
vasopressin, leading to water retention. This is a feature of later,
rather than early, cardiac failure.

Atrial natriuretic peptide. Distension of the atria leads to the
release of this peptide which has natriuretic and vasodilator properties. Its role in cardiac failure is still unclear.

The regional circulations in cardiac failure

There is a redistribution of blood flow to different organs and
tissues in cardiac failure, as there is on exercise. This redistribution is mediated through vasoconstriction in certain areas, notably
the renal arterioles. The renal blood flow falls disproportionately,
and may be reduced to one-quarter of normal. There is little
reduction in the coronary or cerebral blood flow, but there is
vasoconstriction of the skin and splanchnic vessels.

Salt and water retention

An almost invariable feature of cardiac failure is the retention of
sodium and water. This leads to a substantial increase in extracellular and plasma volume and plays a large part in the production
of the clinical features of cardiac failure. Some of the factors
responsible for the fluid and salt retention are discussed above,
but undoubtedly there are still undiscovered mechanisms.

Diminished glomerular filtration. Glomerular filtration is reduced
in cardiac failure, although to a lesser extent than is renal blood
flow. Diminished glomerular filtration may play some part in
sodium retention, but it is probably not an important factor
except when the failure is severe.

Increased tubular reabsorption. There is abundant experimental
evidence that tubular reabsorption of sodium is increased in
cardiac failure. There is no doubt that, in certain patients, there is
increased aldosterone secretion, and that this hormone, by its
action on the distal tubule, promotes the reabsorption of sodium
whilst increasing the excretion of potassium and hydrogen.
However, evidence of hyperaldosteronism is confined to advanced

failure; aldosterone antagonists are relatively ineffective in the treatment of sodium retention in early failure. The enhanced tubular reabsorption of sodium found in cardiac failure seems to be mediated through some mechanism as yet undiscovered.

As mentioned, water retention in heart failure is usually secondary to sodium retention. In some patients with advanced cardiac failure, however, there is a disproportionate retention of water. In these patients, the kidneys can no longer excrete solute-free water and the serum sodium concentration falls as a result of dilution ('dilutional hyponatraemia').

Raised venous pressure in cardiac failure

When the left ventricle fails the pulmonary venous pressure rises, and when the right ventricle fails the pressure rises in the systemic veins. This can be largely explained by the inability of the failing ventricle to discharge the blood presented to it effectively. The increased blood volume resulting from sodium and water retention contributes to the venous return and is thus a factor in producing the raised venous pressure, as is venoconstriction.

The effect of left ventricular failure on the lungs

As explained above, when the left ventricle fails, the diastolic pressure in the left ventricle rises and with it the left atrial pressure. Since the pulmonary veins and capillaries are in continuity with the left atrium, the pressures in these vessels rise concomitantly. In mild left ventricular failure, the pressures in the left atrium and pulmonary veins are within normal limits at rest but rise on exercise. As failure advances, the left atrial pressure progressively increases from its normal level of 5–10 mmHg to one of 25–30 mmHg. The hydrostatic pressure in the capillaries is then close to that needed to overcome the osmotic pressure exerted by the plasma proteins and may lead to an exudation of fluid from the capillaries into the alveolar walls and alveoli. If the pressure in the atrium rises rapidly, there may be a sudden exudation of fluid into the alveoli. If this process takes place slowly, exudation may proceed gradually with a slow build up of tissue tension occurring in the alveolar wall. This restricts further exudation of fluid and limits the risk to the alveoli. In response to this process, some fibrosis may take place in the alveolar wall. The pulmonary congestion caused by the high pulmonary venous pressure and by the changes in the alveolar walls makes the lung more rigid (less compliant). As a result of this, more work must be done by the respiratory muscles to move a given volume of air. The stretch receptors in the lung are stimulated and this leads to hyperventilation.

Left heart failure

Aetiology

The features of left heart failure develop when there is a major obstruction to outflow from the left atrium (e.g. mitral stenosis) or when the left ventricle can no longer cope with the demands upon it. The common causes of left ventricular failure are systemic hypertension, aortic valve disease, mitral regurgitation, myocardial infarction and cardiomyopathy.

Clinical features

The clinical features of left-side cardiac failure are largely the consequence of pulmonary congestion. The symptoms are, there-fore, those of dyspnoea on exertion, orthopnoea, paroxysmal dyspnoea and acute pulmonary oedema. Pulmonary congestion may lead to the physical signs of tachypnoea, crepitations in the lungs and, sometimes, hydrothorax. More direct evidence that the left ventricle is failing is supplied by the presence of pulsus alternans and by a third heart sound.

The chest radiograph shows pulmonary venous congestion and, in the more severe cases, oedema.

The electrocardiogram may be of value although it does not provide direct evidence of left heart failure. For example, it is unusual for hypertension or aortic valve disease to lead to the symptoms of left heart failure without producing ECG evidence of left ventricular hypertrophy first. Again, it is unusual for coronary artery disease to lead to left heart failure if the ECG is normal. This is not, however, true of mitral regurgitation.

The diagnosis of left heart failure is usually not difficult when there is progressive dyspnoea coupled with clinical evidence of advanced left-sided heart disease. However, this evidence may not always be unequivocal and there may be difficulty in dis-tinguishing the symptoms of heart failure from those of pulmonary disease. The dyspnoea of left heart failure is more likely to be provoked by lying down flat. Patients with dyspnoea due to pulmonary disease usually have a history of asthmatic attacks or of chronic cough and sputum.

Paroxysmal nocturnal dyspnoea and acute pulmonary oedema may be difficult to differentiate from acute respiratory attacks. The latter are commonly associated with bronchospasm and purulent sputum. In contrast, the patient with acute pulmonary oedema is usually free of pulmonary infection, has fine crepitations rather than rhonchi and is liable to cough up pink frothy sputum. Furthermore, examination usually reveals the signs of left-sided heart disease. Correct diagnosis is of great importance because the therapy of the two conditions is different. For example, morphine may be lethal in respiratory failure, but invaluable in acute pulmonary oedema. Similarly, high concentrations of oxygen are useful in acute pulmonary oedema but may be dangerous in respiratory failure. The chest radiograph is also helpful in showing signs of oedema or infection. In cases of doubt, estimation of the arterial CO_2 tension is of value because this is usually low in acute pulmonary oedema and high in respiratory failure.

Right heart failure

Aetiology

Failure of the right side of the heart occurs when the right ventricle can no longer cope with the demands upon it, or when there is tricuspid stenosis. Right ventricular failure often follows left ventricular failure, with its consequent effects upon the pulmonary circulation. It also results from right ventricular infarction, pulmonary disease, particularly chronic bronchitis and emphysema, pulmonary valve disease and tricuspid regurgitation.

Clinical features

The characteristic features of right heart failure are those of raised systemic venous pressure and its effects. In the normal individual, the venous pressure in the internal jugular veins does not exceed 2 cm vertically above the sternal angle when the patient is reclining at 45 degrees. In right heart failure this figure is exceeded. Even if normal at rest, it rises on exercise.

Almost as important as the rise in venous pressure is enlargement of the liver which, if chronic, may result in cirrhosis. The third important feature of right heart failure is oedema, which is of the dependent type and usually most evident in the pretibial and ankle regions. Less frequently, ascites occurs.

Other clinical features of cardiac failure

There are a number of common but less specific features of cardiac failure. Fatigue is a frequent symptom which is difficult to evaluate.

The nutrition of patients with cardiac failure is often good in the early stages, but cachexia sets in as disability increases. In the very advanced case, cerebral symptoms may develop with dulling of consciousness, confusion or changes in personality. Patients with cardiac failure are prone to develop venous thrombosis and pulmonary emboli are common. Mild jaundice, due to hepatic congestion or cirrhosis, is quite frequent in right-sided heart failure. Proteinuria due to renal congestion is often present.

Precipitating factors in cardiac failure

Cardiac failure is often precipitated or exacerbated by factors superimposed on the underlying heart disease. Amongst these are arrhythmias, infections, pulmonary embolism, pregnancy, anaemia, excessive sodium intake and over-exertion. The recognition of precipitating factors is of great importance in the management of heart failure, because the correction of these complicating conditions will often result in the abolition of symptoms.

The management of cardiac failure

Ideally, the treatment of cardiac failure is the correction of the cause, but for a variety of reasons this may not be possible, at least initially. In some conditions, such as ischaemic heart disease and the cardiomyopathies, no currently available methods of treatment affect the underlying lesions. In other disorders, the radical treatment necessary for cure, such as major surgery, cannot be safely undertaken until cardiac failure has been corrected.
The principles of treating cardiac failure may be enumerated as follows:

1   the correction or amelioration of the underlying disease;
2   the control of complicating factors;
3   the reduction of demands on the heart by weight loss and the restriction of physical activity;
4   the improvement of myocardial function by the administration of inotropic drugs such as the digitalis glycosides;
5   the correct of sodium and water retention;
6   reduction of preload and/or afterload by vasodilator drugs.

The correction or amelioration of the underlying cause

When heart disease is due to such causes as thyrotoxicosis or hypertension, corrective treatment can be started immediately. In congenital and rheumatic heart disease, surgical management is usually required, but this may have to be deferred until the maximum benefit has been achieved from medical treatment.

The correction of complicating factors

The control of arrhythmias, the correction of anaemia and the treatment of infections play important roles in the management of cardiac failure.

Restriction of activity

Rest reduces the demands on the heart and leads to a fall in venous pressure and a reduction in pulmonary congestion. It allows a relative increase in renal blood flow and often leads to a diuresis. However, bed rest also encourages the development of venous thrombosis and pulmonary embolism.

The degree of physical restriction necessary depends upon the severity of the cardiac failure. When there is severe pulmonary congestion or peripheral oedema, a period of complete rest may be required. At this time, the patient is usually most comfortable propped up by two or more pillows in bed or in an armchair. Complete bed rest is seldom necessary for more than a few days, after which a gradual increase in activity may be encouraged, depending upon the response. In patients with lesser degrees of cardiac failure, there may be no need to enforce bed rest, but excessive activity, particularly walking up hills and stairs, should be temporarily avoided. The degree of physical restriction necessary can be largely determined by the relief of symptoms and the disappearance of the signs of failure.

When the patient has improved, moderate exercise should be encouraged if this does not produce symptoms.

Therapy with inotropic drugs

Drugs which increase myocardial contractility (positive inotropic agents) can augment cardiac output and relieve cardiac failure, but may also increase myocardial oxygen requirement. There is no doubt that in acute myocardial failure such drugs may be beneficial, but their long-term effectiveness is disputed. There are three main groups of inotropic drugs.

1 Digitalis glycosides.
2 Sympathomimetic agents, such as dopamine and dobutamine. These are mainly used intravenously for acute heart failure and are discussed on p. 29.
3 Phosphodiesterase inhibitors. At present, these have little place in therapy, but there are a number of new drugs, such as milrinone, undergoing evaluation.

Digitalis and related compounds. These have, for many years, been regarded as standard therapy for cardiac failure and are the only inotropic agents widely used for its long-term management. They are of undoubted value in the control of supraventricular arrhythmias (especially atrial fibrillation) and if these are of importance in the genesis of cardiac failure, they will quickly relieve it. Their role in cardiac failure in sinus rhythm remains controversial, but they are likely to be beneficial in the dilated heart, because they reduce end-diastolic volume and, thereby, myocardial tension and oxygen requirement.

The inotropic action of digitalis is mediated through the sodium/ potassium-ATPase (sodium) pump, to which it binds. The inhibition of this pump leads to an accumulation of intracellular sodium; because of the sodium–calcium carrier system, this results in an increase in the amount of calcium available to activate contraction. Digitalis also has sympathomimetic and parasympathetic (vagal) effects. The latter is clinically important, in that it causes slowing of the sinus rate and delays conduction through the atrioventricular node. Digitalis reduces the refractory period of atrial and ventricular muscle and, therefore, enhances the risk of ectopic rhythms.

There are many preparations available, but digoxin in one or other of its forms is suitable for most cases. The most commonly used tablet contains 0.25 mg; tablets containing 125 and 62.5 μg are useful in children and the elderly. Suggested dosage schemes are shown in Table 2.1.

Most preparations are well absorbed from the intestinal tract, although with differing degrees of completeness. Digitoxin is almost 100% absorbed in contrast with about 80% in the case of digoxin. Because oral therapy is safest, this route should be used if possible. The intravenous route should be employed only in cases of urgency and should always be avoided if a digitalis preparation has been administered within the previous week.

Intravenous digoxin produces an effect within 15 minutes and has peak activity in about 2 hours. When given by mouth, the effects start in about an hour and are maximal at about 6 hours.

Digoxin is excreted in an unchanged form by the kidneys. This is normally complete in 4–5 days, but is delayed in the presence of renal failure.

Digitalis glycosides may be involved in important drug interactions. Thus quinidine increases the plasma concentrations of digoxin, probably by displacing it from tissue sites. Amiodarone and verapamil seem to have similar effects. When any of these drugs is added the dosage of the glycosides should be reduced. Because hypokalaemia enhances digitalis toxicity, concomitant treatment with potassium losing diuretics must be cautious.

The commonest toxic effects of digitalis therapy are malaise, anorexia, nausea and, later, vomiting. In some patients, there is excessive salivation, yellow vision or diarrhoea.

More serious than these symptoms are the many different types of conduction and rhythm disturbance that may occur. The most frequent are ventricular ectopic rhythms, often taking the form of coupling (bigeminy). This may be well tolerated, but is an indica-

Table 2.1 Some cardiac glycoside preparations.

Intravenous

Preparation	Onset of action (min)	Peak effect (min)	Disappearance (days)	Dose (mg)
Ouabain	5	30–120	3	0.25–0.5
Digoxin	15	120	7	0.25–1.0

Oral

Preparation	Onset of action (h)	Peak effect (h)	Disappearance (weeks)	Initial dose (mg)	Daily maintenance dose (× 1–4) (mg)
Digoxin	1–3	6–12	1	0.5–1.0	0.25
Digitoxin	2–4	6–12	3	0.2–0.4	0.1

Note: Smaller doses are required for children, the elderly and patients with renal failure.

tion for reducing digitalis dosage. Ventricular tachycardia and ventricular fibrillation may also be induced.

Supraventricular rhythm disturbances may be provoked, of which the most important is atrial tachycardia with block (p. 60). Atrioventricular dissociation (p. 75) and junctional rhythms (p. 57) may also occur.

Prolongation of the PR interval is common, as is partial heart block of the Wenckebach type (p. 70). In more severe cases, complete heart block can develop.

Potassium depletion promotes the development of digitalis-induced disturbances of rhythm and conduction, and should be assumed to be present when these occur, in spite of a normal serum potassium. Digitalis should be discontinued immediately and potassium depletion corrected. It is important never to use dc shock therapy in the treatment of digitalis-induced arrhythmias.

Digitalis is indicated in cardiac failure when diuretic therapy alone is inadequate, or if it is required for the control of atrial arrhythmias. It is most likely to be efficacious if there is cardiomegaly with a dilated ventricle and a third heart sound. It is unlikely to be helpful in cases of constrictive pericarditis or in mitral stenosis without atrial fibrillation. It is potentially dangerous in hypertrophic cardiomyopathy (p. 189). Its role in the treatment of arrhythmias is discussed in Chapter 4.

It is relatively easy to assess the therapeutic effectiveness of digitalis therapy in patients with tachycardia due to an arrhythmia. When there is atrial fibrillation, a satisfactory result is usually obtained when the heart rate has been slowed to 70 per minute at rest. If such a rate is difficult to achieve, it suggests some complicating factor, such as infection, pulmonary infarction or thyrotoxicosis. Bradycardia should be avoided. It may be difficult to assess the effectiveness of digitalis therapy in the patient in regular sinus rhythm. However, improvement in symptoms and the disappearance of the tachycardia and gallop rhythm of cardiac failure suggest that an adequate dose is being given.

Measurement of plasma levels plays little role in the use of digitalis glycosides unless toxicity is suspected. The therapeutic level of plasma digoxin (taken some 8 hours after the last dose) is approximately in the range of $1-2$ μg/l, but this provides only a rough guide, because other factors, such as hypokalaemia, may be important.

Toxicity can usually be corrected by withholding the drug and, if indicated, giving potassium. Pacing may be required for heart block, and antiarrhythmic drugs for arrhythmias. In severe cases of digitalis poisoning the fragments of antidigoxin antibodies (Digibind) may be used with effect.

The management of sodium and water retention

Low salt diets effectively counteract cardiac failure. However, with the availability of potent diuretic drugs, no extreme limitation of sodium intake is usually necessary. Nevertheless, some restriction is desirable and inability to control cardiac failure is quite often due to the patient not reducing sodium intake sufficiently. All patients should be advised not to add salt at meals and to avoid obviously salty foods. Occasionally, a strict salt restriction must be applied. It is seldom necessary to practise water restriction, but in cases of dilutional hyponatraemia, limitation to one litre per day may be helpful. These may be identified by a lack of response to conventional treatment for cardiac failure in association with a low serum sodium concentration.

Diuretics are valuable in the treatment of those cases of cardiac failure that do not respond to restriction of activity and limitation of salt intake supplemented, if necessary, by digitalis therapy. All the commonly used diuretics act by promoting sodium excretion, with enhanced water excretion as a secondary effect. There are now a large number of diuretics available, but it is necessary for the physician to be familiar with only three or four varieties.

The loop diuretics: frusemide, bumetanide and ethacrynic acid. These drugs prevent reabsorption at multiple sites including the proximal and distal tubules and the ascending limb of the loop of Henle. They produce a profound diuresis with the excretion of large quantities of sodium and chloride. When given by mouth, action commences in about 1 hour and is complete in 6—8 hours. If given intravenously, the onset of action is almost immediate.

Because these drugs are very potent, their use should be reserved for situations of urgency and for those patients who are resistant to less powerful diuretics.

Frusemide may be given in a dosage of 20—40 mg intravenously, but this occasionally produces hypotension. The oral dose is usually 40—80 mg, but 120 mg or more may be necessary. Bumetanide (1 or 5 mg) is another potent diuretic with a similar action.

Ethacrynic acid is helpful in some patients with severe heart failure who have failed to respond to other drugs. An oral dose of 50 mg may be adequate, but 100 mg once or twice a day may be necessary. Supplements of potassium chloride should be given to all patients receiving these drugs for heart failure.

Thiazide diuretics and chlorthalidone (Table 2.2). The many drugs in this group are essentially similar except in their potency and duration of action. Most of the thiazide diuretics act for 12—24 hours whereas polythiazide and chlorthalidone exert their effect for 48 hours or more. They may have several sites of action, but the main mechanism is the inhibition of sodium reabsorption in the distal convoluted tubule.

These diuretics are less potent than the loop diuretics, but are rather more likely to produce hypokalaemia. If the serum potassium is low, or if the drugs are being given more than once a week, supplements of slow release potassium chloride should be used.

These drugs sometimes cause hyperglycaemia and hyperuricaemia, and may precipitate diabetes and clinical gout. Other occasional undesirable effects include agranulocytosis, thrombocytopenia, nausea, abdominal discomfort, impotence and skin rashes.

Aldosterone antagonists. In some cases of cardiac failure, particularly when there is advanced right-sided heart failure, there is excessive aldosterone secretion. This results in sodium retention and potassium excretion, which can be mitigated by the aldosterone antagonist spironolactone.

It is relatively ineffective when given alone and is best prescribed in combination with a thiazide diuretic. There is a risk of hyperkalaemia; in most cases potassium supplements should be

Table 2.2 Diuretics.

Drug	Tablet size (mg)
Thiazide diuretics	
Chlorothiazide	500
Hydrochlorothiazide	25, 50
Hydroflumethiazide	50
Chlorthalidone	50
Bendrofluazide	2.5, 5
Methyclothiazide	5
Polythiazide	1
Cyclopenthiazide	0.5
Aldosterone antagonists and similar drugs	
Triamterene	50
Triamterene (50 mg) with Hydrochlorothiazide (25 mg) (Dyazide)	
Spironolactone	25, 100
Spironolactone with hydroflumethiazide (Aldactide) (25 or 50 mg of each)	
Amiloride	5
Amiloride (5 mg) with hydrochlorothiazide (50 mg) (Moduretic)	
Loop diuretics	
Frusemide	20, 40
Ethacrynic acid	50
Bumetanide	1, 5

omitted. Some 3 days is necessary before its full effect is produced. Because of its expense, its use should be restricted to cases with refractory heart failure, and it should be discontinued when a good diuresis has been achieved. Gynaecomastia is a common side-effect. The usual dose of spironolactone is 100 mg daily, but occasionally up to 400 mg per day is required.

Triamterene resembles spironolactone in its behaviour, but is not an aldosterone antagonist. Like spironolactone it encourages potassium retention. The usual daily dosage is 100–200 mg. It is best combined with a thiazide diuretic.

Amiloride is similar but more potent; 5 mg daily is usually effective. Combinations of the aldosterone antagonists with thiazide preparations are available (see Table 2.2).

Other less commonly used diuretics. Acetazolamide acts by inhibiting carbonic-anhydrase activity in the renal tubular cells. As a consequence there is an increased excretion of sodium bicarbonate and a retention of hydrogen. This eventually leads to a metabolic acidosis which has the effect of preventing further diuretic action. It is therefore a mild diuretic which can only be used for a few days at a time. The usual dose is 250 to 375 mg daily. It may have a special role in preventing high altitude pulmonary oedema.

Several new diuretics, such as clopamide, mefruside and xipamide have become available, but their place in therapy has yet to be defined.

Diuretic therapy should be employed in virtually all cases of symptomatic heart failure whether or not digitalis is also given. As a rule, thiazide diuretics are indicated in moderate cardiac failure and for long-term maintenance, whereas frusemide, ethacrynic acid or bumetanide are required in acute situations and for patients resistant to thiazide therapy. In resistant cases, particularly if there is hepatic congestion, spironolactone, triamterene or amiloride may be added.

Vasodilator therapy (Table 2.3)

Constriction of the arterioles and veins is a characteristic feature of cardiac failure. In early cardiac failure, the reduction in vascular bed may be beneficial in ensuring an adequate venous return and maintaining the blood pressure, but frequently, particularly in more advanced failure, the arteriolar constriction imposes an excessive afterload and a venoconstriction too high a preload. Depending upon the pathophysiology of the individual case, it may be desirable to reduce preload or afterload or both. Generally, in cardiac failure, it has been found that the optimal filling (or end-diastolic) pressure of the left ventricle is between 15 and 20 mmHg. If the pressure is higher than this, pulmonary congestion will result. The administration of a venodilator will cause the filling pressure to fall, but the cardiac output either stays the same or increases. Ideally, before using a venodilator, the left ventricular end-diastolic pressure should be measured indirectly from a pulmonary wedge pressure recording. Venodilator drugs should not be given to patients with filling pressures of less than 15 mmHg; the administration of venodilating drugs should be discontinued when such a pressure has been achieved. The increased arteriolar resistance that results in excessive afterload imposes a burden on the heart which leads to a fall in cardiac output with or without a rise in end-diastolic pressure. Arteriolar vasodilators usually result in a brisk rise in cardiac output.

Angiotensin converting enzyme (ACE) inhibitors, such as captopril and enalapril, have a unique mechanism in that they block the enhanced activity of the renin–angiotensin system (see

Table 2.3 Some vasodilator drugs.

Venous:
  Isosorbide dinitrate 10−40 mg 4- to 6-hourly orally or 2−7 mg
    per hour intravenously

Arterial:
  Hydralazine 25−50 mg three or four times daily

Venous and arterial:
  Sodium nitroprusside 15−400 µg/min intravenously
  Prazosin 0.5−5 mg four times daily orally

ACE inhibitors:
  Captopril 6.25−12.5 mg three times a day initally rising, if
    necessary, to a maximum of 150 mg daily
  Enalapril 2.5 mg daily initially rising, if necessary, to 10−20 mg
    daily

Therapy should start with the lowest dosage quoted and be increased
cautiously.

p. 265), but have additional vasodilator properties. They seem to
be superior to other orally administered vasodilators in their
effectiveness and, at low dosages, in their lack of side-effects
apart from the occasional occurrence of hypotension and renal
impairment. These adverse effects can be largely avoided by
reducing diuretic therapy for 2−3 days before starting and by
using very small doses of the ACE inhibitor initially, e.g. 6.25 or
12.5 mg of captopril or 2.5 mg enalapril. Isosorbide dinitrate may
be used as a venodilator drug and hydralazine as an arteriolar
dilator. A combination of veno- and arteriolar dilatation can be
achieved by prescribing both these drugs or by the use of prazosin
or nitroprusside. In addition, there are drugs which combine
vasodilatation as a result of the activation of beta$_2$-receptors with
a positive inotropic action. These include salbutamol.

The role of vasodilator therapy in the management of heart
failure is still not clearly defined. At present, it would seem wise
to restrict it to patients with severe failure. Vasodilators are of
considerable value in the management of acute left-sided failure,
with pulmonary oedema, and as an adjuvant to other forms of
therapy in patients who are severely incapacitated by dyspnoea.

Recently, it has been found that life may be prolonged in patients
with heart failure, by the use of either ACE inhibitors, or the
combination of nitrates and hydralazine.

Mechanical removal of effusions and oedema fluid

Hydrothorax and actites usually respond well to conventional
treatment for cardiac failure. In a few cases, however, they cause

considerable discomfort and it is then appropriate to remove 0.5—1.0 litre of fluid. When peripheral oedema is intractable, one may employ peritoneal dialysis or utilize Southey tubes, which are inserted into the oedematous tissues of the legs after the patient has been positioned for several hours with the lower limbs dependent.

The treatment of acute left ventricular failure

Acute left ventricular failure (paroxysmal dyspnoea and acute pulmonary oedema) is an emergency requiring vigorous treatment. Morphine 10—20 mg should be given subcutaneously, intramuscularly or intravenously, if it is not contraindicated on the grounds of respiratory failure. Aminophylline 0.25—0.5 g administered slowly intravenously often provides relief. The patient should receive oxygen therapy, if possible under slight positive pressure. Venous return may be reduced by the application of tourniquets to three limbs at a time, with the serial removal from one to another extremity every 15 minutes. A diuretic such as frusemide 20—40 mg intravenously is also of value as is vasodilator therapy.

If there is no contraindication, and more particularly if there is known to be an atrial arrhythmia with a rapid ventricular response, digoxin in a dosage of 0.5—1.0 mg may be given intravenously. If severe hypertension is present, it may be treated by labetalol, nitroprusside or diazoxide (see p. 278).

Acute circulatory failure (shock)

The terms acute circulatory failure, low output state, and shock are used to describe a syndrome comprising arterial hypotension, cold, moist and cyanosed extremities, a rapid weak pulse, a low urine output and a diminished level of consciousness. This clinical pattern is common to a number of disorders such as severe blood or gastrointestinal fluid loss, burns and acute myocardial infarction. As yet, physiological studies have not clearly defined the nature of the changes responsible for the clinical syndrome, but a common factor is a sudden fall in cardiac output associated with tissue hypoxia. In a substantial proportion of cases, the fall in cardiac output is a consequence of reduction in blood volume and venous return ('hypovolaemic shock'). Such a situation is exemplified by haemorrhage, the loss of fluids from burns, vomiting and diarrhoea. Other causes include acute pancreatitis, anaphylactic shock, and bacteraemia (septic shock). In another group of cases, the cause of the fall in cardiac output is clearly cardiac in origin and the shock may then be designated 'cardiogenic'. This may be due to many different causes, including myocardial infarction, massive pulmonary embolism, dissecting aneurysm, pericardial tamponade, rupture of a valve cusp, and arrhythmias. In cardiogenic shock, the central venous pressure is usually raised, in contrast to hypovolaemic shock, in which it is characteristically low.

Although the fall in cardiac output and blood pressure is an essential feature of shock, these abnormalities are insufficient to account for the syndrome. Falls of the same magnitude may be seen in some patients in whom the clinical features of shock are not seen and in whom the prognosis is good. In the first stage of shock, there is a fall in cardiac output and blood pressure, due to either a diminution in venous return or to an inability of the myocardium to expel an adequate stroke volume. As a consequence of the hypotension, there is a fall in renal blood flow, with oliguria. Reflex tachycardia takes place. Compensatory mechanisms follow, with arteriolar constriction affecting particularly the kidneys, abdominal viscera, muscle and skin. Vasodilatation of the cerebral and coronary vessels permits the maintenance of a relatively good blood flow in these territories. If the vasoconstriction is sufficiently great, the blood pressure may be kept at or close to normal levels but at the expense of producing tissue hypoxia with consequent acidosis. If the underlying process can be corrected quickly, recovery may ensue, but if shock persists untreated for many hours, the stage of irreversibility may be reached. At this time, the correction of the original cause fails to prevent death. The nature of irreversible shock remains undetermined, but has been attributed to the production of endotoxins, and to irreparable cellular changes as a result of hypoxia in the liver, kidney, heart or brain.

Aetiological Diagnosis

Although the condition responsible for shock is often obvious, there is sometimes no evident cause. In such cases, no effort must be spared in identifying it quickly, for successful therapy depends upon this.

Cardiac causes, provided they are thought of, can usually be recognized by a combination of clinical examination, ECG, x-ray and echocardiography. The cause of hypovolaemic shock may be difficult to establish; this applies particularly to intra-abdominal haemorrhage and to occult infection.

Treatment

General management. If the patient is in severe pain or distress, opiates should be given intravenously (provided there is no contraindication) and high-flow oxygen administered, preferably by a tight-fitting face mask making use of the Venturi principle, or by mechanical ventilation. Unless there is pulmonary oedema, the patient should be laid flat, with the legs slightly raised. A catheter should be introduced to measure urinary output. Arterial blood gases and pH should be monitored. Although central venous monitoring may be adequate for the less severe cases of traumatic shock, a Swan−Ganz balloon-tip catheter should be used to obtain pulmonary artery and 'pulmonary capillary wedge' pressures, particularly if a cardiac or pulmonary cause is known or suspected. As measurement of blood pressure by a sphygmomanometer is unreliable in severe shock, direct arterial pressure monitoring should be undertaken, when possible.

Correction of hypovolaemia. This is essential in shock which is not cardiogenic, but may also be of importance in myocardial infarction when prior diuretic therapy has caused fluid depletion, or in right ventricular infarction. One should aim to raise the central venous pressure to between 10 and 15 mmHg, and keep the pulmonary wedge (or pulmonary artery diastolic) pressure between 15 and 20 mmHg. Immediate replacement may be with saline or Ringer's lactate; subsequently, the amount and nature of the fluid infused should be determined by estimates of that lost.

Inotropic agents. These drugs enhance myocardial contractility, but at the expense of increased oxygen consumption. The sympathomimetic drugs isoprenaline and noradrenaline were much used in the past, but they have been largely superseded by dopamine and dobutamine.

The effects of dopamine, a natural precursor of noradrenaline, depend upon the dose. Administered intravenously in a dosage of 2−5 μg/kg per minute, it causes dilatation of renal and mesenteric vessels; at doses of 5−10 μg/kg per minute, it increases myocardial contractility and cardiac output. At higher doses, it causes vasoconstriction (it should not be infused directly into a peripheral vein as leakage may cause local necrosis). Dopamine may induce nausea and vomiting, and can lead to an excessive tachycardia and arrhythmias.

Dobutamine is synthetic sympathomimetic agent whose predominant action is one of stimulating beta$_1$ activity. It is less likely to cause vasoconstriction or tachycardia than dopamine. It is given by intravenous infusion at a rate of 2.5−10 μg/kg per minute.

Both these drugs need to be given with careful monitoring of intravascular pressures.

Vasodilator therapy. Vasodilator drugs are contraindicated in the presence of hypotension. However, when pulmonary oedema complicates shock, they may be combined with inotropic drugs, if the latter succeed in maintaining the blood pressure at a viable level.

Mechanical support. The intra-aortic balloon pump is of value in acute myocardial infarction if shock has been caused by a surgically correctable lesion, such as a ventricular septal defect or papillary muscle rupture.

Further reading

Braunwald, E. (1988) Pathophysiology of heart failure. In Braunwald, E. (Ed.) *Heart Disease.* Philadelphia: Saunders.

Chatterjee, K. & Parmley, W.W. (1983) Vasodilator therapy for acute myocardial infarction and chronic congestive heart failure. *Journal of the American College of Cardiology 1:* 133.

Dollery, C.T. & Corr, L. (1985) Drug treatment of heart failure. *British Heart Journal 54:* 234.

Harris, P. (1983) Evolution and the cardiac patient. *Cardiovascular Research 17:* 313.373.437.

Julian, D.G. & Wenger, N.K. (Eds.) (1986) *Management of Heart Failure.* London: Butterworths.

Lant, A. (1985) Diuretics: clinical pharmacology and therapeutics. *Drugs 29:* Part I: 57; Part II: 162.

Maclean, D. & Tudhope, G.R. (1983) Modern diuretic treatment. *British Medical Journal 286:* 1419.

Packer M. (1987) Do vasodilators prolong life in heart failure? *New England Journal of Medicine 316:* 1471.

The Electrical Activity of the Heart: the Electrocardiogram

Electrical activity is a basic characteristic of the heart and is the stimulus for cardiac contraction. Disturbances of electrical function are common in heart disease. Their registration on an electrocardiogram (ECG) plays an essential role in the diagnosis and management of myocardial infarction, and of rhythm and conduction abnormalities. The ECG also provides important information about the presence of atrial and ventricular enlargement and can contribute to the detection of electrolyte disorders and drug intoxication.

The ECG is best understood by first considering some electrical and chemical features of the myocardial cell. Resting cells have a potassium concentration (about 150 mmol/l) which is high in comparison with that in the extracellular tissues (about 5 mmol/l), whereas extracellular sodium concentration is much greater than intracellular. This ionic disequilibrium between the cell and its environment is maintained by a 'sodium pump' which actively excludes sodium from the cell. The cell membrane is, in fact, relatively permeable to potassium, but this ion is retained within the cell, thus ensuring overall ionic balance. The intra-extracellular potassium gradient results, however, in a difference in electrical potential across the cell membrane so that there is a relative negative potential within the cell of the order of 90 mV — the *transmembrane resting potential.* Cells at rest are therefore 'polarized', and may be regarded as having positive charges on their external surface and negative charges within.

When the cell membrane is injured or electrically stimulated, membrane permeability is increased so that sodium ions enter the cell (Fig. 3.1A). This reduces the membrane potential; when this reaches a certain level ('threshold potential'), further changes take place in the membrane permeability that allow a further rapid influx of sodium accompanied by a slower influx of calcium. Extremely rapid depolarization results, the interior of the cell transiently becoming positive relative to the exterior (phase 0). This is followed by a plateau phase, during which the transmembrane potential is close to zero; this is largely dependent on the continued influx of calcium. Repolarization follows until the resting potential is reached.

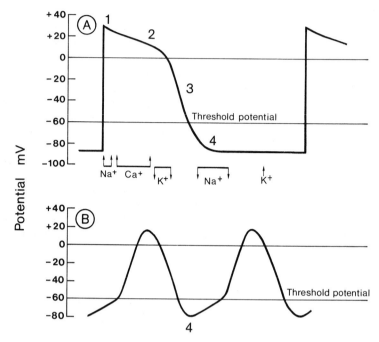

Fig. 3.1 (A) Transmembrane potential. Phase 0 corresponds with depolarization, and phases 1, 2 and 3 with repolarization. Phase 4 is the period of diastolic rest. When the cell is electrically stimulated, the transmembrane potential is reduced to the threshold potential, after which the process of depolarization is self-perpetuating. (B) Transmembrane potential in a pacemaking cell. In these cells, phase 4 is a period of slow depolarization. When the threshold potential is reached, the cell rapidly becomes depolarized.

In a pacemaking or automatic cell (Fig. 3.1B) diastole is not stable; a slow leak of sodium into the cell during this time produces slow depolarization. When the transmembrane potential reaches its threshold, the cell automatically becomes depolarized. This characteristic forms the basis of automaticity.

The groups of automatic cells, which are present in the sinus node, the junctional tissue in the neighbourhood of the atrioventricular (AV) node, the AV bundle of His, the bundle branches and the Purkinje cells of the ventricles vary from each other in their rate of spontaneous depolarization. In the normal heart, the cells of the sinus node have the shortest spontaneous depolarization time (phase 4) and so have the fastest firing rate. The sinus node dominates the heart because impulses spreading from it discharge the other potential pacemakers before they are ready for spontaneous depolarization. If, however, the sinus node discharge rate is reduced for any reason, or if one of the other areas develops a faster rate, a new 'ectopic' focus assumes the role of pacemaker.

A single resting cell may be represented by a square with a positive charge on the outside and a negative one within. A muscle strip can be represented diagrammatically as a series of such squares (Fig. 3.2). If a cell at one end is stimulated, it becomes depolarized and its surface is negatively charged in relation to its fellows. As the electrical impulse spreads from one cell to the next, there is a progressively advancing negative charge. Immediately in front of it is a positive charge of equal magnitude. This combination of negative and positive charges in close proximity is termed a *dipole* with, in this case, the positive charge preceding the negative. The advancing dipole sets up an electrical field which can be detected by an exploring electrode

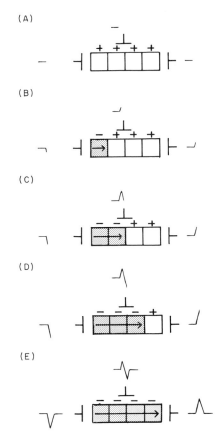

Fig. 3.2 The recording produced from electrodes during depolarization of a muscle strip. By convention, an upstroke (a positive deflection) is recorded as depolarization proceeds towards that electrode, and a negative deflection is obtained from an electrode facing the opposite direction.

paired with an indifferent electrode. By convention, relative positivity in the exploring electrode is represented by an upright deflection and negativity by a downward one. Therefore, as the positive front of the dipole approaches the electrode, an upright deflection is recorded; as it retreats, the deflection is negative.

The whole heart can be regarded as a large number of muscle strips arranged in a complex fashion. At any one time in the cardiac cycle there are numerous dipoles moving in different directions; as viewed from a single electrode many of these cancel each other out. The total electrical activity at any one moment in time can be summated and represented by a single electrical force of a certain magnitude and in a certain direction which is termed the *instantaneous vector*. All the instantaneous vectors occurring throughout the cardiac cycle form the *cardiac vector*.

The pathways of conduction

The sinus node is situated in the right atrium close to the entrance of the superior vena cava. The AV node lies in the right atrial wall immediately above the tricuspid valve. The fibres of the AV bundle (of His) arise from the AV node and run along the posterior border of the septum between the ventricles (Fig. 3.3). On reaching the muscular part of the septum, they split into right and left bundle branches and then spread out in the subendocardium of the ventricles as the Purkinje system. The right bundle is a slender, compact structure. The left bundle soon splits into two or more divisions or fascicles, one of which proceeds anteriorly, sharing the same blood supply as the right bundle, and another is directed posteriorly.

In the usual sequence of events, the electrical impulse arises in the sinus node and spreads across the atria to reach the AV node. It can then only reach the ventricles by passing into the rapidly conducting AV bundle and its branches.

The first part of the ventricles to be activated is the septum, followed by the endocardium. Finally, the impulse spreads outwards to the epicardium.

The electrocardiogram

Electrodes and leads

A conventional electrocardiogram (ECG) consists of tracings from twelve or more leads. The term 'lead' refers to the ECG obtained as a result of recording the difference in potential between a pair of electrodes.

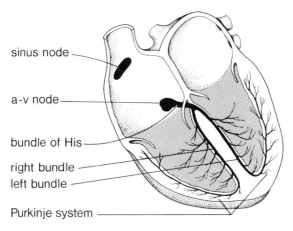

Fig. 3.3 The pathways of conduction.

The bipolar (standard) leads. In these leads, the electrodes are attached to the limbs. In lead I the positive electrode is attached to the left arm and the negative to the right arm. In lead II the positive electrode is attached to the left leg and the negative to the right arm. In lead III the positive is attached to the left leg and the negative to the left arm. They may thus be depicted as:

Lead I = left arm minus right arm (LA−RA)
Lead II = left leg minus right arm (LL−RA)
Lead III = left leg minus left arm (LL−LA)

It can be deduced from these equations that lead II should be equal to the sum of leads I and III.

The position from which the heart is viewed by each of these leads is shown in Fig. 3.4.

Einthoven regarded each limb used in the recording of the bipolar ECG as an apex of an equilateral triangle, equidistant electrically from the heart at the centre. Although useful, this hypothesis is only approximately true, as it assumes that the body is a homogeneous sphere, which it clearly is not.

Unipolar leads. These have an exploring electrode placed on a chosen site linked with an indifferent electrode with a very small potential. In an attempt to obtain a central terminal with 'zero potential', Wilson connected all three limb electrodes through 5000 ohm resistances to form the indifferent electrode.

Unipolar chest leads. When unipolar leads are recorded from the chest wall, the exploring electrode is connected to the positive

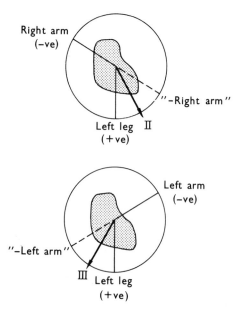

Fig. 3.4 Diagram of the effective position of the bipolar (standard) leads. In lead I, the positive electrode is attached to the left arm and the negative to the right arm. In effect, lead I is the sum of the potentials from the left arm with those that would be obtained from an electrode diametrically opposite the right arm. The resultant force is directed midway between these two points. Similar principles can be applied to derive the effective direction of the leads II and III.

pole of the ECG and the negative to the central terminal of Wilson (Fig. 3.5). By convention, the following sites are normally selected:

V1, the fourth intercostal space just to the right of the sternum.
V2, the fourth intercostal space just to the left of the sternum.
V3, midway between V2 and V4.
V4, the fifth intercostal space in the mid-clavicular line.
V5, the left anterior axillary line at the same horizontal level as V4.
V6, the left mid-axillary line at the same horizontal level as V4.

Additional leads can be taken from V3R and V4R, sites on the right side of the chest equivalent to V3 and V4. Occasionally, leads may be placed at higher levels, e.g. the second, third or fourth intercostal spaces or further laterally (V7 and V8).

Fig. 3.5 The attachments of unipolar chest leads.

Unipolar limb leads. In these leads, the exploring electrode is placed on one limb, and the negative pole is connected to Wilson's central terminal, modified by the omission of the connection from the limb under study to the central terminal (Fig. 3.6). This modification augments the voltage of the ECG, and the leads so derived are referred to as 'a' leads. They are designated as follows:

aVR, Right arm lead; aVL, Left arm lead; aVF, Left foot lead.

The normal electrocardiogram

The normal electrocardiogram (Fig. 3.7) shows a series of deflections from the base-line which are designated P,Q,R,S,T and U (Fig. 3.8). The base-line is referred to as the iso-electric line and the intervals between deflections are described as segments.

Normally, ECGs are recorded at a rate of 25 mm per second and the ECG paper is printed with thin vertical lines 1 mm apart and thick vertical lines 5 mm apart. The interval between the thin lines represents 0.04 sec and that between two thick lines 0.20 sec. If the heart rhythm is regular, the rate can be counted by dividing the number of small squares between two consecutive R waves into 1500 or large squares into 300. If the rhythm is irregular, one can multiply the number of complexes in 6 sec (i.e. 15 cm) by 10. Special rulers simplify the calculation of rate.

There are also thin horizontal lines at 1 mm intervals and thick horizontal lines at 5 mm intervals. An ECG recording is

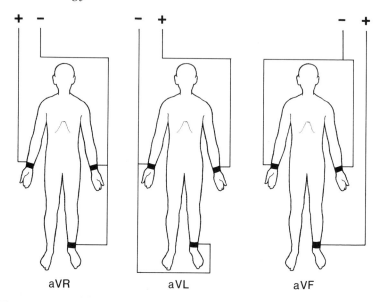

Fig. 3.6 The attachment of unipolar limb leads. Note that the limb under study is not attached to the central (negative) terminal.

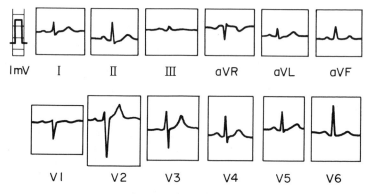

Fig. 3.7 Normal 12-lead electrocardiogram. Note the progression in the upright deflection from 'r' over the right ventricle (V1) to an 'R' over the left ventricle (V6).

standardized so that 1 mV gives a deflection of 10 mm on the paper. The height of a deflection therefore indicates its voltage.

The P wave. The normal P wave results from the spread of electrical activity across the atria (the activity of the sinus node itself cannot be detected in the ECG). Because the impulse spreads from right to left, the P wave is upright in leads I, II and aVF, is

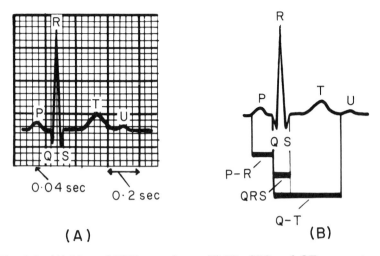

Fig. 3.8 (A) Normal ECG complexes. (B) PR, QRS and QT segments.

inverted in aVR and may be upright, biphasic or inverted in lead III, aVL and V1. It should not be higher than 3 mm in the bipolar leads or 2.5 mm in the unipolar leads, or greater than 0.10 sec in duration.

When abnormal, it may be:

1 Inverted (i.e. negative in the leads in which it is usually positive). This indicates depolarization of the atria in an unusual direction, and that the pacemaker is not in the sinus node, but is situated either elsewhere in the atrium, in the AV node or below this; or there is dextrocardia.

2 Broadened and notched, due to delayed depolarization of the left atrium when this chamber is enlarged (P mitrale) (Fig. 3.9B). In V1, the P wave is then usually biphasic with a small positive wave preceding a deep and broad negative one.

3 Tall and peaked, exceeding 3 mm, as a result of right atrial enlargement (P pulmonale) (Fig. 3.9C).

(A)   (B)   (C)

Fig. 3.9 P wave appearances in lead II. (A) Normal. (B) Broadened and notched (P mitrale). (C) Tall and peaked (P pulmonale).

4 Absent or invisible due to the presence of junctional rhythm or sinu-atrial block.
5 Replaced by flutter or fibrillation waves.

PR interval. This is measured from the beginning of the P wave to the beginning of the QRS complex (i.e. to the onset of the Q wave if there is one, and to the onset of the R wave if there is not). This interval corresponds to the time taken for the impulse to travel from the sinus node to the ventricular muscle. There is an iso-electric segment between the end of the P wave and the beginning of the QRS, whilst the impulse is passing through the AV node and the specialized conducting tissue, as an insufficient amount of tissue is being electrically stimulated to produce a deflection detectable on the body surface.

The PR interval varies with age and with heart rate. The upper limit in children is 0.16, in adolescents 0.18 and in adults 0.20 sec, although it may be even longer in a few normal individuals. The faster the heart rate the shorter is the PR interval. It is regarded as abnormally short if it is less than 0.10 sec. A shortened PR interval is seen when the impulse originates in the junctional tissue and in the Wolff–Parkinson–White syndrome (see p. 74). The PR interval is prolonged in some forms of heart block (see p. 70).

The QRS complex. The QRS complex represents depolarization of the ventricular muscle. The components of the QRS complex are defined as follows (Fig. 3.10):

The R wave is any positive (upward) deflection of the QRS. If there is more than one R wave, the second is denoted R′; an R wave of small voltage may be denoted r.

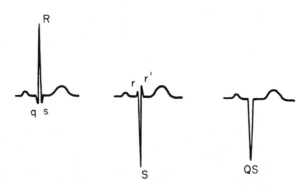

Fig. 3.10 Variations in the QRS complex (see text).

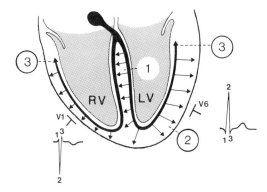

Fig. 3.11 Genesis of QRS complex. Note that the first phase, directed from left to right across the septum, produces a Q wave in V6 and an R wave in V1. The second phase, due mainly to depolarization of the left ventricle from endocardium to epicardium, results in a tall R wave in V6 and a deep S wave in V1. Finally, depolarization of the basal parts of the ventricles, may produce a terminal S wave in V6 and a terminal R wave in V1.

A negative (downward) deflection preceding an R wave is termed Q, and a negative deflection following an R wave is termed S. If the ventricular complex is entirely negative (i.e. there is no R wave), the complex is termed QS. The whole complex is often referred to as the QRS complex irrespective of whether one or two of its components are absent.

Ventricular depolarization starts in the middle of the left side of the septum and spreads across to the right (phase 1 of ventricular depolarization) (Fig. 3.11). Subsequently, the main free walls of the ventricles are activated, the impulse spreading from within outwards and from below upwards. Because of the dominating bulk of the left ventricle, the direction of the vector of phase 2 is to the left and posteriorly. Finally, the base of both ventricular walls and the interventricular septum are stimulated. The appearances of the QRS in different leads can be largely explained by the major vectors of these phases as is seen in Fig. 3.11. In leads facing the left ventricular surface, there is a small Q wave due to septal depolarization and a large R wave due to left ventricular depolarization. On the right side of the heart, as seen from V1, there is usually an r wave due to septal depolarization and a large S wave due to left ventricular forces directed away from the electrode.

As mentioned, small, narrow Q waves are normally to be found in leads facing the left ventricle, e.g. lead I, aVL, aVF, V5 and V6. These Q waves do not normally exceed 2 mm in depth, or 0.03 sec in width. It should be noted that QS waves are normal in aVR, and are common in V1. Abnormally broad and deep Q waves are often a feature of myocardial infarction (see p. 160). Q waves in lead III are difficult to evaluate but can be ignored if there are no Q waves either in lead II or in aVF, or if they do not exceed 0.03 sec. Usually, a 'normal' Q wave in lead III diminishes or disappears on deep inspiration because of an alteration in the position of the heart, whilst the 'pathological' Q wave of infarction persists.

The QRS complex should not exceed 0.10 sec in duration, and usually is in the range 0.06 to 0.08 sec. Broad QRS complexes occur in bundle branch block (p. 73), in ventricular hypertrophy and in ventricular ectopic beats.

The T wave. The wave is due to repolarization of the ventricles. If repolarization (the T wave) occurred in the same direction as depolarization (the QRS complex) the T wave would be directed in an opposite way to that of the QRS (Fig. 3.12). In fact, depolarization takes place from endocardium to epicardium, whereas repolarization takes place from epicardium to endocardium. Because of this, the T wave usually points in the same direction as the major component of the QRS complex. Thus, the T wave is normally upright in leads I and II as well as in V3 to V6, is inverted in aVR, and may be upright or inverted in lead III, aVL, aVF and V1 and V2.

The T waves are usually not taller than 5 mm in standard leads and 10 mm in precordial leads. Unusually tall and peaked T waves may be seen in hyperkalaemia and in early myocardial infarction. Flattened T waves are seen when the voltage of all complexes is low, as in myxoedema, as well as in hypokalaemia and in a large number of other conditions in which it may be regarded as a non-specific abnormality. Slight T wave inversion is also often non-specific, and may be due to such influences as hyperventilation and smoking. More important causes of T wave inversion are myocardial ischaemia and infarction, ventricular hypertrophy and bundle branch block. Detailed descriptions of T wave changes will be found in the subsequent section on abnormalities of the ST segment, and also under the subheadings dealing with ventricular hypertrophy, bundle branch block and myocardial infarction.

The U wave. The U wave is a broad, low-voltage wave present in most normal ECGs. Its cause is unknown; it may become unusually prominent in hypokalaemia and with digitalis therapy.

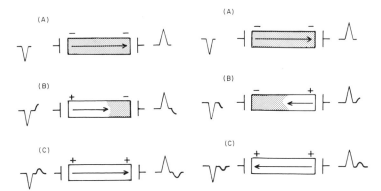

Fig. 3.12 The genesis of the T wave. (A) shows the situation at the end of depolarization. Repolarization produces a negative deflection in the electrode towards which it is proceeding. Thus, as illustrated on the left, if depolarization occurs in the same direction as repolarization, the T wave is negative. If, as is usual, repolarization occurs in the reverse direction to depolarization, an upright T wave is inscribed, as illustrated on the right.

The QT interval. The QT interval represents the total time from the onset of ventricular depolarization to the completion of repolarization. It is measured from the beginning of the Q wave (or the R wave if there is no Q wave) to the end of the T wave. Its duration varies with heart rate, becoming shorter as the heart rate increases. In general, the QT interval at heart rates between 60 and 90 per minute does not exceed in duration half the preceding RR interval. The measurement of the QT interval is often difficult as the end of the T wave cannot always be clearly identified, and the relationship between heart rate and duration of the QT is a complex one. Tables are available in textbooks of electrocardiography giving normal QT intervals. In practice, the main importance of a prolonged QT interval is that it is associated with a risk of ventricular tachycardias (particularly torsade de pointes), and sudden death. A long QT is sometimes an inherited abnormality but may result from such drugs as quinidine, procainamide, disopyramide, amiodarone and tricyclic antidepressants.

The ST segment. The ST segment is that part of the electrocardiogram between the end of the QRS complex and the beginning of the T wave (Fig. 3.13). The point of junction between the S wave and the ST segment is known as the J point. The ST segment occurs during a period of unchanging polarity in the ventricles, corresponding with phase 2 of the action potential (see Fig. 3.1).

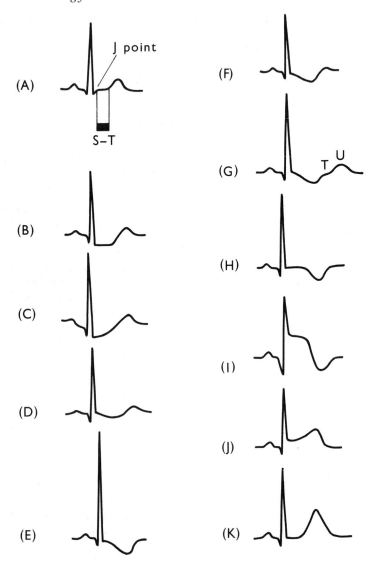

Fig. 3.13 Normal and abnormal ST segments and T waves. (A) Normal ST segment with J point. (B) Horizontal ST depression in myocardial ischaemia. (C) ST segment sloping upwards in sinus tachycardia. (D) ST sagging in digitalis therapy. (E) Asymmetrical T wave inversion associated with ventricular hypertrophy. (F) Similar pattern sometimes seen without voltage changes in hypertrophy-'strain'. (G) ST sagging and prominent U waves of hypokalaemia. (H) Symmetrically inverted T wave of myocardial ischaemia or infarction. (I) ST elevation in acute myocardial infarction. (J) ST elevation in acute pericarditis. (K) Peaked T wave in hyperkalaemia.

The normal ST segment is situated on the iso-electric line but curves upwards.

Displacements of the ST segment and variations in its shape are of great importance in electrocardiographic diagnosis. The characteristic abnormalities of the ST segment are illustrated in Fig. 3.13. In some normal individuals, particularly young blacks, slight ST elevation is seen. This may be up to 1 mm in standard leads and 2 mm in the right precordial leads. Depression of more than 0.5 mm is abnormal. When ST elevation occurs in normal individuals, it is often preceded by a slight notch on the down-stroke of the R wave. In acute myocardial infarction, the ST segment is elevated with a curve which is convex upwards in the leads facing the infarct. At a later stage ST segment elevation becomes less pronounced as T wave inversion develops. These changes are considered in more detail in Chapter 8, p. 160. In pericarditis there is also ST elevation, but the ST segments are concave upwards and the changes are widespread rather than localized as in myocardial infarction. Digitalis therapy depresses the ST segment, particularly in leads II and III, so that there is a gentle sagging, but the T wave remains upright or flattened. In left and right ventricular hypertrophy, ST segment depression may occur in leads facing the relevant ventricle and be accompanied by asymmetrical T wave inversion. This contrasts with the symmetrical T wave inversion seen in myocardial infarction

29°C

Fig. 3.14 ECG in hypothermia. The arrow indicates the characteristic prominent J wave.

Fig. 3.15 Left ventricular hypertrophy, showing tall R waves in V6 and deep S waves in V1, accompanied by ST depression and T wave inversion in V6.

V1   V6

and ischaemia. In acute myocardial ischaemia the ST segment is horizontally depressed or slightly downward sloping from the J point onwards. In sinus tachycardia there may be ST depression which slopes upwards from the J point. In hypothermia there is a prominent J wave (the junction of the S wave and the ST segment) (Fig. 3.14).

Abnormal ECG patterns

Left ventricular hypertrophy (Fig. 3.15)

Hypertrophy of the left ventricle increases the amplitude of R waves in left chest leads and S waves in right chest leads. Where there is septal hypertrophy, deep but narrow Q waves are seen in left chest leads. When left ventricular hypertrophy becomes advanced, the T wave may become flattened in the leads in

Fig. 3.16 Right ventricular hypertrophy showing tall R waves in the right chest leads associated with T wave inversion.

Fig.3.17 The genesis of left bundle branch block. Note that the initial vector is abnormal in being from right to left across the septum, thus producing an initial r wave in V6 and a q wave in V1.

which the R wave is tall; eventually ST depression and T wave inversion may occur.

Many efforts have been made to lay down criteria for the diagnosis of left ventricular hypertrophy. None is satisfactory as many factors contribute to the amplitude of ECG waves, including the thickness of the chest wall and the age of the patient. The following criteria have gained wide acceptance:

1 R in V5 or V6 plus S in V1 is greater than 35 mm;
2 R and V5 or V6 is greater than 25 mm;
3 R in a VL is greater than 13 mm or the R in aVF is greater than 20 mm.

These criteria apply only in individuals over 25 years of age. In younger persons, R in V5 or V6 plus S in V1 should exceed 40 mm before the diagnosis of left ventricular hypertrophy can be made.

Right ventricular hypertrophy (Fig. 3.16)

When the right ventricle becomes hypertrophied, the leads facing the right ventricle (particularly in V1, V3R and V4R) show dominant R waves instead of the usually dominant S wave, i.e. R larger than S, and at least 5 mm tall. As with left ventricular hypertrophy, ST depression and T wave inversion may develop in the leads with tall R waves.

Left bundle branch block (Fig. 3.17)

When the left branch of the bundle is blocked, the interventricular septum is activated from the right instead of from the left side

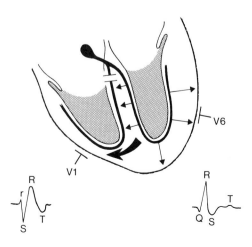

Fig. 3.18 Right bundle branch block.

and the initial vector (phase 1) is directed to the left. Because of this, the normal initial q wave in the left ventricular leads is lost, being replaced by a small r wave. Right ventricular depolarization, which follows, produces an r in V1 and an s in V6. The left ventricle is finally depolarized resulting in an R' in V6 and a broad S in V1. The QRS duration is increased to 0.12 sec or more.

Right bundle branch block (Fig. 3.18)

In this disorder, the right branch of the bundle is blocked, but the septum is activated from left to right, as in the normal heart. The left ventricular q wave is preserved, as is the initial r wave over right chest leads. The left ventricle is then depolarized, producing an S wave in right chest leads and an R wave in left chest leads. Finally, depolarization reaches the right ventricle, and so produces an R' in the right chest leads and a deep broad S wave in the left chest leads. An M pattern is thus seen in the right chest leads, such as V1.

The mean frontal QRS axis

As pointed out on p. 34, the total electrical activity at any one moment of time can be summated and represented by a single electrical force of a certain magnitude and in a certain direction,

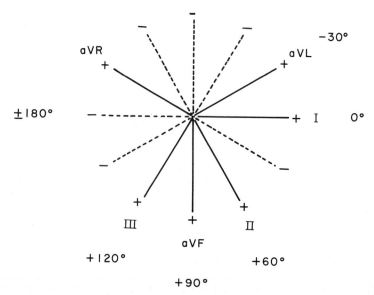

Fig. 3.19 Hexaxial reference system.

termed the instantaneous vector. All the instantaneous vectors occurring during the inscription of the QRS complex can be averaged, the direction of the vector so derived being called the mean QRS axis. It is customary to measure this only in the frontal plane and any two of the ECG leads which view electrical forces in this plane can be used for this purpose. This can be seen from the so-called hexaxial reference system (Fig. 3.19).

An approximate method of deriving the mean frontal QRS axis is to find in which of the leads I, II, III, aVR, aVL and aVF, the deflections of the QRS above and below the line are most nearly equal. The mean frontal QRS axis is at right angles to this lead.

To calculate the QRS axis more accurately, one should plot the difference between positive and negative QRS deflections in lead I on the lead I axis and that in lead III on the lead III axis of Fig. 3.20. By dropping perpendiculars from both points and drawing a line through this intersection from the centre point to the periphery of the curve, the axis may be determined.

Left axis deviation is present when the axis is less than $-30°$ and right axis deviation when the axis is greater than $+110°$.

Calculation of the mean frontal QRS axis is of limited value except in a few conditions such as the differentiation of ostium primum from ostium secundum atrial septal defects (see p. 243).

Left axis deviation is often due to block in the anterior division (fascicle) of the left bundle branch, and when associated with right bundle branch block is a frequent precursor of complete heart block.

Right axis deviation commonly accompanies right ventricular hypertrophy, but may be due to block of the posterior fascicle of the left bundle.

Vectorcardiography

Vectorcardiography is a term applied to the technique by which the movement and magnitude of the cardiac vectors are represented by two-dimensional loops rather than by waves and complexes. The derivation of a vector loop is shown in Fig. 3.21. Vector loops can be obtained in frontal, horizontal and sagittal planes. Unfortunately, vectorcardiography is technically more complex than conventional (scalar) electrocardiography and, except in the hands of experts, contributes little to clinical cardiology at present.

Exercise electrocardiography

The main purpose of exercise electrocardiography is to determine whether a patient has exercise-induced ischaemia, as revealed by

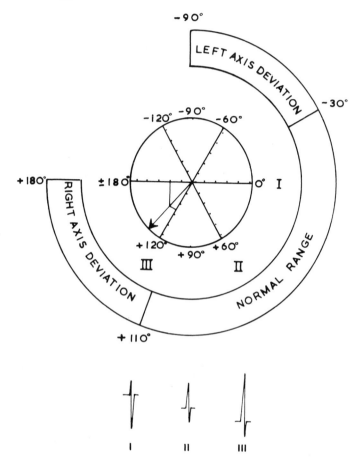

Fig. 3.20 The measurement of the mean frontal plane axis of the QRS complex. In this example, the sum of Q, R and S in lead I is − 2 and in lead III is + 2.5. By drawing a line through the intersection of perpendiculars drawn from these points, the axis may be derived.

ST depression. Exercise tests are carried out on a treadmill or stationary bicycle; if possible, the patient exercises until he develops chest pain (maximal symptom-limited test), but many patients give up because of fatigue or dyspnoea. If angina occurs, ST depression is usually present, but if the test is terminated before it does so, it may be 'false negative'. 'False positives' also occur (i.e. ST depression in the absence of ischaemia), especially in younger women.

Exercise testing is potentially hazardous as hypotension and dangerous arrhythmias (including ventricular fibrillation) may

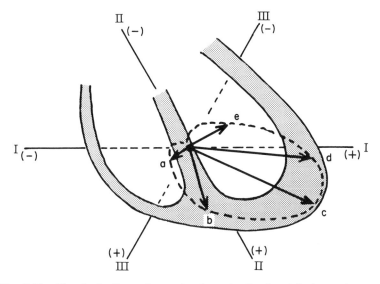

Fig. 3.21 The derivation of a vector loop in the frontal plane. Arrows from a to e indicate the progressive movement of the cardiac vector thoughout the inscription of the QRS.

be induced. The blood pressure should, therefore, be checked regularly throughout this test and full resuscitation facilities (including a defibrillator) should always be available.

Dynamic electrocardiography (Holter monitoring)

With this technique, a continuous tape recording of one or more electrocardiographic leads is obtained, using a small portable tape recorder. Usually, the recording is made over a complete 24-hour period, but some devices allow sampling only in response to activation by the patient, or when they are triggered by an arrhythmia. Special playback apparatus is required, which replays (and may analyse) the recording at many times real speed. It is an invaluable method for the study of transient episodes of arrhythmia which are unlikely to be captured by routine electrocardiography. It is mainly used for the diagnosis of syncope and palpitation of unknown cause, but it is being increasingly employed to detect ST changes in suspected cases of myocardial ischaemia.

Invasive electrophysiology

It is possible to position electrodes in various parts of the heart, having introduced them percutaneously through a peripheral vein (or rarely an artery). Thus, electrodes may be placed in juxtaposition to several sites in the atria and ventricles, and also adjacent to the bundle of His. The sequence of activation of the heart may then be determined, and specific sites found where conduction is accelerated (as in the Wolff—Parkinson—White syndrome) or delayed (as in heart block). Furthermore, by introducing stimuli at an appropriate time and place, an arrhythmia to which a patient is prone may be triggered, and the effect on it of various pharmacological and electrical measures assessed. This technique is particularly valuable in demonstrating the location of the abnormal pathway in the Wolff—Parkinson—White syndrome, and in testing the effectiveness of antiarrhythmic therapy in this condition and in malignant ventricular arrhythmias.

Further reading

Campbell, RWF & Murray A (1986) *Dynamic Electrocardiography.* Edinburgh, Churchill Livingstone.

Goldman, M.J. (1986) *Principles of Clinical Electrocardiography,* 12th edn. Los Altos, Calif.: Lange.

Noble, D. (1979) *The Initiation of the Heartbeat,* 2nd edn. Oxford: Clarendon.

Schamroth, L. (1982) *An Introduction to Electrocardiography,* 6th edn. Oxford: Blackwell.

Task Force on Assessment of Cardiovascular Procedures (1986) Guidelines for exercise testing. *Circulation 74:,* 653A.

Disorders of Rate, Rhythm and Conduction

Introduction

As is discussed in more detail in Chapter 3, there are electrically two types of cell in the myocardium — the automatic and the non-automatic — the automatic cells having the capacity of self-excitation. The group of automatic cells with the most rapid rate of spontaneous depolarization dominates the heart as the pacemaker. This is normally the sinus node, which is under the control both of the vagus and of the sympathetic nervous system. Ectopic rhythms, in which the heart is activated from a pacemaker other than the sinus node, arise from a variety of mechanisms:

Escape of lower centres. An increase in vagal activity reduces the rate of spontaneous depolarization of the sinus node and thereby slows the heart; another group of automatic cells may exhibit a rate faster than that of the sinus node and become the pacemaker.

Increased automaticity of other zones. Increased sympathetic activity increases the rate of discharge not only of the sinus node, but also of other areas, including the ventricles. Ischaemia, digitalis intoxication and electrolyte disorders also enhance ventricular automaticity.

Re-entry. When there are pathways of conduction with differing refractory periods, an impulse may enter an area which is receptive but cannot activate a zone refractory from the previous cycle (Fig. 4.1). When this zone recovers, it may then accept the impulse and act as a pathway back to the area that was initially activated. If this area has had time to recover, it can be stimulated again. In order for there to be time for recovery to take place, the re-entrant pathway must either be long (macro re-entry) or conduction through it must be extremely slow. Re-entry in small areas of atrial or ventricular muscle (micro re-entry) probably also requires that the refractory period is abnormally short. This process can lead to single or repetitive ectopic activity. Supraventricular arrhythmias are frequently associated with anatomically abnormal

Fig. 4.1 The re-entry phenomenon. In (A) the impulse cannot enter a zone which is still in the refractory phase. In (B) this zone has become receptive as adjacent muscle becomes refractory. In (C) the impulse leaves the newly activated zone and re-enters the same tissue as was activated in (A) which has now recovered.

pathways. The most distinctive variety occurs in the Wolff—Parkinson—White syndrome, in which a slender bundle of myocardium forms a bridge between the atria and the ventricles, bypassing the atrioventricular node.

Disturbances of sinus rate and rhythm

Sinus tachycardia is sinus rhythm at a rate faster than is normal. In adults, this is commonly defined as being greater than 100 per minute. In children the heart rate, even at rest, frequently exceeds 100 per minute, and in infants may exceed 150 per minute. Amongst factors associated with disease which cause sinus tachycardia are anaemia, hyperthyroidism and fever. It also occurs as a reflex response to a fall in blood pressure, as in shock, or to a rise in venous pressure, as occurs in heart failure. It may be provoked by such drugs as adrenaline, isoprenaline, ephedrine, propantheline, atropine and thyroxine. Sinus tachycardia is seldom harmful and may be a compensatory mechanism.

The patient with sinus tachycardia may complain of palpitation which is of gradual and explicable onset, unlike the abrupt and unexpected appearance of the symptom in paroxysmal tachycardia. The diagnosis is usually obvious when there is a regular pulse at a rate of more than 100 per minute. Frequently, the tachycardia subsides during the examination as anxiety diminishes. Carotid sinus pressure causes little slowing in contrast to its usually dramatic effect in atrial tachycardia or atrial flutter. The ECG shows P waves having a normal relationship to QRS complexes. The J point may be depressed; the ST then slopes upward (see Fig. 3.13).

Sinus tachycardia does not require treatment.

Sinus bradycardia describes a slow heart in sinus rhythm. This term is commonly applied to heart rates of less than 60 per minute, although such rates are frequently seen in healthy elderly people; in the highly trained athlete the heart rate may be less than 40 per minute. Sinus bradycardia occurs when there is increased vagal tone and can be provoked by carotid sinus or eyeball pressure. Other causes are myxoedema, hypothermia, raised intracranial pressure and certain drugs including digitalis, reserpine, and the beta-adrenergic blocking agents such as propranolol.

Sinus bradycardia seldom gives rise to symptoms or undesirable haemodynamic effects but, occasionally, in the elderly and in acute myocardial infarction, cardiac failure or hypotension may develop if the stroke output cannot be increased to compensate adequately for the slow rate. The heart can be accelerated by atropine 0.6 mg subcutaneously or intravenously, by ephedrine given orally in a dosage of 15—30 mg three times a day or by long-acting isoprenaline 15—30 mg three or four times daily.

Sinus bradycardia is a component of the *sick sinus syndrome*, a condition that occurs transiently in acute myocardial infarction and persistently in some elderly people. The bradycardia may be complicated by paroxysms of atrial arrhythmias (tachycardia, flutter or fibrillation), in which the ventricular rate is very rapid. Syncope may result either from too slow or too fast a heart rate. Treatment is difficult; it may necessitate the combined use of a pacemaker and antiarrhythmic drugs.

Sinus arrhythmia (Fig.4.2)

Normally, the sinus node does not discharge with absolute regularity owing to variations in vagal tone. These variations are related to respiration, and it is characteristic in the young to find acceleration of the heart during inspiration with slowing during expiration. This phasic change in the rhythm of the heart is known as sinus arrhythmia. It is seldom clinically obvious in adults, but is occasionally seen in the healthy old person. It is of no clinical importance, but it must be differentiated from the other types of arrhythmia. Its relationship to respiration usually makes this easy.

Fig. 4.2 Sinus arrhythmia. Note the gradual change in RR interval, with each QRS complex being preceded by a similar P wave.

Supraventricular arrhythmias

A variety of rhythm disturbances can arise in the atria and AV junctional area (that is, the AV node and adjacent specialized tissues). These may result from either increased automaticity or re-entry.

Atrial ectopic beats (atrial extrasystoles, atrial premature beats)

Atrial ectopic beats are common in normal individuals, but seldom give rise to symptoms, apart from an awareness of heart irregularity from time to time. They cause an occasional irregularity in an otherwise normal pulse, and are usually abolished by exercise. The diagnosis is readily confirmed from the ECG (Fig. 4.3) which shows a premature beat occurring earlier than the next anticipated sinus beat. The P wave differs in configuration from that of a sinus beat, because depolarization of the atria takes place in an abnormal direction. The accompanying QRST complex is usually similar to that of previous beats of sinus origin because the pathway of ventricular depolarization is normal. Occasionally, the QRST complex is abnormally broad ('aberrant') because the impulse passes down only one of the bundle branches, the other still being refractory from the preceding beat. It then simulates the appearance of a ventricular ectopic beat (see p. 64) but is usually preceded by a P wave.

Atrial ectopic beats may presage the appearance of other atrial arrhythmias but they require no treatment.

Junctional (nodal) ectopic beats (Fig. 4.4)

Ectopic beats deriving from the junctional tissue are quite common and, like atrial ectopic beats, usually benign. They are responsible for an occasional irregularity in an otherwise regular pulse and cannot be diagnosed without an electrocardiogram, which shows the same features as with atrial ectopic beats except that the P wave is inverted in lead II and is either buried in the QRS complex, or precedes or follows it by a very short interval.

Fig. 4.3 Atrial ectopic beat. Note the premature P wave followed by a QRST of normal appearance.

Fig. 4.4 Junctional ectopic beats. Note that the P wave may precede, follow or coincide with the QRS complex.

Junctional (nodal) rhythm

In this condition the junctional tissue is acting as the pacemaker of the heart and the ECG appearance is that of a succession of junctional ectopic beats. It is usually a transient condition resulting from a depression of sinus node activity. It occurs in some normal individuals and may be provoked by digitalis or ischaemic heart disease. The heart rate is usually in the region of 50—60 per minute and no treatment is required. If the heart rate is undesirably slow, it can be accelerated by the use of atropine.

Supraventricular tachycardias (Fig. 4.5)

Tachycardias which arise in atrial or AV junctional tissue can be described collectively as supraventricular. They share certain characteristics — starting abruptly, usually being regular at a rate of 140—220 per minute, and being associated with narrow QRS complexes, closely resembling those seen in sinus rhythm. Aberrant conduction with broadening of the QRS may, however, occur as may rates above and below those quoted. Atrial tachycardias are often the consequence of an accelerated automatic focus in the atria, whereas junctional tachycardia is usually due to a re-entry mechanism — the commonest form involving dual pathways within the AV node which have different rates of conduction and refractoriness.

Fig. 4.5 Supraventricular tachycardia showing QRS complexes of normal width at a rapid rate and with regular RR intervals.

Normal atrioventricular (AV) conduction is usually preserved. The attacks may last only seconds, but they often persist for minutes or hours or, much less commonly, for days. They may recur at short intervals or be separated from one another by weeks, months or even years. It is sometimes possible to identify provoking factors such as tobacco, coffee, and alcohol. Supraventricular tachycardia is a frequent complication of the Wolff—Parkinson—White syndrome (see p. 74).

Paroxysms are most often encountered in otherwise normal people in whom they give rise to palpitation, but no serious haemodynamic effects. These tachycardias can, however, produce cardiac failure and hypotension in the presence of heart disease because of the increased workload of the heart and the inadequate filling time during diastole.

The patient usually complains of attacks of rapid regular palpitation of abrupt onset, sometimes accompanied by dizziness or even syncope. When the attack is prolonged or when it occurs in those with heart disease, there may be dyspnoea and ischaemic chest pain. There may also be polyuria.

The episodes are often so brief and infrequent that no doctor ever sees them; if the patient is observed at the time, the pulse is found to be regular at a rate between 140 and 220. Carotid sinus massage frequently terminates the attack, but if it fails to do so, it has no effect upon the pulse rate. The ECG usually reveals QRST complexes of normal or near normal configuration occurring rapidly and regularly (Fig. 4.5); P waves, if they can be seen, often appear abnormal. They may precede, coincide with, or follow the QRS. In some instances, the QRST complexes are abnormally broadened and conform to a bundle branch block pattern, the appearances simulating ventricular tachycardia. Differentiation may often be made on the basis of the reaction to carotid sinus stimulation to which ventricular tachycardia does not respond, or to the identification of P waves associated with each QRS complex, for in ventricular tachycardia the P waves usually occur independently of, and at much slower rate than, the ventricular complexes.

It is difficult to obtain conventional ECG recordings of the attacks because of their unpredictability and brevity; the capture of episodes is aided by dynamic electrocardiography (Holter monitoring).

The ECG between attacks is usually normal, but the appearances of the Wolff—Parkinson—White syndrome, the 'short PR syndrome' (with a normal QRS), or other abnormalities of conduction may be seen.

Because of the repetitive paroxysmal nature of the tachycardia, prevention is often of greater importance than the treatment of

Table 4.1 Diagnosis of tachycardias.

	Atrial rate	Atrial complexes (P)	Effect of carotid sinus massage	Ventricular rate	Ventricular complexes (QRS)	Relation of atrial (P) to ventricular complexes (QRS)	Additional clues
Sinus tachycardia (p. 54)	Seldom more than 130	Normal	Slight slowing	Seldom more than 130 at rest	Unchanged	Normal relationship	Gradual changes in rate
Atrial tachycardia with block (p. 60)	140–220	Abnormal	Increases block, slows ventricle	70–220, usually half atrial	Usually unchanged	Long PR or dropped beats	P waves seen best in V1
Supraventricular tachycardia (p. 57)	140–220	Abnormal	Abolishes arrhythmia or has no effect	140–220, regular, same as atrial	Usually unchanged, may be broad and bizarre	Normal or P superimposed on QRS or ST	Sudden onset
Atrial flutter (p. 61)	Usually 280–320	'Sawtooth'	Increases block, slows ventricle	Usually 140–160, regular	Usually unchanged	2 or more atrial (f) waves to each QRS	Suspect when pulse regular at 150
Atrial fibrillation (p. 62)	300+	Irregular	Slight slowing of ventricle	Usually 100–150, irregular	Usually unchanged	No relationship	Complete irregularity
Ventricular tachycardia (p. 65)	60–100	Normal	None	140–220, regular	Broad and bizarre	P waves usually regular and independent of QRS complexes	Preceding ventricular ectopic beats

the individual attack. When possible, a provoking factor such as strong coffee or tobacco should be identified and avoided. Some patients are satisfied by reassurance that there is no serious heart disease, but in those in whom anxiety is important both as a causative factor and as a symptom of the paroxysms, a sedative such as diazepam 2–5 mg orally, thrice daily is helpful. When the attacks are prolonged or if they complicate organic heart disease, either disopyramide (100–150 mg thrice daily), a beta-adrenergic blocking drug, verapamil, or digoxin in the usual doses may be of value. Occasionally, it may be necessary to use quinidine.

In the treatment of the individual attack, the patient may be taught to carry out the Valsalva manoeuvre and the doctor can use carotid sinus massage. If this is not effective, sedation is often all that is necessary. If the patient is in great distress, treatment is more urgent. Verapamil (2–10 mg slowly), digoxin or a beta-adrenoceptor blocking drug may be administered or electrical shock applied.

In intractable cases, an antitachycardiac device may be used, or ablation of the bundle of His undertaken.

Atrial tachycardia with block (Fig. 4.6)

This resembles paroxysmal atrial tachycardia of the type previously described in that there is an ectopic atrial focus discharging at a rate of 140–220 per minute; it differs in that there is some degree of AV block. It is rare in the absence of serious organic heart disease, and is usually due to advanced digitalis intoxication. There is nearly always cellular potassium depletion, but the serum potassium is not necessarily low.

The ventricular rate depends upon the degree of AV block. Commonly, this is 2:1 and there are no adverse haemodynamic effects as the ventricular rate is about 80–100 per minute.

The clinical recognition of this rhythm disturbance is virtually impossible and the diagnosis must be made from the electrocardiogram (Fig. 4.6), in which P waves are seen to occur at a rate of 140–220 per minute; there is either a prolongation of the

Fig. 4.6   Atrial tachycardia with block. This is often most easily recognized in V1. Commonly there are two P waves to each ventricular complex, but greater or lesser degrees of block may occur. It may be difficult to identify those P waves which are superimposed on T waves.

PR interval or some of the P waves are not followed by QRS complexes. Carotid sinus pressure produces a transient increase in the atrioventricular block with a corresponding fall in the ventricular rate — a response quite unlike that of paroxysmal supraventricular tachycardia without block (see p. 58).

Atrial tachycardia with block is seldom dangerous in itself but is associated with a high risk of death from digitalis intoxication. Digitalis should be stopped and potassium supplements given. Electrical shock should not be used unless it is certain that digitalis intoxication is not responsible, as it may induce more serious arrhythmias.

Atrial flutter (Fig. 4.7)

In this arrhythmia, the atria beat regularly at a rate of 250–350 per minute — usually close to 300 per minute. The exact mechanism of atrial flutter remains unclear. The theory of circus movement proposes that the excitation wave moves in a circular fashion around the orifices of the superior and inferior venae cavae and is therefore self-perpetuating (macro re-entry).

Some degree of AV block is almost invariable. In most instances the ventricles beat regularly because of a 2:1, 3:1 or 4:1 response to the regular atrial activity, but it is irregular if the degree of block varies from cycle to cycle. The commonest variety is that of 2:1 block with a ventricular rate of 140–160.

Atrial flutter is almost always a complication of serious organic heart disease. The most common association is with rheumatic heart disease, but it is seen in hyperthyroidism, ischaemic heart disease, myocarditis and other disorders. It may be persistent or occur in paroxysms which are usually self-limited to hours or days, but it may progress to atrial fibrillation. The symptoms resemble those of atrial tachycardia, with palpitation, dizziness or syncope. The arrhythmia often provokes cardiac failure.

The pulse is usually regular at a rate of 140–160 minute. It may be possible to see venous 'flutter' waves in the neck. Carotid sinus massage leads to a transient increase in the atrioventricular block, with a slowing of the ventricular rate only as long as the pressure is maintained.

CSP   F F F F F

Fig. 4.7 Atrial flutter. Note that flutter waves are difficult to discern until carotid sinus pressure is applied.

The electrocardiogram is diagnostic with 'flutter' waves of a sawtooth appearance, best seen in leads II and III occurring at approximately 300 per minute (Fig. 4.7). The sawtooth nature of the complexes may be obscured by the QRS complexes when there is 2:1 block, but it is readily revealed when carotid sinus massage is applied.

As mentioned, atrial flutter is usually self-terminating, but because of its deleterious effects, treatment should be initiated without delay. Digitalis increases the AV block, brings the heart rate under control, and sometimes abolishes the arrhythmia. Treatment should be started with this drug, but electric shock is indicated if immediate correction is necessary and is almost invariably effective (see p. 78). In the patient liable to paroxysms of atrial flutter, digitalis should be continued indefinitely.

Atrial fibrillation (Fig. 4.8)

In this arrhythmia, irregular atrial impulses occur at rates over 300 per minute. It may be due to multiple foci of ectopic activity or to wavelets of excitation following variable courses through the atrial myocardium depending upon the location of patches of excitable and refractory muscle. Some degree of AV block is invariable; the ventricular rhythm is slower than the atrial but it is also irregular.

The presence of atrial fibrillation suggests that there has been either a pathological process involving the atria, as in rheumatic heart disease, or that there has been a rise in pressure with atrial dilatation secondary to mitral valve or left ventricular disease. There is usually an obvious organic lesion, most often rheumatic mitral valve disease. Other causes include ischaemic heart disease, especially acute myocardial infarction, thyrotoxicosis, hypertension, acute infections, particularly when these affect the lungs, and cardiopulmonary surgery. It is a rare complication of many other types of heart disease. In about 5% of patients, no evidence of organic heart disease can be found — 'lone' atrial fibrillation.

Atrial fibrillation may be paroxysmal, with attacks lasting for a few minutes or hours. This is particularly likely in acute myocardial infarction, in chest infections, and in the early stages of thyrotoxicosis and mitral valve disease. In rheumatic cases, the

Fig. 4.8 Atrial fibrillation, with complete irregularity of atrial and ventricular rhythms.

arrhythmia usually becomes established eventually and persists for the rest of the patient's life.

Atrial fibrillation leads to untoward effects for three major reasons (Table 4.2). First, the ventricular response is usually so fast that there is inadequate time for diastolic filling and the cardiac output falls. Secondly, the atrial contribution to ventricular filling is lost. Thirdly, stasis in the ineffectively contracting atrium encourages thrombosis. As a consequence, embolism is common, particularly in patients with mitral valve disease. Emboli from the right atrium produce pulmonary artery obstruction; those from the left atrium may lodge in cerebral, renal or other peripheral vessels.

The first symptom may be that of irregular palpitation, but in many patients atrial fibrillation leads to the sudden development of left ventricular failure and pulmonary oedema. The onset may also be insidious with gradually increasing dyspnoea.

The diagnosis is usually easy because the arterial pulse is totally irregular. The ventricular response to atrial fibrillation appears random. Because of the varying times available for filling of the ventricles, the output of the heart and the volume of the pulse alter from beat to beat. This chaotic pulse serves to differentiate atrial fibrillation from atrial or ventricular ectopic beats, which are the arrhythmias most likely to be confused with it. In these latter conditions some periods of regularity are usually observed, and often the irregularity will be noted to occur every second, third or fourth beat. The venous pulse in atrial fibrillation is also irregular. The heart rate at the apex ('the apex rate') is usually higher than the radial pulse rate because the heart expels so little blood in some beats that no pulsation can be appreciated in the peripheral arteries.

In the electrocardiogram, the P wave disappears but atrial activity produces an irregular undulation of the base line (Fig. 4.8). The QRS complexes are totally irregular in timing, except in the rare situation of atrial fibrillation complicated by complete heart block. In most cases of untreated atrial fibrillation, the ventricular rate lies between 100 and 160 per minute, but rates above or below this are not uncommon.

Although patients with the arrhythmia may survive for many years with few symptoms, atrial fibrillation is frequently a serious

Table 4.2 Adverse effects of atrial fibrillation.

1. Fast ventricular rate may precipitate heart failure.
2. Loss of atrial contribution to ventricular filling.
3. Stasis in the atria leads to thrombosis.

complication because of the risks of heart failure and embolism.

There are three components of the treatment of atrial fibrillation: the control of ventricular rate, the restoration of sinus rhythm and the prevention of embolism. The control of the ventricular rate comes first because it is the fast ventricular rate that is most deleterious, rather than the atrial fibrillation *per se*, and also because the arrhythmia may terminate spontaneously. Depending upon the severity of the clinical situation, digoxin or one of the other cardiac glycosides may be given intravenously or orally. In most cases, oral administration is satisfactory, and brings the heart rate under control within 2 or 3 hours. When full digitalization has been achieved, the ventricular rate at rest should be held at about 70 to 80 per minute. If the heart rate cannot be reduced to this level, a beta-adrenoceptor blocking drug or verapamil may be added. Amiodarone is useful in intractable cases.

When atrial fibrillation has developed recently in a patient with mitral valve disease, heparin should be given as the risk of embolism is particularly high at this time; oral anticoagulants should be continued subsequently for at least a year.

When atrial fibrillation has been present for many years, and there is associated and untreatable severe heart disease, there is little to be gained by trying to restore normal rhythm because this is not likely to be maintained. Even if it is, the atrial muscle has usually atrophied and is functionally ineffective. When the arrhythmia is of relatively recent onset, and particularly when the heart disease has been alleviated or some complicating condition such as thyrotoxicosis or pulmonary infection corrected, the patient is likely to benefit from its termination. Therefore, if sinus rhythm has not returned within a few days, but it seems probable that it would be maintained were the atrial fibrillation terminated, electric shock therapy (p. 78) should be employed. This is effective in most instances, at least initially. However, there is a considerable relapse rate within the succeeding months whether or not prophylactic drugs, such as quinidine, are used. Because of this, it is advisable in most instances to keep the patient on digitalis therapy after restoration of sinus rhythm, as a subsequent recurrence of atrial fibrillation may be associated with a dangerously fast ventricular rate.

Fig. 4.9 Ventricular ectopic beats. Note bizarre pattern of QRST, and succeeding compensatory pause.

Ventricular ectopic rhythms

Ventricular ectopic beats (extrasystoles, premature beats)

An ectopic focus in the ventricles may arise because of ventricular escape, enhanced automatic activity, or re-entry. Ventricular ectopic beats are not uncommon in normal individuals but are encountered frequently in organic heart disease, especially in myocardial infarction. If they occur every second beat (bigeminy or 'coupling') they are usually due to digitalis therapy.

Patients are seldom aware of ventricular ectopic beats, but may complain of the heart seeming to stop briefly, or of an occasional heavy beat. The diagnosis may be suspected from an irregularity of the pulse interrupting an otherwise regular rhythm, but cannot be made without an ECG, in which there are bizarre and broadened QRS complexes followed by T waves pointing in the direction opposite to that of the main QRS component (Fig 4.9). The QRST complexes are not preceded by a P wave and are usually succeeded by a long period (the compensatory pause) before the next sinus-activated beat appears.

The importance of ventricular ectopic beats depends upon their context. In normal individuals they are virtually of no consequence. They are associated with an impaired prognosis in ischaemic heart disease but it is not established that the outlook is improved by their suppression.

Ventricular tachycardia (Fig. 4.10)

In this condition a tachycardia arises in the ventricles at a rate of 120 to 220 per minute; the atria usually remain under the control of the sinus node. It may be a consequence of either re-entry or enhanced automaticity of ventricular pacemaker cells. It is nearly always a complication of serious heart disease, although occasionally seen in an otherwise normal individual. The attacks are liable to occur in paroxysms lasting for seconds or minutes, but

Fig. 4.10 Ventricular tachycardia reverting to sinus rhythm with ventricular ectopic beats. Note similar broad bizarre QRS complexes in ectopic beats and tachycardia.

may continue for several hours. Ventricular tachycardia frequently causes or aggravates heart failure and the shock syndrome.

As with supraventricular tachycardia, the first symptom may be that of rapid and regular palpitation, but because of the more serious effects on the circulation, acute breathlessness and ischaemic chest pain tend to be more severe. On examination there is a rapid, regular but small pulse. The independent atrial activity may be responsible for dissociated 'a' waves in the venous pulse and a variation in the intensity of the first heart sound, but these physical signs are difficult to elicit. The ECG shows rapidly occurring broad QRS complexes resembling those of bundle branch block (Fig. 4.10). P waves may be identified at a rate different from that of the ventricles. They may be difficult to identify unless a 12-lead ECG is recorded. The RR intervals are usually equal, but may vary by up to 0.03 sec from one another. The lack of response to carotid pressure assists in the differentiation from atrial tachycardia with bundle branch block (see also p. 68).

In the patient with good underlying heart function, urgent treatment may not be necessary. Most instances of ventricular tachycardia, however, call for immediate action, particularly in the context of acute myocardial infarction. Lignocaine, 50 to 100 mg, may be given intravenously and repeated if necessary. Alternative therapy includes disopyramide, mexiletine or the beta-adrenoceptor blocking drugs. If these drugs fail to control the arrhythmia, electric shock may be used.

The drugs mentioned above may be used to prevent recurrences, as may amiodarone.

Torsade de pointes (Fig. 4.11)

This distinctive type of ventricular tachycardia is associated with a long QT, and may be idiopathic, due to hypokalaemia, or the result of the toxic action of such drugs as tricyclic antidepressants and type 1a antiarrhythmics. Its characteristic ECG feature is 'twisting of the points' of the QRS complexes. It usually occurs in

Fig. 4.11   Torsade de pointes. This is a progressive change in the direction of the QRS, with a 'twisting of the points'.

repetitive bursts lasting a few seconds; it may progress to ventricular fibrillation. The underlying cause should, if possible, be corrected; pacing often succeeds in abolishing it.

Ventricular fibrillation (Fig. 4.12)

In this condition there is a chaotic electrical disturbance of the ventricles, with impulses occurring irregularly at a rate of 300−500 per minute. Ventricular contraction is uncoordinated and ventricular filling and emptying cease. The cardiac output falls precipitously to zero.

Ventricular fibrillation is a common complication of acute myocardial infarction and ischaemia, and may also result from drowning, electrocution and overdosage of drugs including digitalis, adrenaline and isoprenaline. Self-terminating episodes are rare but may complicate complete heart block.

Because of its catastrophic effects, ventricular fibrillation gives rise to the clinical features of cardiac arrest, with sudden disappearance of arterial pulses, cessation of respiration, loss of consciousness and dilatation of the pupils. Although it cannot be diagnosed clinically, it is to be suspected in any patient dying with apparent suddenness, particularly in the context of acute myocardial infarction. On the electrocardiogram, there is a chaotic rhythm with ventricular complexes of varying amplitude and rate (Fig. 4.12). Eventually asystole ensues.

Ventricular fibrillation is almost invariably fatal, and immediate treatment is necessary if death is to be prevented. As with other forms of cardiac arrest, an effective circulation and ventilation must be obtained within 4 minutes if irreversible brain damage is not to occur. Sinus rhythm can usually only be restored by electric shock, which should be administered as soon as possible. If an electical defibrillator is not immediately available, the standard treatment of cardiac arrest should be started with closed-chest cardiac compression and artificial ventilation (see p. 79).

Recurrences of ventricular fibrillation should be prevented in the same way as ventricular tachycardia.

Fig. 4.12 Ventricular fibrillation. Note broad, bizarre and irregular complexes.

The differentiation of supraventricular from ventricular ectopic rhythms

It may be difficult to differentiate supraventricular (atrial or junctional) from ventricular ectopic rhythms even with an ECG.

Ectopic beats

The QRS complexes of ectopic beats of atrial or junctional origin are usually identical to those of preceding sinus beats. However, they may be broad and bizarre due to *aberration* (Fig. 4.13). Conduction through the bundle branches is aberrant if one branch is still refractory from the preceding beat, when the other has recovered. Usually, the right bundle takes longer to recover than the left and the aberrant beat has the appearance of right bundle branch block. Aberration should be suspected when the ectopic beat is preceded by a P wave different from that of normal sinus beats, or if it is of right bundle branch block type (RSR' in VI), or when the initial part of the QRS is the same in the ectopic beat as it is in the normally conducted beats.

Tachycardias

It may be possible to determine the nature of a tachycardia clinically because the activity of the atria is usually dissociated from that of the ventricles in ventricular tachycardia. There may be irregular cannon waves in the jugular veins (see p. 103) and variation in the intensity of the first heart sound. In junctional tachycardia, cannon waves may occur with every beat.

The response to carotid sinus stimulation is even more diagnostic, for this manoeuvre frequently abolishes supraventricular tachycardia but leaves ventricular tachycardia unaffected. However, one should delay applying this test if possible until an ECG is available, as one may otherwise miss the opportunity of verifying the nature of the arrhythmia by obtaining a graphic record.

Supraventricular tachycardia can be diagnosed easily on the ECG if the QRS complexes resemble, as they usually do, those that

Fig. 4.13 Supraventricular ectopic beats with aberration. Note that the ectopic beats are preceded by a P wave.

the patient exhibited during sinus rhythm. Difficulty arises when supraventricular tachycardia is accompanied by aberrant bizarre complexes. Carotid sinus pressure may quickly resolve this problem, but if it does not, the diagnosis largely depends on identifying P waves on a 12-lead ECG. If these are dissociated from the QRS, ventricular tachycardia is probable. Additional evidence may be provided by the occurrence and nature of ectopic beats in previous tracings. Sometimes the diagnosis requires the insertion of electrodes into the heart to determine the origin and spread of the arrhythmia.

The carotid sinus and arrhythmias

The carotid sinus is situated at the bifurcation of the common carotid artery and is sensitive to changes in arterial pressure. Impulses arising from the stretch receptors in the carotid sinus pass to the medulla and reflexly slow the heart by stimulating the motor nucleus of the vagus nerve and by inhibiting cardiac sympathetic action. Usually, external pressure on the carotid sinus leads to a slight slowing of the heart rate by reducing the activity of the sinus node. In some individuals in whom the carotid sinus is hypersensitive, external pressure leads to extreme bradycardia and hypotension with resulting syncope.

Carotid sinus pressure plays an important part in the recognition and management of cardiac arrhythmias. It is best to locate the carotid artery on one side first and then to stroke it gently, but firmly. If this is ineffective, the manoeuvre should be repeated on the other side. Carotid sinus massage causes only slight slowing of the ventricular rate in patients with sinus tachycardia and with atrial fibrillation. If it has any effect in the patient with supraventricular tachycardia, it causes an abrupt termination of the arrhythmia. In atrial flutter and in atrial tachycardia with block, it produces an increase in atrioventricular block, temporarily decreasing the ventricular rate which rises again when the massage is discontinued. It has no effect in ventricular tachycardia. It is best to carry out carotid sinus massage with ECG control, as excessive bradycardia and even ventricular arrhythmias may result from this procedure. Other dangers include reflex hypotension and cerebrovascular insufficiency.

Disorders of conduction

Sinu-atrial block and sinus arrest

In sinu-atrial block, an impulse from the sinus node fails to activate the atria. This results in a dropped beat; on the electrocardiogram a complete PQRST complex is absent, but the next sinus beat comes in at the predicted time (Fig. 4.14). It is of little clinical importance except that it may be a manifestation of intoxication by digoxin or other antiarrhythmic drugs. It may be a component of the sick sinus syndrome (see p. 55). If it is prolonged, syncope occurs. In sinus arrest, the sinus node fails to initiate an impulse; after a pause, junctional or ventricular escape occurs. Its significance is similar to that of sinu-atrial block.

Atrioventricular (heart) block

The term atrioventricular (AV) block implies that there is some defect in conduction of the impulse from the atria to the ventricles. In first-degree AV block, all the impulses reach the ventricles but they are delayed in their passage and the PR interval exceeds 0.20 sec (Fig. 4.15). In second-degree block, some impulses reach the ventricles while others fail to do so (Fig. 4.16). In complete heart block, no impulses reach the ventricles from the atria, and the ventricles are under the control of a lower pacemaker situated in the junctional tissue, bundle of His, the bundle branches or Purkinje tissue (Fig. 4.17). In bundle branch block, AV conduction is maintained through one branch, the other being blocked.

First-degree AV block (Fig. 4.15). First-degree AV block occurs occasionally in normal individuals, is a characteristic feature of the carditis of acute rheumatic fever, and digitalis overdosage. It cannot be diagnosed clinically and its recognition depends on observing a PR interval of greater than 0.20 sec in the ECG. Its only importance is as an index of digitalis intoxication and as a precursor of the more advanced degrees of AV block.

Second-degree AV block. One of the commonest varieties of second-degree block is the Wenckebach phenomenon in which the PR interval becomes progressively more prolonged from beat to beat until one P wave is not succeeded by a QRS complex (Fig. 4.16). The next atrial complex is followed at a normal or near normal interval by a QRS complex and the cycle of events recurs.

Fig. 4.14 Sinu-atrial block. Note complete absence of PQRST, with the next beat coming in at the predicted time.

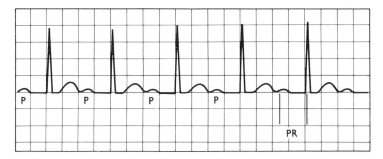

Fig. 4.15 First-degree heart block. The PR interval is prolonged to 0.36 sec, but each sinus impulse is conducted to the ventricles.

The pulse is correspondingly irregular. In 2:1 block, every second atrial beat is followed by a ventricular complex. This may be suspected clinically by a regular slow ventricular rhythm and is confirmed on the electrocardiogram (Fig. 4.16). The Wenckebach phenomenon is frequently the result of digitalis intoxication, but both this and the other varieties of second-degree heart block are often due to ischaemic heart disease, particularly myocardial infarction, and to many other types of cardiac disease. The main significance of second-degree heart block lies in the liability of the patient to develop complete heart block and the Adams—Stokes syndrome. However, if the ventricular rate in second-degree heart block is sufficiently slow, cardiac failure or hypotension may be precipitated.

If the AV block is due to digitalis, this drug must be temporarily discontinued. If other causes can be implicated, the patient must be carefully observed, and if the slow heart rate is responsible for clinical deterioration the heart must be accelerated. This may be achieved by administering atropine or isoprenaline, or by artificial pacing.

Fig. 4.16 (A) Partial heart block of the Wenckebach type. Note that the PR interval increases from beat to beat until a beat is dropped, following which the cycle restarts. (B) Second-degree heart block — 2:1 block. Note that only every second P wave is followed by a QRS.

Fig. 4.17 Complete heart block. Note that both P waves and QRS complexes are regular, but have no fixed relationship to one another.

Complete AV (heart) block (Fig. 4.17). The ventricular rate is slow (25 to 50 min). There are cannon waves in the venous pulse (see p. 103) and a varying first heart sound (see p. 108).

Acute complete heart block is most commonly a complication of myocardial infarction, but may also result from cardiac surgery and myocarditis. In myocardial infarction, it usually follows occlusion of the right coronary artery which is responsible for the blood supply of the junctional tissue and bundle of His (see also p. 157). The severely damaged heart may not be able to compensate adequately for the bradycardia by increasing its stroke volume; heart failure and hypotension may ensue. There is also a considerable risk of ventricular asystole. The bradycardia may be controlled by infusing isoprenaline in a dose of 2—5 mg in 500 ml of 5% laevulose or dextrose, or by an artificial pacemaker (see p. 76). If the patient survives, normal AV conduction is usually restored within a week.

In most cases of chronic complete heart block there is fibrosis of both bundle branches of unknown cause. This variety is most commonly seen in the elderly. A congenital form occurs either as an isolated finding or in association with other congenital heart defects. Heart block can also complicate rheumatic or ischaemic heart disease, or follow trauma to the conducting tissue at surgery. A proportion of patients with chronic complete heart block survive for years with no symptoms, but once heart failure or syncopal attacks of the Adams—Stokes variety develop, the expectation of life is usually only a few months. For this reason, treatment is indicated when symptoms arise. The heart rate may be accelerated by the use of long-acting isoprenaline in a dosage of 15—60 mg three or four times a day but this therapy may provoke dangerous arrhythmias. An artificial pacemaker is indicated in virtually all cases.

The Adams—Stokes attack

In an Adams—Stokes attack the patient loses consciousness for a period of some seconds because of transient cardiac arrest. It usually occurs in patients with second-degree or complete heart

block who develop sudden loss of ventricular activity. It is particularly common during the progression from second-degree to
complete heart block because the ventricular pacemaker necessary
for survival may not have become firmly established. In some
cases, the Adams–Stokes attack is due not to ventricular asystole
but to a short burst of ventricular tachycardia or fibrillation.

The presenting symptom is syncope with or without a preceding
period of dizziness. The attack usually lasts some 10 to 30 seconds
and convulsions may occur. During the attack the patient is
pulseless, pale or cyanosed. Consciousness returns rapidly with
reappearance of the heart beat, the patient then flushing as blood
courses through capillaries dilated by the hypoxia of the attack.
Attacks of the Adams–Stokes variety may be separated from one
another by a number of months, but occasionally a series occurs
over a period of minutes or hours. Sooner or later, the patient is
likely to die of ventricular asystole or ventricular fibrillation.

The diagnosis should be considered in any patient presenting
with syncope, but is unlikely to be the explanation in the absence
of bundle branch block, second-degree block, or complete AV
block between the episodes.

During an attack a blow over the cardiac apex may restore the
heart action, but if it does not do so, the usual therapy for cardiac
arrest should be undertaken (p. 79) with closed-chest cardiac
compression and artifical ventilation. Adams–Stokes attacks can
be prevented by an artificial pacemaker.

Bundle branch block

In this condition, either the right or the left branch of the bundle
of His is not conducting impulses.

Block of the right bundle branch gives rise to a characteristic
electrocardiographic appearance (Figs. 3.18 and 4.18A). This is
often an isolated congenital lesion of no importance but may be
associated with other congenital heart defects, particularly atrial
septal defect; in middle or advanced age, it is usually due to
ischaemic heart disease or idiopathic fibrosis. Right bundle branch
block may be partial, with QRS width of less than 0.12 sec, or
complete, in which the QRS is of 0.12 sec duration or more. It
may be suspected clinically because the block leads to a delayed
activation, and therefore contraction, of the right ventricle. This
results in late closure of the pulmonary valve which can be
recognized by a wide splitting of the second heart sound (p. 108).
Right bundle branch block is of little clinical significance, except
as an indicator of possible heart disease and as a precursor of
complete heart block (especially if associated with left or right

Fig. 4.18A Right bundle branch block.

Fig. 4.18B Left bundle branch block.

axis deviation indicating block in one of the fascicles of the left bundle).

Left bundle branch block is rare in the otherwise normal individual and is most commonly seen in ischaemic heart disease. It is difficult to recognize clinically, although there may be reversed splitting of the second heart sound (p. 108); it is readily identified on the ECG (Figs. 3:17 and 4.18B). Because it is associated with severe ventricular disease (usually ischaemic) it carries a more serious prognosis than right bundle branch block, but patients with this lesion may survive for many years.

Neither form of bundle branch block requires treatment.

Pre-excitation (Wolff–Parkinson–White syndrome)

In this condition, an anomalous conduction pathway bypasses the AV node. This permits the abnormally early activation of part of one ventricle, the remaining ventricular muscle receiving its impulse normally. This leads to a short PR interval (less than 0.11 sec) and a widened QRS (Fig. 4.19).

The normal and abnormal conduction pathways are able to form part of a re-entry circuit. This facilitates the occurrence of

Fig. 4.19 Pre-excitation (Wolff–Parkinson–White syndrome). Note short PR interval, and broad QRS complex with notch (delta wave) on the upstroke.

paroxysmal tachycardia. The combination of pre-excitation and paroxysmal tachycardia constitutes the Wolff–Parkinson–White syndrome.

In most cases, no underlying heart disease is present. The paroxysms of supraventricular tachycardia may respond to a variety of drugs including disopyramide, verapamil, quinidine, and beta-adrenoceptor blocking drugs. If atrial fibrillation develops, the anomalous pathway conducts impulses to the ventricles at an extremely fast rate (sometimes more than 250 per minute). Digoxin is dangerous in this situation. Amiodarone is particularly effective in controlling the arrhythmias associated with the Wolff-Parkinson–White syndrome.

Increasingly, surgery is being used to interrupt the abnormal pathway.

Atrioventricular dissociation (Fig. 4.20)

This term is used to describe a form of rhythm disturbance in which a pacemaker in the atrium is controlling atrial activity and another pacemaker situated in the junctional tissue or the ventricle is controlling the ventricular activity. Although there is dissociation of atria and ventricles in complete heart block, AV dissociation often occurs in the absence of any abnormality of conduction. It is always secondary to some other abnormality, with either slowing of the sinus node or acceleration of a lower pacemaker, or a combination of the two. When the two pacemakers are initiating impulses almost synchronously the territory of one is refractory to stimulation from the other. Sooner or later, the two foci cease to fire at the same time; the territory of one is then captured by the other (Fig. 4.20). It is a not uncommon complication of digitalis therapy and of acute myocardial infarction. It is important to differentiate this from organic heart block as it carries a much less sinister prognosis and requires no specific therapy.

Fig. 4.20 Atrioventricular dissociation. Note the varying relationship between P waves and QRS complexes. When atrial and ventricular activity is almost synchronous, the atria and ventricles are activated independently, i.e. they are dissociated. However, when the two foci cease to fire at approximately the same time, the territory of one can be captured by the other. Thus the third atrial complex (P wave) is followed by a QRS complex and the atrium has 'captured' the ventricle. Subsequently, there is a return to atrioventricular dissociation.

Electrical therapy

When a brief electrical shock of high energy is applied to the heart, all parts of the heart are usually depolarized simultaneously; the sinus node subsequently recommences cardiac rhythmicity. If, however, the shock falls during the 'vulnerable' period of ventricular repolarization (i.e. on the T wave) (Fig. 4.21), depolarization of the ventricles is incomplete, the re-entry phenomenon may occur and lead to ventricular tachycardia or fibrillation.

Electrical pacing

Control over the electrical activity of the heart may be obtained by the use of an artificial pacemaker (Fig. 4.22). A pacemaking system consists of a pulse generator (containing batteries and electronic circuitry) and one or more electrodes. If pacing is to be maintained for only a short perid of time, an external power source is used; if long-term pacing is necessary, the pulse generator is implanted.

Electrical pacemaking is potentially hazardous. If the electrical impulse is of sufficient magnitude and falls during the period of ventricular repolarization, i.e. on the T wave of the ECG, ventricular fibrillation may be induced. This problem is overcome by the use of a 'demand' pacemaker which operates only when there is no ventricular complex generated by the patient's own heart. In the absence of a complex, the pacemaker discharges after a selected interval. Some pacemakers detect or stimulate atrial activity as well; these allow the atria and ventricles to function in the normal sequence. This produces 'physiological' pacing, and allows the heart rate to increase on exercise. Other adaptive pacemakers increase heart rate when muscular activity is detected. Numerous varieties of pacemaker are now available;

Fig. 4.21 The vulnerable period of ventricular repolarization is illustrated by the hatched area. Electrical impulses of sufficient magnitude occurring during the upstroke of the T wave may initiate ventricular fibrillation.

P   Q R S   T

P   P   P   P   P

Fig. 4.22 Electrical pacing. A thin vertical pacing impulse, indicated by the arrow, immediately precedes the broad QRS resulting from ventricular stimulation. The P waves continue independently, due to heart block.

many of them are 'programmable', i.e. the cardiologist can choose the particular type of pacing programme that is most suitable for an individual patient. Hazards of pacemaking include infection and failure of the components of the pacemaking unit, such as batteries, circuitry and electrodes.

When pacing is employed in the treatment of heart block in acute myocardial infarction, it is customary to introduce the electrode through a peripheral vein and to position its tip in the apex of the right ventricle. The other end of the electrode is attached to a portable battery-operated demand pacemaker. The electrode is withdrawn when the risks of atrioventricular block seem to have disappeared.

In chronic heart block, an electrode of a similar type is positioned with its tip in the right ventricle, but with its proximal end attached to a pacemaker buried under the skin of the axillary region or the anterior chest. Pacing with the electrode tip in the right atrium can be used for patients with the sick sinus syndrome, provided that atrioventricular conduction is normal. Electrodes may be placed upon the surface of the myocardium at the time of a thoracotomy or laparotomy and the wires passed subcutaneously to a pacemaker positioned in the sheath of the rectus abdominis. Pacemakers should have a life of more than 10 years but regular checking for battery or other failure is necessary.

Electrical stimulators may also be used to terminate tachyarrhythmias (antitachyarrhythmia devices or ATDs). Some of these devices stop the arrhythmia by an intense burst of current (e.g. the internal defibrillator). Others are designed to introduce single or multiple low energy stimuli at a critical time during the arrhythmia cycles; these may be very effective in some cases of troublesome supraventricular tachycardias.

Direct current (dc) shock therapy

The dc shock must be timed to avoid the vulnerable period and it is customary to arrange for the defibrillator to discharge 0.02 sec after the peak of the R wave. A synchronized discharge of this kind is not possible when there is ventricular fibrillation.

Because the procedure is a painful one, an anaesthetic is usually given, except when there is ventricular fibrillation (because the patient is unconscious). A short-acting barbiturate is often used, but an alternative is to supplement an analgesic such as morphine with diazepam 5−10 mg intravenously. One electrode, smeared with electrode jelly, is placed in the right parasternal region and the other either in the left axilla or posteriorly below the left scapula. The machine is charged to the chosen level and discharged by pressing a button on the electrode. For the treatment of ventricular fibrillation, a shock of 200−400 watt seconds (Ws) is usually necessary, but for other arrhythmias it is best to start with a small shock such as 50 or 100 Ws. This may be increased until 400 Ws is reached, but if four or five shocks are ineffective it is unlikely that sinus rhythm will be restored by further shocks.

Apart from slight skin burns, the procedure is usually free from undesirable effects. However, there is a danger of producing serious arrhythmias in the patient with digitalis intoxication, and it is wise to discontinue this drug for one or two days prior to electric shock administration if possible.

The indications for electric shock therapy are discussed under the individual arrhythmias, but in general it may be stated that electric shock therapy is almost invariably effective for all types of tachycardia including the supraventricular tachycardia, atrial flutter, atrial fibrillation, ventricular tachycardia and ventricular fibrillation. Some cases of chronic atrial fibrillation are resistant. Electric shock should not be given if it is thought that the arrhythmia is digitalis- or quinidine-induced.

A relatively new form of antiarrhythmic therapy is 'ablation'. With this technique, a shock is delivered by an electrode positioned against the endocardium with the deliberate intention of damaging subjacent tissue. This has been used particularly for supraventricular arrhythmias which have proved impossible to control. By ablating the bundle of His, heart block is produced. The ventricle is then protected from the fast rate but a pacemaker is needed.

Cardiac arrest

Cardiac arrest may be defined as the sudden cessation of cardiac function. This is usually due to ventricular fibrillation or asystole, but sometimes there is electromechanical dissociation — the ECG shows continuing electrical activity but mechanical function has ceased; this is often due to cardiac rupture but it may be caused by drugs. Cardiac arrest may result from a large number of different factors, and in many cases more than one factor is involved. The commonest cause of cardiac arrest is acute myocardial infarction and ischaemia. Anaesthesia is also important, particularly if there has been underventilation or an obstruction to ventilation. Further problems associated with anaesthesia arise from endotracheal intubation which may cause strong vagal reflexes, and the use of anaesthetic drugs such as cyclopropane and chloroform. Disturbances of electrolytes, particularly potassium, magnesium and calcium, may be responsible, as may drugs including digitalis, adrenaline, isoprenaline and quinidine. Other causes include drowning, hypothermia and electrocution.

Cardiac arrest usually occurs suddenly and without warning. The most important finding is absence of arterial pulsation. Consciousness is soon lost and respiration ceases. After a short interval the pupils dilate. The combination of unconsciousness and loss of pulse should be sufficient for diagnosis.

Treatment should be started immediately; irreversible brain damage will occur if there is circulatory arrest for more than 4 minutes. A blow over the cardiac apex will sometimes restart the heart; if this fails, external cardiac massage should be combined with artificial ventilation. For external cardiac massage, the patient must be lying on a firm surface, either on the floor or on a board placed behind his chest. The heel of one hand should be placed on the lower part of the sternum and the heel of the other hand placed immediately on top of it. The sternum is then rhythmically depressed by about 3—5 cm 60 times or more per minute. The action should be forceful and must be applied only to the sternum. Pressure by the fingers or the hand on the ribs leads to fractures which may cause serious respiratory embarrassment, or damage the liver and spleen. If the cardiac compression is effective, pulses can be felt in the carotid or femoral arteries, and the pupils become smaller. Occasionally, open-chest massage may be more effective than closed-chest, but this technique is only suitable for use by surgeons.

At the same time that external cardiac compression is commenced, ventilation must be ensured. First of all, the neck is extended and the jaw pulled forward. If no apparatus is available, mouth-to-mouth or mouth-to-nose breathing is employed. A Brook airway which has mouthpieces for both patient and resuscitator is a useful method of giving direct ventilatory assistance. Various bags and masks are available for artificial ventilation, but ideally an endotracheal tube should be introduced by someone skilled in the technique as soon as possible and ventilation achieved with oxygen.

The UK Resuscitation Council recommends the strategies in Fig. 4.23. The patient needs to be observed carefully after recovery from cardiac arrest as further episodes may occur. If there has been cerebral damage, hypothermia may be helpful. Renal failure is not uncommon if cardiac arrest has been prolonged. Respiratory function may also be depressed and mechanical ventilation may be needed for some days.

The results of treating cardiac arrest are good provided it has been recognized immediately and the underlying cardiac disease is not severe. Thus, in the operating theatre, nearly all cases are resuscitated, but after myocardial infarction, the prognosis is less good, particularly if cardiac failure or shock have preceded it.

Antiarrhythmic drugs

Anti-arrhythmic therapy is used to:

1 suppress or prevent arrhythmias;
2 slow the ventricular response to supraventricular arrhythmias.

Drugs to suppress or prevent arrhythmias

There are four main classes of antiarrhythmic drug action.

I 'Membrane-stabilizing' drugs, which also have a local anaesthetic action, block the inflow of sodium into the cell and, therefore, the rate of depolarization. This has the effect of reducing the automaticity of ectopic pacemaker foci.

II 'Anti-sympathetic' drugs — notably those which block beta-adrenoceptors.

Fig. 4.23 Strategies for the treatment of ventricular fibrillation and asystole recommended by the UK Resuscitation Council.

III Drugs which prolong action potential. Amiodarone is the only available drug whose main action is of this type.

IV Drugs which block the inflow of calcium into the cell. This affects the activity of certain cells, particularly those of the atrioventricular node, which are dependent more on the calcium inflow than on sodium. Verapamil belongs to this group.

Class I drugs

These are subdivided into three subclasses (see Table 4.3).

Quinidine. This drug has been used for more than 50 years in the prevention and termination of atrial and ventricular ectopic rhythms. When given in adequate doses it is an effective antiarrhythmic agent, but frequently produces nausea, vomiting, headache, tinnitus and diarrhoea. More serious are its cardiotoxic effects, including heart block and asystole, and the provocation of ventricular tachycardia and ventricular fibrillation. Quinidine causes a clinically significant increase in digoxin plasma levels when they are given together; digoxin dosage should be halved in patients on this drug when quinidine is added. Other rarer toxic effects include respiratory depression, thrombocytopaenia

Table 4.3 Vaughan—Williams classification of antiarrhythmic drugs.

Class I: membrane-stabilizing drugs. Inhibit fast sodium channel
  (a) Prolong action potential (QT): quinidine, procainamide, disopyramide
  (b) Shorten action potential: lignocaine, mexiletine
  (c) Prolong QRS: flecainide, encainide, propafenone

Class II: beta-blocking drugs

Class III: prolong action potential (QT)
  Amiodarone, bretylium, sotalol

Class IV: calcium antagonists
  Verapamil, diltiazem

and skin rashes. Because of its toxicity, quinidine has been largely replaced by dc shock and by other antiarrhythmic drugs. However, it remains of value in preventing recurrences of supraventricular tachycardia, flutter and fibrillation, and ventricular tachycardia and fibrillation, particularly when such therapy is required over long periods of time.

Quinidine is usually given orally as the sulphate in tablets containing 0.2 g or 0.3 g. The dose required for maintenance varies from 0.2 g thrice daily to 0.4 g 4-hourly. A sustained action preparation (Kinidin Durules) may be used in a dosage of 0.25—0.50 g twice daily. The dosage required to suppress or prevent arrhythmias varies considerably from patient to patient and therapy must be individualized, preferably with estimation of blood levels of the drug; a plasma concentration of 2—4 μg/ml should be aimed for.

Quinidine produces a variety of ECG effects including a prolonged QT interval, depression of the ST segment and T wave inversion. These do not necessarily indicate overdosage, but the appearance of conduction defects or ventricular arrhythmias (notably torsade de pointes) implies cardiac toxicity and the drug should be discontinued.

Procainamide. The actions of procainamide are similar to those of quinidine, but it is less effective in the treatment of atrial arrhythmias and is less toxic when used intravenously.

Procainamide may be administered intravenously, intramuscularly and orally. When given intravenously, it may produce a marked hypotensive effect due to peripheral vasodilatation, but this can be avoided with care. It should be given at a rate not exceeding 100 mg per minute; an ECG should be recorded and the blood pressure taken every minute. Further procainamide should not be given if the systolic pressure falls below 90 mmHg, or if the QRS complex becomes more than 25% wider than it had been, or if the arrhythmia has been controlled. If parenteral treatment with procainamide is necessary, but there is no urgency, procainamide can be given by the intramuscular route in doses of 250–500 mg 6-hourly.

By the oral route, a total daily dose of some 3 g, which may be as 500 mg 4-hourly or in a long-acting preparation (Durules) 1 g thrice daily, is required. In this dosage, nausea, vomiting and anorexia are common; nightmares, depression and convulsions are rare. Long-term oral procainamide therapy may lead to depression of the bone marrow, skin rashes and a syndrome simulating systemic lupus erythematosus.

Disopyramide. Disopyramide resembles quinidine in its anti-arrhythmic effects but has atropine-like actions which cause a dry mouth and urinary retention and, rarely, glaucoma. It has a negative inotropic effect and should be avoided in cardiac failure. It may provoke arrhythmias including torsade de pointes. The oral dosage is 100–150 mg three to four times daily. Intravenously it may be given in a dosage of 0.5 mg/kg.

Lignocaine. This drug resembles quinidine and procainamide in its mode of action, but is relatively ineffective in controlling atrial arrhythmias and has virtually no myocardial depressant effect in therapeutic doses. It is therefore safer to give intravenously than quinidine, procainamide and disopyramide. However, it should not be given in the presence of AV block, which it may aggravate. The drug is used mainly intravenously, and by this route its duration of action is only 10–20 minutes. Initally, a dose of 50–100 mg (i.e. 5–10 ml of the 1% solution) can be given over a period of 1–2 minutes and repeated, if necessary, 2 minutes later. This may be followed by an intravenous infusion of 4 mg per minute for 30 minutes, 3 mg per minute for a further 30 minutes and thereafter 2 mg per minute for 24–48 hours, if necessary. Serious toxic effects from lignocaine are unusual, but include confusion, convulsions, respiratory depression and coma.

Mexiletine. Mexiletine resembles lignocaine in its structure and actions but is well absorbed orally and is therefore useful in the chronic treatment of ventricular arrhythmias. Toxic effects include nausea, vomiting and tremor. The oral dosage is usually 200–250 mg thrice daily.

Flecainide. Flecainide is one of the most effective antiarrhythmic drugs, and usually abolishes all ventricular ectopic activity. Like other class Ic drugs, it prolongs the PR interval and QRS duration, and has a relatively high risk of provoking ventricular arrhythmias. It is also negatively inotropic, and it is liable to provoke or aggravate cardiac failure. Oral flecainide is given in a dosage of 100 mg twice daily, increasing to 200 mg twice daily, if required.

Propafenone. Propafenone, which is not available in many countries including the United Kingdom is a class Ic drug, which has been found particularly useful in the management of the Wolff−Parkinson−White syndrome. It is also effective in many cases of ventricular tachycardia but, like other drugs in its class, it is also prone to provoke ventricular arrhythmias. Oral pro-pafenone is given in a dosage of 150−300 mg thrice daily.

Beta-adrenoceptor blocking drugs (Table 4.4)

Beta-adrenoceptor blocking drugs oppose the effects of cate-cholamines on the beta-adrenoceptors.

Some block the receptors in the heart selectively (beta$_1$-receptor blocking agents). Others also block receptors in the bronchi and peripheral vessels. Consequently, they may induce bronchospasm in susceptible subjects and impair the circulation to the limbs.

Propranolol and similar drugs antagonize the ability of sym-pathetic substances to increase the rate and contractility of the heart. These drugs are sometimes effective in abolishing ven-tricular and atrial arrhythmias and are of value in slowing the ventricular response to atrial arrhythmias.

There is little to choose between propranolol and the other beta-adrenergic blocking drugs except in their effect on the bronchi. A selective preparation should be used for patients with airways obstruction. Intravenous preparations of most of these drugs are available; they must be used with great caution.

Unwanted effects of beta-adrenergic blocking drugs include lethargy, cardiac failure, bronchospasm, nightmares, impotence, cold extremities and rashes.

These drugs are also used to prevent angina and to treat hyper-tension. For these conditions, larger doses may be required.

Amiodarone. This drug prolongs the action potential and the refractory period; it is therefore of value in blocking re-entrant pathways. It has proved particularly effective in the Wolff−Parkinson−White syndrome, but also in many resistant supraven-tricular and ventricular arrhythmias. Its toxic effects have pre-cluded its widespread use. It causes corneal deposits, but these appear to be benign and reversible and seldom give rise to symptoms. Other side-effects include a bluish discoloration of

Table 4.4 Beta-adrenoceptor blocking drugs.

Drug	Tablet size (mg)
Non-selective:	
Propranolol	10, 40, 80, 160
Oxprenolol	20, 40, 80, 160
Sotalol	40, 80, 160, 200
Nadolol	40, 80
Pindolol	5
Timolol	10
Selective:	
Acebutolol	100, 200, 400
Atenolol	100
Metoprolol	50, 100
Alpha- and beta-adrenergic blockade	
Labetalol	100, 200, 400

* NB. Sustained action formulations of some of the above drugs are available.

the skin following exposure to the sun and thyroid disorders, especially thyrotoxicosis. More rarely, a pneumonitis may occur, which may be fatal. Oral amiodarone may not exert its anti-arrhythmic action for up to a week and on stopping the drug may take several weeks for the effects to disappear. The usual dosage is 200 mg thrice daily for a week, gradually reducing thereafter to 200 mg daily.

Bretylium. Bretylium is an adrenergic blocking agent, which was at one time used in the management of hypertension, but was abandoned because of undesirable side-effects and tachyphylaxis in long-term use. It prolongs action potential without affecting the fast sodium current and is, therefore, categorized as a class III drug. It is relatively ineffective at suppressing ventricular ectopic activity but quite often prevents recurrences of ventricular tachycardia and ventricular fibrillation when other drugs have failed. It is given as 5 mg/kg intramuscularly, or as a slowly administered intravenous infusion, in a dosage of 500 mg every 6–8 hours.

Verapamil. This calcium antagonist, when used intravenously in a dosage of 2–10 mg is usually effective in abolishing supraventricular tachycardia. It must be administered slowly and should be avoided in those receiving beta-blocking drugs, and given cautiously to patients with compromised ventricular function. Oral verapamil (40–120 mg three times a day) is useful in slowing the ventricular rate in atrial fibrillation.

Drugs used to slow the ventricular response to atrial arrhythmias

Digitalis and allied drugs. These are the mainstay of therapy designed to slow the ventricular response to atrial arrhythmias such as atrial flutter and atrial fibrillation. They are considered in detail in Chapter 2.

Beta-adrenergic blocking drugs. These are of value in combination with digoxin when it alone slows the heart rate inadequately (see above). Verapamil is also of value in this context, but should not be given with beta-blockers.

Further reading

Bennett, D.H. (1985) *Cardiac arrhythmias*, 2nd edn. Bristol: Wright.

Bloomfield, P. & Miller, H.C. (1987) Permanent pacing. *British Medical Journal* 295: 741.

Camm, A.J. (1986) Asystole and electromechanical dissociation. *British Medical Journal* 292: 1123.

Chamberlain, D. (1986) Ventricular fibrillation. *British Medical Journal* 292: 1068.

Fisher, J.M. (1986) Recognising a cardiac arrest and providing basic life support. *British Medical Journal* 292: 1002.

Kulbertus, H.E. (1986) *Medical management of Cardiac Arrhythmias*. Edinburgh: Churchill Livingstone.

Mason, J.W. (1987) Amiodarone. *New England Journal of Medicine 314:* 455.

Opie, L. (1984) *The Heart*. London: Grune and Stratton.

Parsonnet, V. & Bernstein, A.D. (1986) Pacing in perspective: concepts and controversies. *Circulation 73:* 1087.

5

The Symptoms of Heart Disease

Dyspnoea

Dyspnoea — difficulty with breathing — is the commonest symptom of heart failure. The term implies discomfort in the act of respiration, a consciousness of laboured breathing. It is, of course, also a symptom of respiratory disease and occurs in normal individuals on exercise.

No single explanation so far advanced accounts for all cases of dyspnoea. Furthermore, because it is subjective the degree of distress depends, in part, upon the personality of the patient. Thus some patients do not complain of breathlessness in spite of obviously laboured respiration, whereas others claim to be short of breath although their capacity for exercise is normal.

Mechanisms

The dyspnoea of cardiac disease may be due to the following factors:

Increased work of breathing

It is probable that in most cases of cardiac failure the discomfort arises in overworked respiratory muscles. In left-sided cardiac failure, engorgement of the pulmonary veins and capillaries occurs; if the pulmonary capillary pressure exceeds 25 mmHg, fluid may exude into the alveolar walls or even into the alveoli. These changes make the lung more rigid (less compliant) and require more respiratory work for a given volume of air inspired.

Reduced vital capacity

This is due to pulmonary venous congestion and, occasionally, to hydrothorax or ascites.

Reflex hyperventilation

The pulmonary stretch receptors may be abnormally stretched by congestion of the lungs.

Bronchial narrowing

Bronchial narrowing by spasm or fluid may occur in cardiac failure and adds to the work of breathing.

Hypoxaemia and carbon dioxide retention

These may both contribute to dyspnoea. They are seldom important factors in patients with left-sided heart failure, in whom the carbon dioxide tension is normal or low as a result of hyperventilation, and there is little hypoxaemia except when there is pulmonary oedema. In cyanotic congenital heart disease, hypoxaemia is severe.

Clinical features

The patient with cardiac dyspnoea breathes rapidly and shallowly. This pattern contrasts with that of the anxious individual who has deep and sighing respiration, and 'is unable to take a deep breath' or 'fill his lungs with air'. It also differs from the deep breathing of patients with diabetic keto-acidosis or renal failure.

Dyspnoea in patients with cardiac disease is usually slowly progressive, although it may be suddenly exacerbated by the onset of atrial fibrillation or the occurrence of pulmonary infarction or infection. At first it occurs only on effort, but as the disease process advances, less and less exercise is required to provoke breathlessness until it may eventually be present at rest.

Orthopnoea. This is dyspnoea when lying flat. There are several possible explanations for its occurrence in left heart failure.

1   When an individual lies flat there is increased venous return, which in the patient on the verge of failure may increase pulmonary venous congestion, and thereby decrease pulmonary compliance and vital capacity.
2   The vital capacity is reduced in the recumbent posture by the relatively high position of the diaphragm, which may be further displaced upwards by ascites or an enlarged liver.

Orthopnoea usually occurs when there is already a considerable limitation of exercise tolerance, but is occasionally an early symptom. Many patients learn for themselves that they are more comfortable propped up by three or four pillows.

Paroxysmal dyspnoea

In patients with left-sided cardiac failure, attacks of dyspnoea may develop without an obvious precipitating cause. They are most apt to occur during sleep (paroxysmal nocturnal dyspnoea). The mechanism is probably the same as that of orthopnoea, but the sensory unawareness of the sleeping state prevents the patient from correcting the situation by sitting up. The victim wakes up intensely short of breath and frightened. He sits on the side of the bed or struggles to the window. The attack may pass off spontaneously within a few minutes, or progress to acute pulmonary oedema.

Acute pulmonary oedema

In this condition, fluid accumulates in the alveoli as a result of a high pulmonary capillary pressure. Such attacks occur in patients with mitral stenosis, acute myocardial infarction and other left-sided cardiac lesions. There is often a provoking factor such as an arrhythmia or respiratory infection.

The patient is intensely dyspnoeic with noisy breathing, cough and frothy sputum which is often blood-tinged. The skin is usually moist, cold and cyanosed. The pulse is fast and may be irregular. Crepitations may be heard throughout the chest in a severe attack. In some patients, rhonchi, due to fluid in the bronchi, predominate and the clinical picture may resemble bronchial asthma. Pulmonary oedema is usually visible on a chest radiograph (see p. 122).

Cheyne–Stokes respiration

In Cheyne–Stokes respiration, there is a periodic waxing and waning in the depth of respiration, over a period of about one minute. As William Stokes wrote in 1854:

It consists in the occurrence of a series of inspirations, increasing to maximum, and then declining in force and length, until a state of apparent apnoea is established. In this condition the patient may remain for such a length of time as to make his attendants believe that he is dead, when a low inspiration, followed by one more decided marks the commencement of a new ascending and then descending series of inspirations.

This pattern of breathing is seen during sleep in some normal individuals, but its occurrence in the conscious patient suggests advanced left ventricular failure. It also occurs in patients with cerebral vascular disease, particularly if they have received morphine.

The cause of Cheyne–Stokes breathing is not yet established but it seems likely that the prolonged lung-to-brain circulation time disturbs the normal feedback mechanisms for respiratory control.

Cardiac pain

There are two major causes of cardiac pain: myocardial ischaemia and pericarditis.

Myocardial ischaemia and infarction (see also Chapter 8)

A transient and reversible inadequacy of the coronary circulation gives rise to that type of chest pain known as angina pectoris. If the reduction in coronary blood flow is such as to cause death of an area of myocardium (myocardial infarction), the pain is usually more severe and prolonged.

The term angina pectoris was adopted by William Heberden, who described the characteristics of the syndrome in 1768. He wrote:

There is a disorder of the breast marked with strong and peculiar symptoms, considerable for the kind of danger belonging to it, and not extremely rare which deserves to be mentioned more at length. The seat of it, and the sense of strangling, and anxiety with which it is attended, may make it not improperly called angina pectoris.

They who are afflicted with it, are seized while they are walking (more especially if it be uphill, and soon after eating) with a painful and most disagreeable sensation in the breast, which seems as if it were to extinguish life, if it were to increase or continue; but the moment they stand still, all this uneasiness vanishes.

In all other respects the patients are, at the beginning of this disorder, perfectly well, and in particular have no shortness of breath, from which it is totally different. The pain is sometimes situated in the upper part, sometimes in the middle, sometimes at the bottom of the os sterni, and often more inclined to the left than to the right side. It likewise very frequently extends from the breast to the middle of the left arm.

Heberden clearly described the four cardinal features of angina pectoris, namely its location in the retrosternal region and its radiation particularly to the left arm, its relationship to exertion, its relatively short duration (usually 1 to 10 minutes), and the strangling quality. For a more detailed description of the characteristics of angina pectoris, see p. 144.

Angina pectoris most commonly occurs in response to exercise in patients with coronary artery disease. The same symptom can be provoked by paroxysmal tachycardia, when there is insufficient time during diastole for the coronary arteries to fill and meet the increased oxygen demands of the tachycardia. Angina is a frequent symptom in aortic stenosis because of the inability of the coronary circulation to match the oxygen requirements of extreme left ventricular hypertrophy. Other conditions which may cause or exacerbate angina pectoris are coronary arterial spasm, aortic regurgitation, syphilitic aortitis, anaemia, hyperthyroidism and mitral stenosis.

There seems little doubt that the cause of angina pectoris is myocardial hypoxia secondary to inadequate coronary blood flow. The site of angina appears to be the myocardium; the stimulus to the pain has not been determined but may be due to a chemical substance related to oxygen lack or to a phenomenon analogous to cramp. The impulses arising in the myocardium pass through afferent sympathetic fibres to reach the upper thoracic sympathetic ganglia and are then directed to the upper four or five thoracic spinal nerves. In this way, the same segments of the spinal cord receive sensations from the heart as receive sensory impulses from the anterior chest wall and the inner aspect of the arm, forearm and hand. The pain is perceived as arising in the territory supplied by the corresponding spinal somatic nerves, rather than in the organ itself.

The pain of myocardial infarction is similar to that of angina pectoris in its location and character, but its duration is longer (usually more than 30 minutes), it is usually more severe, and it has no relationship to exertion.

Pericarditis (see also Chapter 9)

Pain is a characteristic feature of pericarditis, and appears to arise in the parietal pericardium, the visceral pericardium being insensitive. It is usually sharp, but may be of an aching nature. It is situated in the retrosternal region, and radiates to the neck, back or upper abdomen, but rarely the arms. It may be exacerbated by inspiration, swallowing and by lying down flat.

Palpitation

Palpitation may be defined as an awareness of the heart beat. It takes several different forms includings a thumping sensation in the chest, a throbbing in the neck, a consciousness of missed or extra beats, or a racing of the heart. Anxious individuals are often distressed by the sinus tachycardia associated with emotion. Even normal individuals may be disagreeably conscious of their heart action when lying on the left side. Palpitation is, therefore, a common symptom in those without heart disease, but it is also an important complaint in patients with arrhythmias or abnormal heart action. Ectopic beats frequently give rise to the sensation of jumping of the heart, missed beats or extra beats. Patients with supraventricular tachycardia are aware of the sudden onset of rapid regular beating of the heart, whereas those with atrial fibrillation may be conscious of its irregularity.

Patients with a vigorous cardiac action due, for example, to thyrotoxicosis or aortic regurgitation, may feel the regular forceful beating of their hearts.

Oedema

Oedema — the accumulation of fluid in the interstitial tissues — is an important but relatively late manifestation of cardiac failure. It does not usually occur except in the presence of a raised venous pressure, and salt and water retention. Oedema is preceded by a gain in body weight of some 3—5 kg due to an increase in the extracellular fluid.

Normally, fluid exudes into the tissues at the arterial ends of capillaries because the hydrostatic pressure of approximately 30 mmHg exceeds the colloid osmotic pressure of 25 mmHg. Fluid is reabsorbed at the venous ends because the hydrostatic pressure at this point is approximately 12 mmHg. Oedema occurs when there is inadequate reabsorption of fluid from the tissues. A high venous pressure alone can, by increasing the hydrostatic force at the venous ends of the capillaries, cause oedema, as it does, for example, in vena caval obstruction. Raised venous pressure is nearly always a factor in cardiac oedema, but is seldom the sole explanation, for the retention of salt and water almost invariably antedates the appearance of the oedema.

The location of oedema in cardiac failure is determined by local factors, particularly gravity. In the ambulant patient, it occurs bilaterally in the lower legs and feet; in those kept in bed, it accumulates in the sacral area. When the oedema is very great, it may affect the whole of the lower limbs, the genitalia, the abdominal and chest walls and even the face (anasarca).

In the oedema of cardiac failure, the tissues dimple ('pit') when pressure is applied to them by the thumb.

Ascites

The intraperitoneal accumulation of fluid is a manifestation of advanced heart disease, usually occurring later than peripheral oedema but for similar reasons. In some conditions, however, such as tricuspid valve disease and constrictive pericarditis, ascites may be even more evident than oedema and is probably then, in part, a consequence of portal hypertension secondary to cardiac cirrhosis of the liver.

Cyanosis

Cyanosis, a blue discoloration of the skin or mucous membranes, is more a sign than a symptom of heart disease and is often first noticed by relatives when the affected individual exercises or is exposed to cold temperatures. It is usually due to a large proportion of reduced haemoglobin in the superficial capillaries and venules. It has been observed that cyanosis appears when the amount of reduced haemoglobin in the blood of these vessels exceeds 5 g/100 ml. Cyanosis results either from oxygen desaturation of the arterial blood or from an unusually large extraction of oxygen in the peripheral tissues. When the cyanosis is due to arterial oxygen desaturation, it is considered to be 'central' in origin because it is caused by a disorder in the heart or lungs. When the cause of the cyanosis is high oxygen extraction in the tissues, it is said to be 'peripheral'.

Central cyanosis is due either to blood bypassing the lungs as it is shunted from the venous side of the circulation to the arterial, as a result of congenital heart disease, or to inadequate oxygenation of the blood in the lungs, as in some varieties of lung disease. Clubbing of the digits is a common accompaniment of cyanotic congenital heart disease.

Peripheral cyanosis, a consequence of diminished blood flow through the skin and mucous membranes, occurs in normal people when they are cold, and in patients with a low cardiac output due to such conditions as mitral stenosis and acute circulatory failure.

The differentiation of central from peripheral cyanosis is usually not difficult. In peripheral cyanosis the skin is cold, and the cyanosis does not affect the warm mucous membranes such as those of the tongue. Furthermore, peripheral cyanosis can be abolished by warming the skin. The central origin of the cyanosis can be confirmed by measuring the arterial oxygen saturation which is usually less than 85%.

Rarely, central cyanosis may be due not to arterial oxygen desaturation but to methaemoglobinaemia or sulphaemoglobinaemia as a result of taking certain drugs.

Haemoptysis

The expectoration of blood is not uncommon in patients with heart disease. Several mechanisms are involved; examination of the sputum may help to determine which of them is responsible.

Frank haemoptysis — the coughing up of pure blood — occurs

in mitral stenosis, due to the rupture of pulmonary or bronchial veins, or to pulmonary infarction. When there is pulmonary infection, the sputum may be purulent or rusty in appearance. In pulmonary oedema, the frothy sputum may be pink or streaked with blood.

Of course, patients with heart disease may also have haemoptysis due to other types of lung disease such as tuberculosis, bronchiectasis and bronchial neoplasm.

Syncope

Syncope is a transient loss of consciousness due to inadequate cerebral blood flow or perfusion pressure. Cerebral blood flow and perfusion pressure depend upon the cardiac output, the arterial blood pressure and the resistance of the cerebral circulation. Cerebral arteries are relatively uninfluenced by the autonomic system but are dilated by carbon dioxide.

The commonest type of syncope is that of the simple faint (*vasomotor* or *vasodepressor syncope*). It is often a response to emotion, but various physical factors such as blood loss, debility after infection and pain may contribute to its occurrence. It is believed to result mainly from dilatation of the arterial resistance vessels in the muscles. The fall in blood pressure causes a diminished perfusion pressure in the brain and loss of consciousness. Fainting of this kind usually develops when standing, rarely when sitting and virtually never when lying or walking. The first symptom is usually a sense of weakness, accompanied by yawning or sighing, sweating, nausea and 'a sinking feeling' in the stomach. After seconds or minutes, unconsciousness ensues; this is transient because the subject usually falls flat on the ground and this posture leads to an improvement in cerebral blood flow. In a severe attack, the face is pale, the pupils are dilated and respiration is slow. The heart rate is usually diminished and the radial pulse difficult to feel, although carotid artery pulsation can be detected without difficulty.

Micturition syncope occurs in adult men with nocturia. Consciousness is lost immediately after passing urine. It is particularly likely after considerable alcohol consumption. It may be due to reflex vasodilatation secondary to sudden relief of distension of the bladder combined with the vasodilator effects of alcohol and a warm bed.

Heart disease may be responsible for syncope. A catastrophic fall in cardiac output may result if the heart rate is either extremely slow or very fast. In supraventricular and ventricular tachycardias the ventricular rate sometimes exceeds 180 per minute, leaving insufficient time for adequate filling of the heart. A more important and dangerous form of syncope is the *Adams–Stokes attack,* which is a brief episode of cardiac arrest due to either asystole or ventricular fibrillation. This characteristically occurs in patients with heart block in whom either the ventricular pacemaker suddenly fails, or in whom ventricular arrhythmias are superimposed on the heart block. In most cases, effective cardiac action returns in 10 to 15 seconds, but if the attack is more prolonged convulsions may occur. The return of consciousness is accompanied by flushing as flood flows once more through vessels dilated by hypoxia.

Syncope on exertion. This is a characteristic feature of severe aortic stenosis (see p. 222), and may be due to an inability of the heart to supply an adequate blood flow in the face of the increased demands of the muscles. Patients with aortic stenosis are also susceptible to syncope due to heart block or ventricular arrhythmias.

Carotid sinus syncope. This is a rare condition occurring in elderly individuals in whom light pressure on the carotid sinus produces extreme cardiac slowing or reflex hypotension.

When a normal individual stands up, pooling of blood in the legs is prevented by arteriolar and venous constriction, and there is an acceleration of the heart rate together with an increase in plasma catecholamine levels. *Postural syncope,* due to orthostatic hypotension, occurs in patients with autonomic disorders, including diabetic neuropathy and tabes dorsalis, as well as in some otherwise normal elderly individuals in whom these compensatory mechanisms do not function. Some hypotensive agents, particularly anti-adrenergic drugs such as guanethidine, lead to orthostatic hypotension.

Syncope of cardiac origin also occurs in other conditions in which there may be a sudden fall in cardiac output such as massive pulmonary embolism, acute myocardial infarction and mitral valve obstruction due to left atrial myxoma or ball-valve thrombus.

Functional capacity

On the basis of recommendations of the New York Heart Association, patients may be divided into four classes depending upon the severity of their symptoms.

In class 1, the patients, although they have heart disease, can withstand normal physical activity without symptoms. If the patient develops symptoms on moderate or severe exertion but not at rest or with mild exertion, then he is classified as class 2. In class 3, symptoms are present even on mild exertion. In class 4 it is impossible to undertake any physical activity without distress, which may be present even at rest.

Such a classification is of value provided its limitations are borne in mind. Thus, many patients with severe heart disease have few or no complaints, whereas those who have an anxiety neurosis, or are anaemic or pregnant may have dyspnoea in the absence of heart disease.

Further reading

Criteria Committee of the New York Heart Association (1964) *Diseases of the Heart and Blood Vessels (Nomenclature and Criteria for Diagnosis).* Boston: Little, Brown.

The Physical Signs of Heart Disease

Signs are small measurable things but interpretations are illimitable.

George Eliot *Middlemarch*

The arterial pulse

The elastic structure of the aorta and its major branches enables them to act as both reservoirs and conduits. As a consequence, they are able to convert the highly pulsatile discontinuous blood flow from the ventricles into a more continuous flow in the peripheral vessels. The pressure pulse recorded a short distance above the aortic valve shows a sharp upstroke, produced by the rapid ejection of blood from the left ventricle, followed by a slower downstroke, as the rate of flow into peripheral arteries exceeds that from the left ventricle into the aorta (Fig. 6.1). This descending limb of the pulse wave is interrupted by the *dicrotic notch*, as the column of blood, briefly retreating towards the ventricle at the onset of diastole, is halted by aortic valve closure. As the main wave of the pulse travels peripherally, secondary waves are produced at the points of branching of the arteries. These are reflected backwards and summate with the main wave. Consequently, the peak systolic pressure in a peripheral artery may be higher than that in the central aorta.

When the arterial pulse is examined, the following characteristics should be noted: rate, rhythm, amplitude and quality or wave form. It is customary to feel the right radial artery to determine the rate and rhythm of the heart, but the amplitude and quality of the pulse is better appreciated in the carotid arteries. One should also search for pulsation in the radial, brachial, carotid, femoral, dorsalis pedis and posterior tibial arteries on both sides.

The *rate* of the pulse, if regular, can be calculated by multiplying the number of beats in 15 seconds by 4. If it is irregular, the number of beats in 30 seconds should be doubled. The pulse rate in normal resting adults ranges from 60 to 100 per minute. A rate of less than 60 per minute is most commonly due to sinus brady-cardia (see p. 54), but may also be due to junctional rhythm or

Fig. 6.1 The normal arterial
pulse wave.

Dicrotic
notch

heart block. Rates in excess of 100 per minute (tachycardia) are
most often due to sinus tachycardia associated with emotion or
exercise; the heart rate may exceed 200 beats per minute on
vigorous exercise. If the rate exceeds 120 per minute at rest in
adults, some form of arrhythmia is likely (see Chapter 4).

The normal pulse is regular or exhibits sinus arrhythmia. An
occasional irregularity in an otherwise regular pulse suggests
ectopic beats, and a coupling of beats (pulsus bigeminus or
bigeminy) is due to the alternation of normal and ectopic beats.
A totally irregular pulse suggests atrial fibrillation.

The *amplitude* of the pulse depends on the pulse pressure, i.e.
the difference between the systolic and diastolic pressures. The
pulse is of small volume when the pulse pressure is small. This is
the case when there is a low stroke volume and peripheral
vasoconstriction as occurs in acute myocardial infarction, the
shock syndrome, mitral stenosis and pericardial constriction or
tamponade. In aortic stenosis, the pulse is small and prolonged
and has a slow upstroke. This is called an *anacrotic* pulse if the
wave has a notch on its upstroke (Fig. 6.2). *Pulsus bisferiens* is a
pulse of moderate or large volume in which a double beat can be
felt. This sign suggests a combination of aortic stenosis and
regurgitation but is not diagnostic.

A large pulse, associated with a large stroke volume occurs in
aortic regurgitation, anaemia, pregnancy and thyrotoxicosis. When
a large volume pulse rises rapidly and collapses suddenly (Fig.
6.2) it is described as a *collapsing* pulse; this is also called a
waterhammer pulse, after a Victorian toy of this name. This type
of pulse is encountered when there is a rapid runoff of blood
during diastole as in aortic regurgitation, persistent ductus
arteriosus and arteriovenous fistulae. It is best felt by placing the
palm of the hand on the patient's vertically elevated forearm,
thereby increasing the retrograde flow of blood during diastole.

(A)   (B)

Fig. 6.2   (A) The pulse of
severe aortic stenosis. (B)
The rapidly rising and
collapsing pulse of aortic
regurgitation.

A reduction in systolic pressure of up to 10 mmHg may occur on inspiration in normal people, probably because the capacity of the pulmonary vascular bed enlarges and reduces the return of blood to the left ventricle. This is partly compensated for by a simultaneous increase in right ventricular output. A more substantial inspiratory fall, which occurs in obstructive airways disease, especially asthma, and pericardial constriction, produces *pulsus paradoxus*. In obstructive lung disease the reduction in arterial pressure is the consequence of the increased negativity of the intrathoracic pressure. In pericardial constriction and tamponade, this may be due to the right ventricle being unable to compensate for the augmented pulmonary vascular capacity by increasing its output. Another and probably more important explanation is that an inspiratory increase in the right ventricle occurs at the expense of left ventricle, as they are both confined within an indistensible pericardium.

In *pulsus alternans,* the beats are evenly spaced in time but are alternately large and small in volume. This is most readily detected when the blood pressure is being measured, for as the cuff is being deflated only alternate beats are heard at first. After a fall of a further 5 or 10 mmHg, every beat is audible. The mechanism of pulsus alternans is not well understood, but is usually associated with left ventricular failure.

The *absence* of a peripheral pulse indicates an anatomical aberration, or narrowing or occlusion of the artery proximal to it. In coarctation of the aorta, pulsation of the femoral arteries is delayed compared with that of the radial arteries.

Blood pressure recording

Precise recording of blood pressure can be obtained only by intra-arterial catheterization but a sufficiently accurate estimate may be made using a sphygmomanometer. This instrument consists of a manometer linked to an inflatable bag, surrounded by an inelastic cuff. The size of bag and cuff is of importance in ensuring accuracy, large cuffs being required for the obese and small for children. The cuff must fit around the arm snugly, being neither loose nor touching any article of clothing. It should be applied about 2 cm above the antecubital space with the rubber bag over the medial aspect of the arm.

Manometers are of two types: mercury and aneroid. The mercury type requires care in ensuring that there is no loss or oxidation of mercury and that the air vent at the top of the tube is open. Aneroid manometers are as accurate as mercury instruments, provided they are calibrated regularly.

It is best for the patient to be reclining comfortably, but the blood pressure can be taken satisfactorily with the patient sitting or standing provided the limb is supported and at the same level as the heart. Using a mercury manometer, one's eye should be in line with the top of the meniscus.

The patient should be warm, confortable and in a quiet environment. He should have stayed in the same position for 5 minutes before the blood pressure recording; if in doubt, several recordings should be made.

The cuff should be inflated until the pulsations of the brachial artery can no longer be felt. The pressure is then raised by a further 20 mmHg and released at a rate of about 2 mmHg a second. As the pressure falls, sounds (Korotkoff sounds) are heard as blood begins to pass through the artery which has been occluded. At first these are faint and tapping; then a swishing quality is noted. The sounds become crisper and more intense and, as the pressure falls further, there is an abrupt muffling (fourth phase) and, finally, the sounds disappear altogether (fifth phase). Sometimes there is a period of silence after the first appearance of the sounds before they reappear, known as the auscultatory gap, which is particularly common in the presence of hypertension.

The systolic pressure is that at which the sounds are first heard. Intra-arterial pressure recordings suggest that the fifth phase usually represents the diastolic pressure better than the fourth but in some individuals, particularly if they are vasodilated, the sounds may never disappear; this may also be due to over-extension of the elbow. To avoid inconsistency between different observers and repeated observations, the pressures both at muffling and disappearance should be noted.

When blood pressure measurements are taken in the leg, the patient should be lying on his abdomen, with a large cuff covering the mid-thigh region, and the stethoscope placed in the popliteal fossa.

Certain circumstances make blood pressure estimations difficult. In the shock syndrome, blood pressure readings from a sphygmomanometer may be grossly inaccurate. In atrial fibrillation and other arrhythmias, the blood pressure may vary from beat to beat; the average of a number of beats should be taken for both the systolic and diastolic pressures.

The venous pulse and pressure (Fig. 6.3)

Inspection of the veins in the neck is an essential but often neglected part of cardiac diagnosis. The external jugular vein is easily seen, but is so often obstructed as it passes through the

Fig. 6.3 The venous pulse. Note the 'a' wave due to atrial systole and the 'c' wave occurring at the time of tricuspid valve closure. The upstroke of the 'v' wave occurs as the atrium is filling passively during ventricular systole; the descent from the peak of 'v' to 'y' occurs as blood flows from the atrium to the ventricle after tricuspid valve opening.

fascial plane that it cannot be relied upon as a guide to the true venous pressure. The internal jugular vein cannot be directly visualized, but it imparts a broad pulsation to the tissues of the neck overlying it. Its undulations can be seen in virtually all individuals, if the correct technique of examination is used; occasionally, especially in the obese or bull-necked, it cannot be identified. There are normally three peaks, 'a' corresponding to atrial systole, 'c' occurring at the time of tricuspid valve closure, and 'v' at the time of tricuspid valve opening. The 'x' trough corresponds to the descent of the tricuspid valve ring as the right ventricle contracts, and the 'y' trough represents the fall in pressure as blood flows into the right ventricle. As it is usually not possible to see the 'c' wave in the jugular pulse, the normal venous pulse in the neck is composed of two positive and two negative waves (Fig. 6.3).

It is essential to observe both the *waveform* and the *pressure level* of the jugular venous pulse. The pressure should not be determined until the characteristics of the wave form have been identified. The patient should be reclining with the chest, head and neck at 45°, and with the muscles of the neck relaxed. If venous pulsation cannot be seen with the patient at 45°, he should be placed more horizontally until it can.

In differentiating venous from arterial pulsation the following points are important: the venous pulse normally shows two positive pulsations in each cardiac cycle compared with the single pulsation in the arteries; the venous pulse cannot usually be felt, although it can be readily seen, whereas the arterial pulsation is more easily felt than seen; the venous pulse wave can be obliterated by light pressure at the root of the neck. Pressure on the abdomen, by increasing venous return to the thorax, increases the venous pressure in the neck transiently and permits it to be visualized more easily.

With the patient is the semi-recumbent position, the vertical height of the top of the venous column above the sternal angle is observed. In normal individuals, this does not exceed 2 cm; it is increased by factors which augment venous return including pregnancy, anxiety, exercise and anaemia. If these causes cannot be invoked, raised venous pressure is usually due to right-sided cardiac failure; it is important to exclude non-pulsating engorgement due to obstruction of the superior vena cava.

Hepato-jugular reflux. If pressure is exerted on the relaxed abdomen, venous return to the right atrium is increased, and the jugular venous pressure rises accordingly. In normals this rise is very transient; in patients with heart failure, it may remain high as long as pressure is exerted on the abdomen.

The timing of venous waves may be difficult; it is essential either to feel the carotid artery pulsation on the other side of the neck or to listen for the first heart sound in order to allow identification of the 'a' wave which precedes these two events.

Giant 'a' wave (Fig. 6.4). This develops when the right atrium contracts forcefully against the increased resistance provided by a stenotic tricuspid valve, or hypertrophied right ventricle.

Cannon waves. These are large venous pulsations due to atrial contraction against a closed tricuspid valve. They occur intermittently in complete heart block and in ventricular tachycardia when atrial and ventricular systoles coincide (Fig. 6.4). In junctional rhythms, atrial and ventricular contractions are synchronous and cannon waves occur with every heart beat.

Systolic venous pulsation ('cv' wave). This is due to blood regurgitating into the venous system during ventricular systole and is characteristic of tricuspid regurgitation (Fig. 6.4).

In pericardial constriction, the venous pressure is greatly raised, and there is a sharp 'y' descent as blood rushes into the right ventricle in the early part of diastole (Fig. 6.4). Another feature of this condition is elevation of venous pressure during inspiration because the increase in venous return at this time cannot be accommodated by the constricted right ventricle.

Inspection of the chest

Abnormalities of the thorax and lungs may cause changes in the position of the heart; they may also result from or cause heart disease. Funnel chest (pectus excavatum) and kyphoscoliosis may

(A)

CANNON
WAVES

(B)

(C)

(D)

Fig. 6.4 (A) The giant 'a' wave. (B) Intermittent cannon waves in complete heart block, occurring at the time of synchronous atrial and ventricular contraction. (C) The systolic venous pulsation of tricuspid regurgitation. (D) The venous pulse in pericardial constriction, showing the rapid 'y' descent, followed by a plateau.

lead to displacement of the heart. Cardiac enlargement associated with advanced congenital heart disease in childhood may cause deformity of the sternum and ribs.

The rate and pattern of breathing should be noted. The respiratory rate is often increased in left ventricular failure. Prolonged expiration suggests obstructive airways disease.

The cardiac impulse is frequently visible, particularly when there is heart disease. It is often possible to see the exaggerated apical impulse of left ventricular hypertrophy, the displaced apex of left ventricular dilatation, the left parasternal pulsation of right ventricular hypertrophy or the abnormal pulmonary arterial pulsation in the second and third left interspaces in pulmonary hypertension.

Palpation of the chest

In the normal individual, the maximal thrust of the left ventricle — the apex beat — can be felt at or just internal to the mid-clavicular line in the fifth intercostal space. If it is displaced, one should determine whether this is due to abnormalities of the thoracic

Fig. 6.5 The apex cardiogram. Note 'a' due to atrial systole, 'e' as the ventricle rotates forward with left ventricular systole, the fall from 'e' to 'o' as the ventricle empties, the early rapid filling wave (rfw) in the ventricle, followed by a slow filling wave (sfw).

cage or lungs. After the apex beat has been located and assessed, the whole precordium should be explored with the palm of the hand in the search for abnormal pulsation.

The graphic record of the movements of the apex beat shows a characteristic pattern — the *apex cardiogram* (Fig. 6.5). This commences with an 'a' wave as atrial systole causes ventricular distension. The next wave, which is the major one in the cardiac cycle, corresponds to the forward rotation of the apex due to left ventricular systole. The apex beat starts to retract as soon as the aortic valve opens and continues to do so until the 'o' point is reached, at which time the mitral valve opens and the ventricle distends rapidly. This process then slows and there is little change before the next atrial systole. Normally, only the ventricular systolic component is detectable by palpation, but in left ventricular hypertrophy, the 'a' wave can sometimes be felt immediately before ventricular systole, producing a double impulse. More rarely, one can feel an impulse at the end of rapid filling, corresponding with the third heart sound (see below).

The ventricular impulse may be abnormal in three different ways.

1   Left ventricular hypertrophy produces a sustained heaving or thrusting apex beat.
2   Left ventricular dilatation displaces the apex downwards

and outwards. If there is a large left ventricular stroke volume, as in aortic regurgitation, the impulse is vigorous, but when myocardial contractility is impaired as by ischaemic heart disease, it may be diffuse and feeble.

3   In mitral stenosis, the apex beat often has a characteristic abrupt tapping quality due to the vibrations associated with the loud first sound.

Following myocardial infarction affecting the anterior wall of the heart, there is often an outward movement of the non-contracting area of the left ventricle during systole between the apex and the left sternal edge.

The right ventricular impulse in the left parasternal region is not usually palpable in health, except in children and thin adults. In right ventricular hypertrophy, as occurs in pulmonary stenosis and pulmonary hypertension (particularly secondary to mitral stenosis) there is a sustained lifting impulse along the left sternal edge. When there is right ventricular dilatation associated with a high right ventricular output (as in atrial septal defect), the impulse is vigorous but less sustained. In severe mitral regurgitation, systolic pulsation of the enlarged left atrium may also cause a left parasternal heave.

Pulmonary arterial pulsation can quite often be felt in the second left intercostal space when there is pulmonary hypertension or high pulmonary blood flow. Occasionally, the pulsation of an aneurysm can be detected in the aortic area.

Vibrations may be felt over the precordium corresponding to audible sounds and murmurs. When they are associated with heart sounds, they may be described as 'shocks'. Shocks may accompany any loud heart sound.

'Thrills' are the tactile equivalent of murmurs. They do not occur in the absence of loud murmurs and have no significance beyond that possessed by the murmur. Thrills are usually best felt by the palm of the hand when the patient is sitting upright and holding his breath in full expiration. The commonest thrills are the following:

An apical systolic thrill corresponding with the loud systolic murmur of mitral regurgitation.

A systolic thrill between the apex and the left sternal edge in ventricular septal defect.

A systolic thrill in the second right intercostal space, occasionally over the sternum and the third or fourth left intercostal space, in aortic stenosis. This is often associated with a systolic thrill over the carotid arteries.

A systolic thrill in the second or third left intercostal spaces in pulmonary stenosis.

Diastolic and presystolic thrills at the apex in mitral stenosis.
A continuous systolic and diastolic thrill below the left clavicle in persistent ductus arteriosus.

It is rare for the murmurs of aortic or pulmonary regurgitation to be accompanied by a thrill.

After the chest has been palpated, the opportunity should be taken to palpate the abdomen. Particular attention should be paid to the liver. Enlargement, often tender, is a characteristic feature of right-sided heart failure. Systolic pulsation may be felt in tricuspid regurgitation, and presystolic pulsation in tricuspid stenosis.

Percussion of the heart

A crude estimate of the size of the heart may be made by percussion, but this is much less accurate than radiology and it has little place in diagnosis. It is sometimes of value in the diagnosis of pericardial effusion, as in this condition the area of cardiac dullness may be extended to the right of the sternum and to the second left intercostal space. In emphysema, the area of cardiac dullness may be reduced.

Auscultation: heart sounds and murmurs

Vibrations within the heart give rise to sounds which are loud enough to be audible through a stethoscope and to be registered graphically by a phonocardiogram. If the noise is brief and transient, it is termed a heart sound; if more prolonged, it is a murmur. Careful auscultation, combined with the other methods of physical examination, provides information about the heart which even the most sophisticated modern techniques of investigation can scarcely match. A phonocardiogram is useful, however, in timing murmurs and sounds and is of value in differentiating the various types of added sound such as the opening snap and the third heart sound.

The physician should always use a stethoscope with which he is familiar. The earpieces should fit comfortably; the tubing should be short (not greater than 30 cm) and thick-walled. Both types of endpiece (diaphragm and bell) are necessary. The rigid diaphragm is best for hearing high-frequency sounds and murmurs such as the second heart sound and the diastolic murmur of aortic regurgitation. The bell pressed *lightly* on the chest is superior to the diaphragm for the low-pitched third and fourth heart sounds and the mid-diastolic and presystolic murmurs of mitral stenosis.

Traditionally, there are four areas of auscultation: aortic (right second intercostal space), pulmonary (left second intercostal space), tricuspid (lower sternal) and mitral (apex beat). These designations are misleading, especially with regard to the aortic valve, because aortic murmurs (especially if diastolic) are often maximal at the left sternal edge at the level of the fourth intercostal space. The opening snap of mitral stenosis is also best heard in this area. Auscultation should never be restricted to the traditional areas; one should start on one side of the precordium and gradually move the stethoscope towards the other areas. One may begin in the pulmonary area in order to identify the first and second heart sounds, while palpating the carotid artery whose pulsation occurs just after the first heart sound. The aortic area may be listened to next, before moving obliquely across the sternum to the lower left sternal edge, thence to the tricuspid area, to the mitral area and into the axilla. One should then listen particularly in the aortic, pulmonary and lower left sternal edge areas with the patient sitting up and holding his breath in full expiration. The apical area should be listened to with the patient rotated into the left lateral position. If mitral stenosis is suspected, the patient should exercise by sitting forward and backwards several times, and then lie down again in the left lateral position.

Success in auscultation depends upon listening selectively for individual sounds and murmurs. Initially, the first heart sound should be identified and assessed before turning one's attention to the second heart sound and to any additional sounds. Having noted any normal or abnormal sounds, one should then listen for systolic and, later, for diastolic murmurs.

The heart sounds

The first sound

The first sound occurs at the time of closure of the atrioventricular valves. Although some have attributed the sound to the impact of closure, it seems more likely that it is due to the tensing of the cusps as they are projected into the atrium at the beginning of ventricular systole. Both tricuspid and mitral valves contribute to the sound. As these valves close slightly asynchronously, the first heart sound, in health, may be narrowly split. As the mitral component is louder, the first heart sound is usually best heard at the apex.

The intensity of the first heart sound is related to the extent of upward movement of the cusps when the ventricles contract. In the normal resting heart the valve cusps come into light contact with each other before the onset of ventricular systole which, therefore, projects them only a short distance. If the cusps are well down in the ventricular chamber, ventricular systole forces them rapidly upwards and causes a loud sound. This situation arises when the atrium contracts immediately before the ventricle (short PR interval) and when the left atrial pressure is abnormally high, as in mitral stenosis. In complete heart block, the relationship between atrial and ventricular systole changes from cycle to cycle, and the first sound varies in intensity accordingly. When the cusps are rigid, as in calcific mitral valve disease, the first sound is soft or inaudible.

The second sound

The second heart sound is related to the closure of the semilunar valves. Normally, it is single on expiration but splits into its aortic and pulmonary components during inspiration (Fig. 6.6). This phenomenon is accounted for by the prolongation of right ventricular systole associated with the increased flow into the right side of the heart occurring with inspiration. Splitting is best heard in the second left intercostal space. Abnormally wide splitting of the second sound, due to delay in pulmonary valve closure, occurs when the right ventricle is over-burdened by either a volume load (as in atrial septal defect) or a pressure load (as in pulmonary stenosis), or when there is a delay in electrical activation of the right ventricle (as in right bundle branch block). In atrial septal defect, there is usually 'fixed' splitting of the second heart sound because the increase in venous return on inspiration affects the filling of both ventricles.

When there is left bundle branch block and when the left ventricle is overburdened, as by systemic hypertension or aortic stenosis, the aortic component of the sound may be delayed. This produces 'reversed' splitting; the sound being single on inspiration and split on expiration (Fig. 6.7).

The intensity of the second heart sound may be increased by systemic or pulmonary hypertension, but this is not a reliable sign. The aortic component of the second sound may be reduced or inaudible in aortic stenosis, particularly if the aortic valve is calcified, and the pulmonary component may be soft or absent in pulmonary stenosis. Both first and second sounds may be soft when the heart is separated from the chest wall by fat, pericardial effusion or emphysematous lung, or when the cardiac output is low as in shock.

Fig. 6.6 Normal splitting of the second heart sound during inspiration, with the aortic component preceding the pulmonary.

Fig. 6.7 'Reversed' splitting of the second sound. Due to delay in left ventricular emptying, the aortic component follows the pulmonary component of the second sound on expiration. On inspiration, the pulmonary component is, as usual, delayed and is superimposed on the aortic component.

The third sound (Fig. 6.8A)

The third sound occurs at the end of the period of rapid filling of the ventricles. It is probably due to sudden tensing of the valve structures and ventricular walls at this time. It is usually generated in the left ventricle and is best heard at or internal to the apex. The sound is low-pitched and distant, and is often heard only with the lightly applied stethoscope bell. Although normal in the young, it is a pathological finding in the middle-aged and elderly. Its presence implies either left ventricular failure or abnormally rapid filling of the ventricle, as in mitral regurgitation, pregnancy or anaemia. Occasionally, a third heart sound can be heard over the right ventricle in right ventricular failure. In pericardial constriction, there is a very early third heart sound of higher frequency associated with the sudden limitation to ventricular filling.

The fourth or atrial sound (Fig. 6.8B)

This sound resembles the third heart sound in being low-pitched and best heard at the apex, and probably has a similar mechanism. In this instance, the ventricular distension results from atrial contraction; the fourth sound immediately precedes the first heart sound. It is rarely heard in health, and is usually a sign of either ventricular failure or hypertrophy. Thus, a fourth heart sound is heard over the left ventricle in some cases of aortic stenosis, hypertension and ischaemic heart disease. A right ventricular fourth heart sound may be heard at the left sternal edge in pulmonary stenosis and pulmonary hypertension.

Gallop rhythm

This term is applied to a cadence of three heart sounds which may be heard in the presence of tachycardia. It may be due to a third heart sound, to a fourth heart sound or to the superimposition of the two ('summation gallop').

(A)   (B)

Fig. 6.8   (A) The third heart sound. (B) The fourth or atrial sound. (C) The ejection click (ec). (D) The opening snap.

(C)   (D)

Additional sounds in systole

Early systolic sounds (ejection sounds or clicks) occur at the time of aortic and pulmonary valve opening (Fig. 6.8C). The clicks may arise from sudden tensing of the opening cusps or from distension of the great vessels. Aortic clicks are almost invariable in valvar aortic stenosis provided the cusps are not calcified, and may be present in systemic hypertension. Pulmonary systolic clicks occur under conditions in which the pulmonary artery is dilated, as it is in valvar pulmonary stenosis and in pulmonary hypertension. They are usually heard best in held expiration.

Clicks occurring later in systole are usually due to ballooning of a mitral valve cusp (mitral valve prolapse). A systolic clicking or crunching may occur in pneumothorax.

The opening snap (Fig. 6.8D)

This is one of the most important signs in auscultation and is virtually diagnostic of mitral stenosis. It occurs at the time of mitral valve opening and is presumed to be due to sudden tension of stenosed but pliant cusps. It is soft or absent if the mitral valve is rigid from fibrosis or calcification. It is heard best at the left sternal edge in the fourth intercostal space or between this point and the apex beat and has a snapping quality. Unlike splitting of the second sound and the third heart sound with which it may be confused, it can often be heard widely over the precordium (see Table 6.1).

Heart murmurs

Murmurs appear to result from vibrations set up by turbulent blood flow. Turbulence is encouraged by high velocity of flow, by abrupt change in the calibre of a vessel or chamber and by

Table 6.1 The differentiation of splitting of the second heart sound, the opening snap, and the third heart sound (of the left ventricle).

	Splitting of second sound (normal)	Splitting of second sound (fixed)	Splitting of second sound (reversed)	Opening snap	Third heart sound
Interval between first component of second sound and 'extra' sound	0–0.05 sec (maximal on inspiration)	0.03–0.08 sec (at all phases)	0.01–0.03 sec (maximal on expiration)	0.03–0.12 sec	0.10–0.16 sec
Effect of inspiration	Widens	Unaffected	Narrows	None	None
Character	Abrupt — heard best with diaphragm			'Snap' heard best with diaphragm	Low-pitched heard best with bell
Site of maximal intensity	Second left intercostal space			Lower left sternal edge	At apex
Radiation	Left sternal edge			All cardiac areas	Localized (usually)

reduced blood viscosity. Murmurs therefore develop when there is rapid flow through a valve, valvar narrowing, or anaemia.

The following features of a murmur should be noted: its timing in the cardiac cycle, its location and radiation, its intensity and its quality.

Murmurs may occur either in systole or in diastole; they may continue from one into the other.

Murmurs are usually best heard at the place on the chest wall closest to their site of origin or in the direction of blood flow. Thus, the murmur of aortic stenosis is loudest over the aortic valve (the third left intercostal space), or in the second right intercostal space, or in the neck. On the other hand, the diastolic murmur of aortic regurgitation is usually maximal at the fourth left intercostal space and is less well heard in the 'aortic area'.

The intensity of murmurs may be classified in six grades.

Grade 1   Only just audible, even under good auscultatory conditions
Grade 2   Soft
Grade 3   Moderately loud
Grade 4   Loud
Grade 5   Very loud but not audible with the stethoscope away from the chest
Grade 6   So loud as to be audible with the stethoscope lifted from the chest wall

The quality of a murmur may be 'blowing', 'rumbling', 'harsh' or 'musical'. These are poor descriptions of what is heard; only with experience can one appreciate what is meant by such terms. Murmurs may also be described as low, medium or high-pitched.

Systolic murmurs

These are usually midsystolic or pansystolic (holosystolic) in timing.

Midsystolic murmurs start after the opening of the aortic and pulmonary valves, increase in intensity to a maximum in midsystole and decrease and disappear before the second heart sound (Fig. 6.9A). Because of their configuration, they are sometimes called 'diamond-shaped', and are also termed 'ejection' because they arise during ejection of blood from the ventricles into great arteries. Murmurs arising at the aortic and pulmonary valves are characteristically midsystolic.

The murmur of aortic stenosis, which is often harsh, is usually best heard in the second right intercostal space, although sometimes it is maximal at the lower left sternal edge or even at the

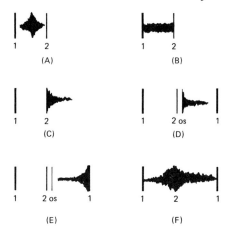

Fig. 6.9 (A) A midsystolic murmur. (B) A pansystolic murmur. (C) An early diastolic murmur. (D) A mid-diastolic murmur, following an opening snap in mitral stenosis. (E) The presystolic murmur of mitral stenosis. (F) The continuous murmur of a persistent ductus arteriosus.

apex. It frequently radiates to the neck. The murmur of subaortic stenosis is loudest at the lower left sternal edge. The murmur of pulmonary valve stenosis is maximal at the second left intercostal space, that of infundibular pulmonary stenosis most intense at the third or fourth left intercostal space. The murmurs of aortic and pulmonary stenosis are often loud and accompanied by thrills.

A systolic murmur due to high flow in the pulmonary artery is characteristic of atrial septal defect but also occurs in conditions associated with a high cardiac output such as pregnancy, thyrotoxicosis and anaemia. These murmurs are usually of no more than grade 3 intensity and are not associated with thrills.

Quite frequently, particularly in children, midsystolic murmurs may be heard in the pulmonary area for which no organic cause can be found. These may be termed 'functional' or 'benign'. Such murmurs are neither intense nor accompanied by a thrill. They usually vary with position and respiration.

Pansystolic (holosystolic) murmurs persist from the first to the second heart sound and only occur as a result of mitral regurgitation, tricuspid regurgitation or ventricular septal defect, for it is only in these conditions that a pressure difference exists across the defective valve or septum throughout systole (Fig. 6.9B). In mitral regurgitation, the murmur is maximal at or just internal to the apex beat, and radiates into the axilla. It may be maximal in late systole.

The murmur of tricuspid regurgitation is usually loudest in the xiphisternal region, or at the lower left sternal edge. It frequently radiates to the apex and may therefore be readily confused with that of mitral regurgitation, but differs in becoming louder on inspiration, due to the increase in venous return at this time.

The murmur of ventricular septal defect is usually loud and is maximal at the lower left sternal edge.

Murmurs may be confined to early or late systole; those associated with a prolapsed mitral cusp characteristically follow a midsystolic click.

Assessing the significance of a systolic murmur

One can usually determine the cause of a systolic murmur by taking into account its location and radiation, its intensity, its character and its association with other abnormal findings. The duration of the murmur is also of value if one can be certain whether it is midsystolic or pansystolic, but even experts may be unsure on this point.

In aortic stenosis, there is usually a loud murmur at the lower left sternal edge and aortic area which is associated with a thrill, a small flat pulse and left ventricular hypertrophy. If the valve cusps are not calcified, there is an early systolic ('ejection') click; if the stenosis is severe, there may be reversed splitting of the second sound.

In aortic valve sclerosis, a common finding in the elderly, there is an aortic systolic murmur in the absence of any of the other features of aortic stenosis.

In pulmonary stenosis, the loud murmur in the pulmonary or lower left sternal area is accompanied by right ventricular hypertrophy, a soft and late pulmonary component of the second sound and a systolic thrill.

In severe mitral regurgitation, the apical systolic murmur, which is well heard from cardiac apex to axilla, is usually accompanied by left ventricular enlargement, a third heart sound and a mid-diastolic flow murmur. In tricuspid regurgitation, the murmur in the tricuspid area is usually increased by inspiration, and is associated with systolic pulsation in the jugular veins.

It is of particular importance to determine whether a systolic murmur is of the 'benign' variety, for the misinterpretation of such a murmur as organic may lead to unwarranted cardiac invalidism. Benign systolic murmurs are seldom of more than grade 2 intensity, are never pansystolic, are usually best heard in the pulmonary area and are not associated with cardiac enlargement or with abnormal heart sounds. Similar murmurs are encountered in pregnancy, thyrotoxicosis and anaemia, and these conditions should be excluded before a murmur is accepted as being of no significance. The pulmonary systolic murmur of atrial septal defect resembles a benign systolic murmur but is accompanied by wide splitting of the second heart sound, and often by a mid-diastolic murmur due to high flow across the tricuspid valve. One can usually be confident of the benign nature of a murmur on physical examination alone. Only if there are other features such as cardiomegaly or abnormal sounds is further investigation with ECG, radiography and echocardiography necessary.

Diastolic murmurs

Diastolic murmurs are of three main varieties: early diastolic, mid-diastolic and presystolic.

Early (immediate) diastolic murmurs

These murmurs occur shortly after closure of the aortic or pulmonary valves at the beginning of diastole (Fig. 6.9C). They are due to regurgitation through one or other of these valves when pressure in the aorta or pulmonary artery exceeds that of the related ventricle. The murmur decreases in intensity as diastole continues. The murmur is usually soft, high-pitched and blowing, and is best heard by using the diaphragm chest piece with the patient sitting forward, in full expiration. The murmur of aortic regurgitation is usually loudest at the third or fourth left intercostal space close to the sternum, but is occasionally maximal in the second right intercostal space.

The uncommon early diastolic murmur of pulmonary regurgitation (the Graham Steell murmur) is best heard in the left second, third and fourth intercostal spaces. It is similar in character to that of aortic regurgitation but is increased by inspiration and is accompanied by signs of pulmonary hypertension.

Mid-diastolic murmurs

Mid-diastolic murmurs are associated with flow through the atrioventricular valves and necessarily start an appreciable time after the second heart sound. The most important cause is mitral stenosis, in which there is a low-pitched murmur maximal in a localized area at or internal to the apex beat. The murmur is most easily heard with the bell of the stethoscope and with the patient lying in the left lateral position, preferably after exercise (Fig. 6.9D). It is frequently associated with an opening snap, a presystolic murmur and a loud first heart sound.

In tricuspid stenosis, a murmur due to a similar mechanism occurs, but in this condition it is maximal in the xiphisternal or lower left sternal region. This murmur is often of a rather scratchy character and is accentuated by inspiration. Mid-diastolic murmurs may also occur when there is a large flow through atrioventricular valves. Such flow murmurs in the mitral area occur in association with mitral regurgitation, ventricular septal defect and persistent ductus arteriosus. A high-flow tricuspid murmur occurs in atrial septal defect. Another mid-diastolic murmur is that due to rheumatic valvulitis (the Carey Coombs murmur). A mid-diastolic murmur may also be heard, in the absence of mitral valve disease, in patients with severe aortic regurgitation (the Austin Flint murmur). This may be due to the aortic regurgitant flow pushing the aortic cusp of the mitral valve across the mitral valve orifice, thereby causing turbulence as blood is also flowing simultaneously from the left atrium to the left ventricle.

Presystolic murmurs

Presystolic murmurs are produced when atrial systole propels blood through narrowed mitral or tricuspid valves. The presystolic murmur of mitral stenosis leads up to the loud first sound of that condition (Fig. 6.9E); it is most easily heard with the patient lying in the left lateral position with the bell of the stethoscope placed at or internal to the apex beat. The presystolic murmur of tricuspid stenosis is maximal in the xiphisternal region or at the lower left sternal edge and is accentuated by inspiration.

Continuous murmurs

The term 'continuous' is applied to a murmur which starts during systole and continues into diastole; it is not necessarily continuous throughout the cardiac cycle. The commonest types are the venous hum and the murmur of persistent ductus arteriosus.

The venous hum is common in childhood, but may be heard in anaemic or pregnant adults. It is due to high blood flow in the jugular veins and can be diminished or abolished by lying the patient flat, or by constricting the veins by pressure. It is usually loudest in the neck, but may be audible over the upper chest.

The murmur in persistent ductus arteriosus is caused by the flow of blood from the high-pressure aorta into the low-pressure pulmonary artery. It is maximal in the left second intercostal space or under the left clavicle. It increases in intensity throughout systole, is maximal at the time of the second heart sound, and diminishes during diastole (Fig. 6.9F). It often has a 'machinery' or whirring quality. Similar murmurs are caused by systemic, pulmonary and coronary arteriovenous fistulae, and by rupture of an aneurysm of a sinus of Valsalva (see p. 283).

Pericardial friction (or rub)

As roughened visceral and parietal layers of pericardium slide over one another, they produce a harsh creaking sound which may be likened to the noise made by two pieces of sandpaper rubbing together. As the movement occurs during ventricular systole, ventricular diastole and atrial systole, the rub may be present at one or all of these times. It may be heard all over the precordium, or only at a localized site. It usually sounds superficial and can be accentuated by leaning the patient forward or by pressing the stethoscope diaphragm firmly on the chest. It can occur in acute pericarditis of any cause, as well as in uraemic pericarditis and during the course of acute myocardial infarction. In the latter condition, it is often evanescent, lasting for only a few minutes or hours.

Further reading

Perloff, J.K. (1986) *Physical Examination of the Heart and Circulation.* Philadelphia: Saunders.

Turner, R.W.D. & Gold, R.G. (1984) *Auscultation of the Heart.* Edinburgh: Churchill Livingstone.

Radiology and Other Techniques of Investigation

Radiological examination of the heart is an essential part of the full cardiological assessment as are the newer non-invasive investigations, including radionuclide studies and echocardiography.

Plain chest radiography and fluoroscopy

Plain radiographs are usually taken in postero-anterior and lateral views; oblique positions are sometimes used.

In the postero-anterior projection, the patient faces the x-ray cassette. In this view (Fig. 7.1) the right border of the heart consists (from above downwards) of the superior vena cava, the ascending aorta, the right atrium, and the inferior vena cava. The left border of the heart is formed by the aortic arch, the pulmonary artery and its left main branch, and the left ventricle. Between the left ventricle and the diaphragm, there may be a small triangular shadow due to an epicardial fat pad. In this view, the maximum transverse diameter of the heart does not usually exceed 50% of the chest, measured from the inner aspects of the ribs, although 'cardiothoracic ratios' greater than this are sometimes seen in normal individuals.

In the lateral view (Fig. 7.2), the anterior border of the heart is formed by the pulmonary artery and right ventricle and the posterior border by the left atrium and left ventricle.

Enlargement of the left ventricle, which is most frequently due to hypertension, ischaemic heart disease, aortic valve disease and mitral regurgitation, produces depression and elongation of the cardiac apex (Fig. 7.3). Left ventricular enlargement is better seen in the lateral view. A normal left ventricle may be displaced posteriorly by an enlarged right ventricle.

Right ventricular enlargement, usually the consequence of pulmonary hypertension or pulmonary stenosis, produces an elevation of the cardiac apex in the postero-anterior view, and in the lateral views of the heart makes the normally straight anterior border of the heart bulge towards or impinge on the sternum.

The body of the left atrium enlarges posteriorly and to the right,

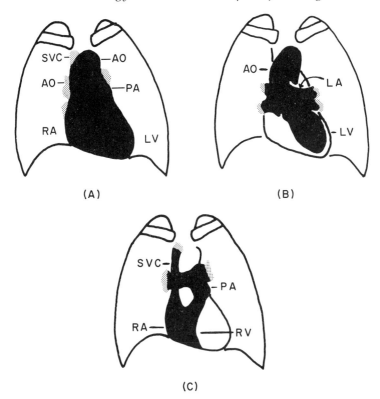

Fig. 7.1 The postero-anterior view. (A) The normal chest radiograph. (B) Appearances of the left side of the heart, after injection of radio-opaque material into the left atrium, showing the positions of the left atrium (LA), the left ventricle (LV) and the aorta (AO). (C) Appearances of the right side of the heart after injection of radio-opaque material into the superior vena cava (SVC). The positions of the right atrium (RA), the right ventricle (RV), and the pulmonary artery (PA), are shown.

but its appendage protrudes to the left. Thus, in the postero-anterior view, the left atrial appendage is seen on the left border of the heart between the pulmonary artery and the left ventricle (Fig. 7.4), whereas the main body of the left atrium forms a dense shadow within the right atrial border, or protrudes to the right above the right atrium on the right side of the heart. Left atrial enlargement is best diagnosed in the lateral view in which it can be seen displacing the barium-filled oesophagus posteriorly.

The right atrium enlarges mainly to the right and, in the postero-anterior view, makes the right border of the heart more prominent.

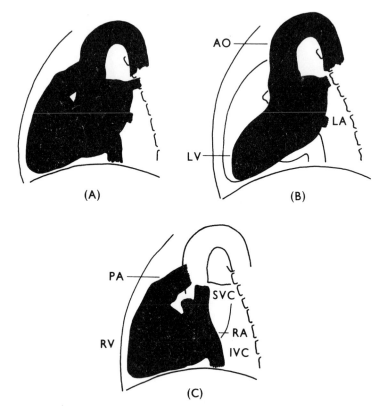

Fig. 7.2 The lateral view. (A) Normal chest radiograph. (B) Appearances of the left side of the heart, after injection of radio-opaque contrast medium into the left atrium, showing the positions of the left atrium (LA), left ventricle (LV) and aorta (AO). (C) Appearances of the right side of the heart after injection of contrast medium into the right atrium showing positions of superior and inferior venae cavae (SVC, IVC), right atrium (RA), right ventricle (RV) and pulmonary artery (PA).

Fig. 7.3 Depression and elongation of the cardiac apex in left ventricular enlargement.

Fig. 7.4 The bulge produced by the left atrial appendage (LA App.) is seen on the left border of the heart between the positions of the pulmonary artery and left ventricle.

LA App.

Fig. 7.5 Dilatation of the ascending aorta (Asc. AO), visible on the right upper cardiac silhouette, in aortic stenosis.

Asc. AO

Enlargement of the ascending aorta, as from post-stenotic dilatation in aortic stenosis or from aneurysm of the ascending aorta, is seen as a projection to the right (Fig. 7.5). The sclerotic 'uncoiled' aorta of the elderly produces a loop above the heart shadow (Fig. 7.6).

A pericardial effusion causes generalized enlargement of the cardiac silhouette, with both lateral borders being smoothly convex (Fig. 7.7).

Calcification within the heart can sometimes be suspected on a plain radiograph (Fig. 7.8), but tomography and fluoroscopy are necessary for confirmation. Calcification in the mitral valve, which is usually rheumatic, is best visualized in the lateral view in which it is seen in the posterior third of the cardiac mass. The aortic valve is located more in the centre of the heart; in the postero-anterior view it is situated just to the left of the spine. Calcification of the pericardium is best seen in a penetrated lateral view (Fig. 7.9).

Fig. 7.6 The appearances of an 'uncoiled' aorta.

Fig. 7.7 The appearances of a pericardial effusion.

Fluoroscopy of the heart is of particular value in showing valve calcification, abnormal movements of the pulmonary artery and aorta, and the systolic expansion of a ventricular aneurysm.

The plain chest radiograph is of great value in demonstrating abnormalities of the pulmonary circulation.

Pulmonary venous hypertension, as occurs in left ventricular failure and mitral stenosis, is revealed by dilatation of the pulmonary veins, particularly those draining the upper zones.

Oedema of the lungs is at first interstitial and causes haziness around the vascular shadows, with thin horizontal lines at the bases (Kerley's lines), due to fluid in the interlobular septa and distended lymphatics. Alveolar oedema produces a fluffy opacification spreading out from the hilar region, often providing a 'butterfly' appearance. Occasionally, pulmonary oedema is predominantly unilateral.

In moderate pulmonary arterial hypertension, the main right and left pulmonary arteries are enlarged, although the more

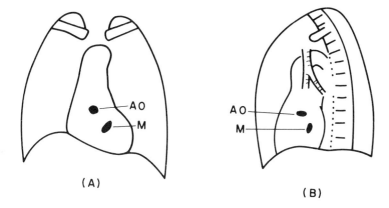

Fig. 7.8 The position of the aortic (AO) and mitral (M) valve calcification in: (A) the postero-anterior view and (B) the lateral view.

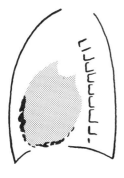

Fig. 7.9 Calcification of the pericardium, outlining the ventricles, in the lateral view.

peripheral arteries may be normal. In severe pulmonary hypertension, the major pulmonary arteries, which are greatly dilated, contrast with narrowed peripheral pulmonary arteries; the major arteries appear to be 'cut off'.

When there is increased pulmonary blood flow, as in atrial septal defect, ventricular septal defect and persistent ductus arteriosus, both main and peripheral pulmonary arteries are dilated (Fig. 7.10). Fluoroscopy may show a vigorous pulsation (the 'hilar dance').

When the pulmonary blood flow is decreased, as in pulmonary stenosis, the pulmonary arteries are poorly seen. However, the main and left pulmonary arteries may be dilated by the jet of blood emerging from the stenosis (Fig. 7.11)

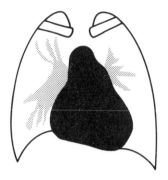

Fig. 7.10   Radiological appearances in atrial septal defect, showing enlarged pulmonary arteries and right side of the heart.

Fig. 7.11   Dilatation of the main and left pulmonary artery in pulmonary valve stenosis.

Cardiac catheterization and angiocardiography

These techniques are undertaken in order to establish a precise diagnosis and to assess the severity of the disorders present.
  Cardiac catheterization permits:

1 the recording of pressure within the heart and great vessels (see Table 7.1) for normal pressures;
2 the sampling of blood for blood gases;
3 the injection of indicators for the measurement of cardiac output;
4 the injection of radio-opaque substances which can delineate abnormalities of anatomy or function in the cardiovascular system;
5 the introduction of a balloon-tipped catheter for therapeutic purposes, e.g. the Rashkind procedure and angioplasty;
6 the introduction of a bioptome, to obtain a sample of endocardium or myocardium.

Table 7.1 Normal cardiovascular pressures (mmHg).

	Mean	Range
Right atrium — mean	4	0−8
Right ventricle		
systolic	25	15−30
end diastolic	4	0−8
Pulmonary artery		
systolic	25	15−30
diastolic	10	5−15
mean	15	10−20
Pulmonary artery wedge — mean	10	5−14
Left atrium — mean	7	4−12
Left ventricle		
systolic	120	90−140
end diastolic	7	4−12
Aorta		
systolic	120	90−140
diastolic	70	60−90
mean	85	70−105

Right heart catheterization

Under local anaesthesia, a catheter is introduced percutaneously or by cutdown into a basilic, saphenous or femoral vein, and advanced to the right atrium. It is manoeuvred with fluoroscopic control through the tricuspid valve to the right ventricle, thence to the pulmonary artery and finally wedged in a distal pulmonary artery. The pulmonary arterial wedge (pulmonary capillary) tracing so obtained is an indirect measurement of pressure in the left atrium.

If appropriate radiological facilities are not available, a catheter (Swan−Ganz) with a balloon close to its tip may be used. If the balloon is inflated when the right atrium is reached, the tip will 'float' into a pulmonary artery. If the balloon is impacted in the artery, a pulmonary artery wedge tracing is obtained.

If there is a septal defect, the catheter may be passed through this into the left side of the heart; if there is a persistent ductus arteriosus, this may be traversed.

As the catheter is withdrawn from the pulmonary artery, blood samples can be obtained from each vessel and chamber. When a left-to-right shunt is present, the blood is found to be more oxygenated in the affected chamber and beyond than it is in the great veins. In a persistent ductus arteriosus the oxygen saturation in the left pulmonary artery exceeds that in the right ventricle, whereas in a ventricular septal defect, the oxygen saturation in the right ventricle and pulmonary artery is greater than that in the right atrium. In an atrial septal defect, the oxygen saturation in the right atrium exceeds that in the superior and inferior venae cavae.

Pulmonary stenosis can be confirmed by demonstrating a systolic pressure difference between the pulmonary artery and right ventricle; in tricuspid stenosis the diastolic pressure in the right atrium is higher than that in the right ventricle.

Left heart catheterization

Although it is possible to obtain an indirect left atrial pressure from the pulmonary arterial wedge position, the left atrium and ventricle must be entered when more precise and detailed information is required about the left side of the heart. There are several techniques which can be used.

Trans-septal technique. A catheter containing a special needle is advanced from the femoral or saphenous vein to the right atrium. The needle is used to perforate the inter-atrial septum. Subsequently, the catheter is advanced over the needle into the left atrium and manoeuvred into the left ventricle.

Retrograde aortic technique. A catheter is introduced into the femoral or brachial arteries and advanced retrogradely until it reaches the aortic valve. In most cases it is possible to pass the catheter through the aortic valve into the left ventricle.

Direct left ventricular puncture. The left ventricle is punctured directly by a needle inserted through the chest wall.

Angiocardiography

By the injection of contrast medium it is possible to demonstrate the anatomy of the chambers of the heart and the great arteries, and to observe the patterns of blood flow. Cine films are taken at 50−150 frames per second in one or two planes.

The contrast medium is injected at the site most appropriate for the delineation of the suspected abnormality. Therefore, in ventricular septal defect and mitral regurgitation, the injection is made into the left ventricle; in aortic regurgitation it is made into the aorta. When coronary angiography is performed, selective injections are made into each of the two main coronary arteries (see p. 147).

Indications for and risks of cardiac catheterization and angiocardiography

Cardiac catheterization and angiocardiography are procedures which require considerable skill and experience on the part of the physician and entail some discomfort and hazard for the patient. The natural anxiety of patients prior to the procedure is best allayed by previous preparation and explanation, combined with the use of a sedative if necessary. Anaesthesia may have to be employed in children, but should be avoided if possible because of its effects on haemodynamics and blood gases.

Right heart catheterization entails little danger, although arrhythmias may be provoked when the catheter tip is in the right ventricle. Left heart catheterization imposes a greater risk both from arrhythmias and from perforation of the myocardium by a transthoracic or trans-septal needle, which may produce haemopericardium and tamponade. The injection of radio-opaque contrast medium in angiocardiography often provokes transient ventricular arrhythmias and, occasionally, ventricular fibrillation. Apart from the mortality of the procedures, there is a morbidity due to complications which include thrombosis of the catheterized artery or vein, pulmonary and systemic embolism, haemorrhage from puncture sites and toxic reactions to the contrast medium.

These techniques are mainly used to evaluate the nature and extent of the heart disease prior to cardiac surgery, but they are also of value when doubt exists as to the nature of a murmur, or the cause of chest pain. In recent years, echocardiography and Doppler ultrasound have rendered cardiac catheterization unnecessary in many cases of congenital and valvar heart disease, but it is still required when these techniques provide an equivocal result or when coronary arteriography is also needed.

The severity of a stenotic lesion is best determined by measuring both the pressure difference and the blood flow across the valve. This requires the simultaneous recording of pressures on both sides of the valve and the estimation of cardiac output. Thus, measurements must be obtained in the left ventricle and aorta in aortic stenosis, and in the left atrium (or pulmonary artery wedge position) and left ventricle in mitral stenosis. The severity of regurgitation is best evaluated by cine-angiography at the appropriate site.

The measurement of cardiac output

The cardiac output can be measured by one of two techniques: the Fick principle and the indicator-dilution method.

The Fick principle. Fick pointed out that:

1 The quantity of blood traversing the lungs in a given period of time equals the cardiac output.
2 The change in oxygen (O_2) concentration between pulmonary arteries (PA) and pulmonary veins (PV) depends upon the O_2 uptake in the lungs, and the volume of blood into which it is absorbed, i.e. the cardiac output (CO).
   Therefore,

$$PVO_2 - PAO_2 = \frac{O_2 \text{ uptake}}{CO} \quad \text{and} \quad CO = \frac{O_2 \text{ uptake}}{PVO_2 - PAO_2}$$

Oxygen uptake is derived from the analysis of expired air. Blood samples are obtained by catheterization, arterial blood being used instead of pulmonary venous blood.

Indicator-dilution method. This is based on a similar principle, namely that the concentration of an injected substance in the blood is dependent upon the amount of that substance injected and the volume of blood in which it is diluted.

Currently, the most popular technique is to use cold saline and to measure the change in temperature with a thermistor attached to a catheter tip. An injection of cold saline, of known volume and temperature, is injected into a vein or the right atrium and the temperature is sampled in the pulmonary artery.

Radionuclide studies

Nuclear imaging is of value in two major contexts which particularly relate to ischaemic heart disease: the demonstration of abnormalities of myocardial perfusion and the evaluation of left ventricular function.

Myocardial perfusion studies

Certain radiopharmaceuticals, of which thallium-201 is the one most commonly used, are taken up into the myocardium in proportion to the regional blood flow. They therefore do not concentrate in areas of ischaemia or fibrosis. Thallium imaging has been found to be of greatest value in the detection of transient myocardial ischaemia in patients with suspected angina pectoris. If the radio-isotope is injected intravenously during an exercise test at the time when the patient develops chest pain or ST depression, a 'cold spot' will be seen corresponding to the area of ischaemia, while the rest of the myocardium will take up the isotope. If nuclear imaging is repeated some 4 hours later, when no ischaemia is present, the 'cold spot' will be seen to have disappeared. This is a relatively sensitive and specific test, but unfortunately the cost of thallium and the degree of skill and experience necessary for optimal interpretation limits its application.

Radionuclide ventriculography

The most common technique for the imaging of left ventricular function involves the use of technetium-labelled red cells so that the pool of blood in the left ventricle can be detected. By using the ECG to 'gate' the images ('gated pool scan'), segments of the cardiac cycle from successive beats can be superimposed. By obtaining 20 or more exposures during each cardiac cycle, it is possible to record the radionuclide equivalent of a cine-angiogram. This technique allows the evaluation of several aspects of left ventricular function including contractility of the ventricle, end-systolic and end-diastolic volumes and the detection of regional wall abnormalities including ventricular aneurysms.

Echocardiography

When an ultrasonic beam encounters a boundary between structures of different acoustic densities, some of the waves are reflected. These can be detected and used to provide an electrical signal. The procedure of echocardiography exploits this principle to identify many cardiac structures and to study their movements (Figs. 7.12A and B).

A piezo-electric crystal which acts both as transmitter and receiver, is used to generate high frequency pulses of very short duration. These travel through body tissues at known velocity: the 'echoes' which occur from interfaces are detected by the transducer, amplified and then displayed either on an oscilloscope or on a strip-chart recorder. Bone and lung both interfere with ultrasonic transmission, so that the views that can be obtained of the heart are limited.

The transducer is usually placed in the fourth left intercostal space close to the sternal edge. As can be seen in Figs. 7.12A and B, by rotating the probe a sweeping view of many of the intracardiac structures may be obtained.

In cross-sectional (two-dimensional, 2D) echocardiography, an ultrasonic beam is moved rapidly across the heart (or a series of ultrasonic elements are fired in sequence) to allow a real-time

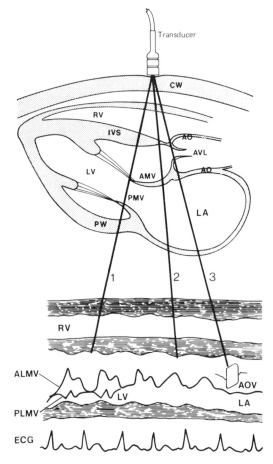

Fig. 7.12A The transducer is angled in different directions to permit study of the various cardiac structures. (1) The beam traverses the right ventricle (RV), interventricular septum (IVS), and anterior and posterior leaflets of the mitral valve (ALMV and PLMV). These leaflets separate abruptly as the blood flows rapidly from the left atrium to the left ventricle. As the flow decreases they approximate only to be separated again when atrial contraction propels more blood into the ventricle. (2) Provides good views of the RV, septum, ALMV and left atrium. (3) Shows separation of the aortic valve cusps in systole.

recording of changes in cardiac shape and movement, which are displayed on a videotape (Fig. 7.13).

Echocardiography has proved particularly valuable in studying disorders of the mitral valve. In the normal valve, the cusps open rapidly in early diastole and return quickly towards the closed

Fig. 7.12B Normal echocardiogram, corresponding to 12A, view (1), showing right ventricular outflow tract, interventricular septum, both cusps of the mitral valve, and the left ventricular cavity. RVOT = right ventricular outflow tract. IVS = interventricular septum. MV = mitral valve. LV = left ventricle.

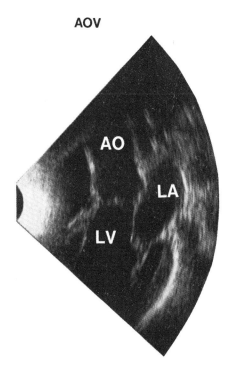

Fig. 7.13 Cross-sectional long axis parasternal view of a normal heart showing the aortic root, aortic valve, left ventricle and left atrium. LV = left ventricle, AO = aorta, LA = left atrium.

position, being further propelled downwards by atrial systole before finally moving upwards before closure. In mitral stenosis, the diastolic closure rate is slow and the posterior cusp, instead of moving away from the anterior cusp during diastole, moves forward with it (Fig. 7.14). Other abnormalities which may be detected are multiple echoes suggesting calcification, and abnormal movements of the leaflets during systole, indicating prolapse of the cusps (Fig. 7.15).

Although calcification of the aortic valve may be readily demonstrated, other abnormalities of this valve are less diagnostic. However, a useful indicator of aortic regurgitation is the fluttering of the mitral valve which may be produced by the regurgitant jet during early diastole.

Another major diagnostic use of echocardiography is the detection of pericardial effusion. Echo-free spaces may be demonstrated in front of and behind the heart.

The technique is also useful in detecting abnormalities in many varieties of congenital heart disease and in demonstrating such abnormalities as an atrial myxoma.

Fig. 7.14 Severe mitral stenosis — an M-mode parasternal echocardiogram. The left atrium (LA) is huge and the mitral valve shows the characteristic slow diastolic closure rate. RVOT = right ventricular outflow tract. MV = mitral valve.

Doppler ultrasound

This technique makes use of the familiar phenomenon whereby the pitch of a sound appears to become higher as its source approaches us, and falls as it goes away. In the body, the blood corpuscles act as moving targets which reflect the ultrasound wave, and alter its pitch, depending upon the direction and velocity of blood flow. In pulse Doppler, a single transducer is used, which first emits a brief ultrasound pulse, and then switches to receive the returning signal. Because ultrasound has a constant velocity in the body, the depth of the target can be determined by the interval between emission and receipt of the signal. The time interval and, therefore, the depth of the target area being examined can be varied as required, and can be correlated with a simultaneously recorded cross-sectional echocardiogram, thus locating precisely the site of the area being examined, Unfortunately, there is a limit to the rate at which pulses can be

Fig. 7.15 Mitral valve prolapse. M-mode echocardiogram showing (arrow) 'hammocking' appearance of mitral cusp as it prolapses posteriorly during late systole.

generated, because one wave may not have returned before the next is generated; this leads to distortion (aliasing) of the signal. This prevents the recognition of high velocities. For identifying these, continuous wave (CW) Doppler is used. In this technique, one transducer continuously emits ultrasound, which is detected by a separate receiver. CW Doppler is particularly useful for evaluating lesions such as aortic stenosis in which there are high velocity jets.

Doppler ultrasound has proved to be of especial value in assessing congenital heart disease and valve lesions. Quite minor degrees of valvular regurgitation can be detected, particularly in the tricuspid area; quantitation of mitral regurgitation is not reliable. The technique can be used to assess the severity of stenotic lesions non-invasively, most successfully in the aortic area (Fig. 11.12).

Further reading

Feigenbaum, H. (1986) *Echocardiography*, 4th edn. Philadelphia: Lea and Febiger.

Gerson, M.C. (Ed.) (1987) *Cardiac Nuclear Medicine*. New York: McGraw Hill.

Grainger, R.G. & Allison, D.J. (Eds.) (1986) *Diagnostic Radiology*. Edinburgh Churchill Livingstone.

Jefferson, K. & Rees, S. (1980) *Clinical Cardiac Radiology*, 2nd edn. London: Butterworth.

Mendel, D. & Oldershaw, P. (1986) *Cardiac Catheterization*, 3rd edn. Oxford: Blackwell.

Task Force on Assessment of Cardiovascular Procedures (1986) Guidelines for clinical use of cardiac radionuclide imaging. *Circulation 74:* 1469A

Diseases of the Coronary Arteries

The coronary circulation

There are two major coronary arteries — right and left (Fig. 8.1). The right coronary artery arises from the right coronary sinus of Valsalva and runs down in the groove between the right atrium and the right ventricle. In most hearts, its branches supply the sinus node, the atrioventricular node and bundle, the right ventricle and the inferior part of the left ventricle. The left coronary artery, which arises from the left coronary sinus of Valsalva, soon divides into two large branches: the anterior descending branch which runs down between the two ventricles anteriorly, and the left circumflex branch which passes around in the groove between the left atrium and the left ventricle. The anterior descending artery supplies the interventricular septum and the anterior wall of the left ventricle. The circumflex supplies the lateral and posterior aspects of the left ventricle. The major vessels traverse the external surface of the myocardium, sending branches perpendicularly into the muscle mass. There are normally many small anastomoses between the coronary arteries, but these are of no functional importance. When an area of the heart becomes ischaemic, the anastomoses enlarge and then provide a collateral blood supply to the affected muscle which is often vital for its survival.

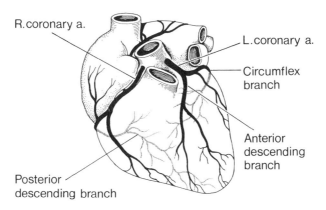

R.coronary a.

L.coronary a.

Circumflex branch

Anterior descending branch

Posterior descending branch

Fig. 8.1 The anatomy of the coronary arteries (see text).

The arteries divide to form arterioles and capillaries similar to those elsewhere in the body, and the venules and veins join to form larger venous channels. Virtually all the blood from the left coronary artery eventually drains into the coronary sinus; that from the right coronary artery drains mainly into the anterior cardiac veins. From these veins the blood passes into the right atrium.

The blood flow in the coronary arteries resembles that in other regions in being dependent on the blood pressure and on the vascular resistance of the arteries and arterioles. A distinctive feature of the coronary circulation is that the arteries are compressed by the contracting myocardium during systole so that the resistance to flow at that time is sharply increased. Consequently, coronary blood flow occurs mainly during diastole. Flow is largely determined by the calibre of the coronary arteries themselves. Certainly, the aortic diastolic pressure is also a determinant of coronary flow; but according to Poiseuille's equation, flow is dependent directly on pressure differences but related to the fourth power of the radius. Therefore, a doubling of aortic diastolic pressure doubles coronary flow, whereas a doubling of the radius of the coronary arteries leads to a sixteenfold increase in flow. In health, variations in coronary blood flow are mainly due to changes in impedance in the small coronary arteries; these dilate in response to a fall in tissue oxygen tension but they are also under the influence of the autonomic nervous system. Variations in tone also occur in the large coronary arteries but these affect blood flow only if these vessels are narrowed by disease or they are extreme (spasm).

In the normal resting heart, almost all the oxygen is extracted during its passage through the capillaries; coronary sinus blood is therefore almost completely desaturated. Unlike other organs, the heart cannot call upon a venous oxygen reserve when faced by increased demands, and is largely dependent upon the ability of the coronary arteries to increase their diameter.

Coronary artery disease

Coronary artery disease is the commonest cause of heart disease and the most important single cause of death in the affluent countries of the world. In the overwhelming majority of cases, disease of the coronary arteries is due to atherosclerosis. However, they may also be involved in other disorders.

Congenital abnormalities such as arteriovenous fistulae and anomalous origin from the pulmonary artery.

Coronary embolism associated with thrombosis arising in the

left atrium or ventricle or from mitral or aortic valve prostheses, or from infective endocarditis.

Syphilitic aortitis involving the coronary ostia (p. 300).

Occlusion of a coronary artery due to dissecting aneurysm (p. 279).

Polyarteritis (p. 307) and other connective tissue diseases.

Coronary artery spasm which may affect both diseased and otherwise normal vessels (p. 138).

Definitions

Atherosclerosis. This has been defined (by a WHO study group) as 'a variable combination of changes of the intima of arteries (as distinguished from arterioles) consisting of a focal accumulation of lipids, complex carbohydrates, blood and blood products, fibrous tissue and calcium deposits, and associated with medial changes'. It is synonymous with *atheroma* but not with *arteriosclerosis*, which is a less specific term used to describe hardening of arteries and arterioles.

Coronary artery disease. This term is used to describe coronary arteries which are affected by a pathological process. Coronary artery disease usually exists for many years before a disorder of myocardial function develops. It is, therefore, not synonymous with ischaemic heart disease.

Ischaemic heart disease. This term is used to describe cardiac disease resulting from myocardial ischaemia. Although myocardial ischaemia also occurs in such conditions as aortic stenosis, ischaemic heart disease is generally applied only to cases of atherosclerotic origin.

Coronary heart disease and *atherosclerotic heart disease.* These are used synonymously with ischaemic heart disease.

Coronary thrombosis. This is used to describe the occlusion of a coronary artery by thrombus. This may or may not lead to myocardial infarction.

Coronary occlusion. This is used to describe occlusion of the coronary artery by any cause. Again, this may or may not cause myocardial infarction.

Myocardial infarction. This is used to indicate necrosis of a portion of heart muscle as a result of inadequate blood supply.

Silent ischaemia. This term is used to describe the occurrence of ischaemia in the absence of symptoms. It is applied particularly to episodes of ST elevation or depression unaccompanied by pain.

Vasospastic angina (Prinzmetal's angina)

This term is used to describe a syndrome of which the essential features are angina pectoris due to an increase in coronary vaso-motor tone and ST elevation in the ECG. The angina is attributable not, as in classical angina, to an increase in myocardial oxygen demand, but to a transient reduction in coronary blood flow. The disorder may occur either in otherwise apparently normal coronary arteries, or in atherosclerotic vessels. In the former case, the increase in tone must be extreme (spasm), but in severely stenotic arteries, even physiological changes in tone can produce a critical reduction in blood flow. The mechanism for coronary spasm is unknown, but it may be provoked by certain drugs, notably ergometrine.

The clinical picture is typically one of anginal pain occurring at rest, particularly in the early morning. The attacks are usually self-limiting, but the pain may be severe, and they sometimes lead on to myocardial infarction. Nitrates and calcium antagonists are effective in the treatment of individual episodes, and also when used prophylactically.

Clinical manifestation of ischaemic heart disease

Coronary atherosclerosis may lead to a variety of syndromes which can affect the same patient at different times. These are: angina pectoris, acute myocardial infarction, unstable angina, cardiac failure, arrhythmias and sudden death.

Pathology of coronary atherosclerosis and its complications

The characteristic lesion is the plaque, whose major components are lipid, much of it extracellular, and arterial smooth muscle cells and their products, such as fibrous proteins and complex carbo-hydrates. Plaques vary from one another in their composition. At one extreme are fatty plaques, containing a large pool of choles-terol and its esters, separated from the lumen by a thin fibrous cap. At the other extreme, are solid plaques, consisting of smooth muscle cells. Calcification may be superimposed. These deposits are focal and are most commonly located at the bends and bifur-cations of arteries.

The atheromatous plaque, which is produced by this process, may itself narrow the lumen of the artery. The fibrous cap is prone to fracture, allowing the necrotic core to ulcerate and trigger off platelet aggregation and fibrin deposition. This is a repetitive process and leads to further narrowing, which may proceed to complete occlusion.

When patients who have experienced *angina pectoris* come to necropsy, there is usually found to be widespread but patchy coronary atherosclerosis and myocardial fibrosis. There is commonly evidence of old coronary occlusion and myocardial infarction. The basic pathological cause for the angina is the coronary arterial narrowing which has reduced the lumen of at least one of the three main coronary arteries by 75%. In most cases, two or all three of these arteries are affected.

Sudden death is often attributed to coronary artery disease when widespread coronary atherosclerosis is present. Recent coronary occlusion or myocardial infarction can be demonstrated in only a minority of cases but plaque rupture and non-occlusive thrombus are common. In most instances, it is probable that acute myocardial ischaemia has provoked fatal ventricular fibrillation.

The essential pathological feature of *acute myocardial infarction* is myocardial necrosis. This is usually, but not always, the consequence of total occlusion of a coronary artery. Plaque rupture is commonly found at necropsy; in most cases there is superimposed thrombosis (see p. 154).

Incidence and prevalence of ischaemic heart disease

The incidence of ischaemic heart disease increases with age. It is relatively uncommon under the age of 40; the frequency rises rapidly after this age in males, but less so in females. Under the age of 45, ischaemic heart disease is more than ten times as common in males as in females; between 45 and 60 it is at least twice as common in males; in the older age groups the incidence is approximately equal in the two sexes. The number of deaths attributed to ischaemic heart disease has increased considerably in the last 40 years; the annual death rate from this cause has, however, recently fallen substantially in a number of countries including the United States, Australia and New Zealand, but little or not at all in some others such as the United Kingdom.

Aetiological factors in ischaemic heart disease and their control

Coronary atherosclerosis is a necessary precursor of ischaemic heart disease but it may require a further pathological process, such as thrombosis, to produce clinical manifestations.

Pathogenesis of coronary atherosclerosis. There are two main theories as to the pathogenesis of atherosclerosis — the lipid-infiltration (or 'insudation') theory and the thrombogenic theory.

The lipid-infiltration theory proposes that the principal factor in the development of atherosclerosis is accumulation of plasma constituents, notably lipids by passage through the arterial wall. This concept is supported by the strong relationship between serum cholesterol levels and the development of atheroma. It seems that the presence of low density lipoproteins stimulates the proliferation of smooth muscle cells, which are the cells mainly involved in atherogenesis. The alternative hypothesis is that the process starts with the formation of thrombi, at a defect in the arterial intima. These are subsequently endothelialized and absorbed as a fibrous lesion into the intima. Even if this latter explanation of the origin of atheroma is incorrect, it is probable that the development of mural thrombi and their incorporation into the arterial wall is a factor of importance in the progression of atherosclerosis.

In addition to the mechanisms mentioned, injury to the endothelium, as may result from hypertension and cigarette smoking, is probably an important factor.

Lipid disorders. There is much circumstantial evidence to incriminate lipid abnormalities in the genesis of atheroma:

1   Deposition of lipid in the arterial wall occurs at an early, if not at the initial, stage of the process.
2   Atheroma can be induced in animals by cholesterol feeding and other means of raising plasma cholesterol levels. However, the lesions differ from those in the human in not being associated with thrombosis.
3   There is a high incidence of ischaemic (atherosclerotic) heart disease in individuals with elevated plasma lipid levels, particularly if they have familial hyperlipoproteinaemia.
4   There is increasing epidemiological evidence that high levels of high density lipoproteins (HDL) are protective against ischaemic heart disease in contrast to the adverse effects of high levels of low density lipoproteins.

Hyperlipoproteinaemias are subdivided into several types, based on whether cholesterol, triglycerides or chylomicrons are increased (see Table 8.1). Only types II and III are clearly associated with coronary atherosclerosis, although a relationship to type IV seems probable. Of particular interest from the genetic point of view is familial hypercholesterolaemia. Homozygotes, who have been found to have absent low density lipoprotein

Table 8.1 Hyperlipoproteinaemias.

Types	Chylomicrons	Cholesterol	Triglycerides	Clinical aspects
I	+++	↑	↑	Rare. Familial. Childhood hepatosplenomegaly. Xanthomata. No definite association with coronary disease.
IIa	—	↑	—	Often familial. Tendinous and tuberous xanthomata associated with early atherosclerosis.
IIb	—	↑	↑	
III	—	↑		Orange and yellow palmar creases. Xanthomata. Peripheral and coronary artery disease.
IV	—	— —	↑	Familial or dietary. Also oral contraceptives. Probable association with atherosclerosis.
V	++	↑	↑	Rare. Abdominal pain. Pancreatis. Not definitely associated with atherosclerosis.

(LDL) receptors, develop coronary disease in childhood or adolescence. Heterozygotes have a reduced number of LDL receptors, and often develop coronary disease as young adults.

Certain other types of disorder which disturb lipid metabolism are associated with a high incidence of coronary disease. These include hypothyroidism and diabetes mellitus. Women who have had bilateral öophorectomy are liable to develop hypercholesterolaemia and premature coronary disease.

Even when these specific disease processes are excluded, there is a strong relationship between hyperlipidaemia and the risk of developing coronary disease at a relatively early age. Thus, in countries such as the United States and the United Kingdom, in which the average plasma cholesterol level of the community is relatively high, there is a much higher incidence of coronary artery disease than in those countries in which hypercholestero-laemia is rare. In long-term studies of whole populations, it has been shown that the higher the level of plasma cholesterol, the greater is the individual's risk of developing coronary artery disease. The cause of the high cholesterol levels is not yet fully established, although it seems likely that it is related in part to dietary factors. A high content of saturated fat (mainly of animal origin) in the diet is particularly suspect but a relative deficiency of polyunsaturated fats (especially the essential fatty acid, linoleic acid) may be important.

Treatment of hyperlidaemia should start with dietary measures. Weight reduction alone substantially reduces hypertriglyceri-daemia; alcohol restriction reinforces this. For hypercholestero-laemia, total fat should be reduced to 25−30% of food energy, polyunsaturated fatty acids, especially linoleic acid, providing 7−10%.

There are several drugs available to correct hyperlipidaemia.

Bile-acid sequestrants are anion-exchange resins, which are not absorbed. Cholestyramine 8−12 g twice daily is effective in hyper-cholesterolaemia, but is unpleasant to take, and may cause dys-pepsia and constipation. A large trial with this drug showed a reduction in myocardial infarction but no effect on total mortality.

Nicotinic acid reduces triglycerides and, to a lesser extent, chol-esterol. The most troublesome side-effect is flushing, but choles-tatic jaundice and aggravation of diabetes may occur. Treatment should start with 100 mg three times daily, and rise slowly to 1−2 g three times daily.

Clofibrate reduces triglycerides, and to a lesser extent, choles-terol. A large trial showed a reduction in myocardial infarction but non-cardiac mortality was higher in the treated group. Other problems include gall-stones and potentiation of coumarin anti-coagulants. The dosage is 500 mg three times daily.

Hypertension. The higher the blood pressure, whether systolic or diastolic, the greater is the risk of developing ischaemic heart disease. Hypertension may contribute to its development in two ways: by accelerating the development of arterial disease and by increasing the work load of the left ventricle. Whilst there is, as yet, little convincing evidence that lowering blood pressure pre-vents myocardial infarction, it seems likely in the long run to slow the progression of atherosclerosis, and diminish the risk of heart failure.

Obesity. Though common in patients with ischaemic heart dis-ease, it cannot necessarily be implicated as a causal factor.

Family history. Coronary artery disease often occurs in several members of the same family but it is likely that both genetic and environmental factors are involved. To some extent, at least, the familial incidence is due to the inheritance of hyperlipidaemia or hypertension.

Cigarette smoking. Heavy consumption of cigarettes is associated with a high incidence of myocardial infarction and sudden death. Giving up smoking reduces the risk of these events.

Physical activity. Physical exercise appears to have some protective effect — perhaps by encouraging the enlargement of the coronary arteries and their anastomoses. Young people should be encouraged to exercise regularly. The middle-aged should also exercise but must return to it gradually if they are out of condition.

Mental stress. It is widely believed that stress contributes to coronary disease. This may well be so, but convincing evidence is not, as yet, available. It must be said that this is a very difficult area of study.

Diabetes. Ischaemic heart disease appears to develop more frequently and at an earlier age in those with diabetes than in other individuals.

Haemostatic factors. It has recently been shown that individuals with high levels of active factor VII and fibrinogen have an enhanced risk of coronary events.

Prevention of ischaemic heart disease

Coronary atherosclerosis and ischaemic heart disease are not the inevitable consequences of ageing, although they increase with age. Both heredity and environment play major roles. The latter is clearly susceptible to modification unlike inborn genetic characteristics. Nonetheless, heredity is related to coronary disease through intermediary factors, such as hyperlipidaemia and hypertension, which can be corrected. It is still not certain that the reduction in risk factors, other than smoking, prevents coronary disease, but it seems probable that the life-style changes that have taken place in, for example, the United States and Australia, have contributed to the fall in ischaemic heart disease deaths that have occurred in those countries.

Two types of strategy have been proposed to prevent coronary disease — a 'high-risk' strategy, involving the identification and treatment of those at high risk, e.g. hyperlipidaemic individuals, or a 'low-risk' strategy, aimed at reducing risk factors in the community at large. The two approaches are not incompatible and both should be pursued, because whilst the high-risk patients are those most likely to benefit, they are relatively few in number and constitute only a small proportion of those who develop coronary disease.

The recommendations of the British Cardiac Society include the following:

1   Every opportunity should be taken to eliminate smoking.
2   Those with blood cholesterol concentrations above 6.5 mmol/l should be given dietary advice. If the level is above 7.8 mmol/l drug therapy may be required. The aim should be to reduce cholesterol towards 5.2 mmol/l.
3   The consumption of fat should be reduced, so that no more than 35% of food energy comes from fat, and 15% from saturated fat. The ratio of polyunsaturated to saturated fat should be increased to at least 0.45.
4   Those with diastolic blood pressure above 100 mmHg should receive treatment.
5   Physical activity should be encouraged.
6   General practitioners are in the best position to identify and counsel those at high risk because of family history, hypertension or smoking.

Angina pectoris

Definition

As originally described by Heberden, angina pectoris was a symptom complex; there was no implied association with the heart. Today, the term is still used to describe a symptom, but one which is the consequence of myocardial ischaemia. As discussed on p. 90, there are many causes but coronary atherosclerosis is much the commonest. Almost invariably, at least one of the major coronary arteries has a reduction in luminal diameter of 70% or more; frequently two or three major arteries are involved. In most patients, there is a clear relationship to exercise, but the threshold for this may vary, presumably due to changes in coronary vasomotor tone.

Anginal pain has four major characteristics: its location, its character, its relation to exercise, and its duration.

The location of angina pectoris

Angina pectoris is most often felt behind the middle or upper third of the sternum. Even when the discomfort may be more obvious in another area, the sternal region is usually involved to a greater or lesser extent. Angina may also be felt in the lower sternal or xiphisternal region, over both sides of the chest, more commonly the left, in the neck and lower jaw and in both arms, again particularly the left. It may affect only the upper arm, but often reaches the elbow, the wrist or the fingers. In some patients the elbow region escapes and the patient is aware of discomfort in the upper arm and a tingling feeling in the fingers. Rarely, it may radiate through to the left scapular region. It is very unusual for the pain to be located predominantly under the left nipple and virtually never is it confined to this area.

The character of angina pectoris

Angina pectoris is most frequently likened to a pressing feeling, a tight band, or a heavy weight. Many patients deny actual pain and refer only to a sense of discomfort. It is not usually severe but can cause much anxiety and distress. It is not stabbing in quality, but the terms 'sharp' (perhaps meaning rather intense) and 'burning' are sometimes used. The sensation appreciated in the neck and arms is often of a different type. In the neck, it is frequently described as 'choking'; in the jaw it is often a dull ache or 'like toothache'. The feeling in the arms is usually one of numbness, heaviness or tingling.

The relationship of angina pectoris to exercise and other provoking factors

Angina pectoris is usually provoked by exertion, nearly always that of walking, particularly up hill. The amount of exercise required to produce angina varies from time to time in any individual, but it is more readily provoked after a heavy meal or in cold weather. Emotion is also an important provoking factor; angina often develops during sexual intercourse and may be induced by anger and irritation.

Some patients experience nocturnal angina, which wakes them up. In some cases this may be due to dreams, but it is probable that increased coronary artery tone, which is maximal in the early morning, is often responsible.

Angina pectoris may be provoked by several different types of tachycardia, particularly paroxysmal tachycardia associated with very rapid ventricular rates. Anaemia also contributes to its development, although it is unusual for it to do so in the absence of coronary atherosclerosis.

The duration of the attack

Most attacks last 1–3 minutes. Their duration is seldom less than

30 seconds or more than 15 minutes, although a vague sensation of discomfort may persist after the pain has stopped.

Other symptoms and signs in angina pectoris

Some patients complain of breathlessness accompanying the anginal pain. Other symptoms include flatulence, feelings of faintness, and acute anxiety. Tachycardia and a rise in blood pressure may be noted during an attack but there are usually no abnormal signs.

The electrocardiogram

In between attacks of angina pectoris, the ECG is usually normal. There may, however, be evidence of old myocardial infarction, or non-specific changes such as flattening or inversion of T waves in the leads in which these are normally upright, or signs of a conduction defect. If the patient is seen during an attack there are usually well-marked abnormalities which take the form of a horizontal or downward sloping depression of the ST segment (Fig. 8.2). Similar changes may be provoked by an exercise test (see below).

Diagnosis

By definition, angina is a symptom complex with a pathophysiological basis of myocardial ischaemia. The diagnosis must, therefore, depend on the history, combined with evidence of inadequate coronary blood flow.

There is usually no problem in determining the location of the pain and the factors that provoke it, but patients often find it difficult to find the words to describe the sensation and estimates of the duration of the attack are often inaccurate. Most weight must therefore be placed on the first two elements. If the pain is located solely in the left sub-mammary region, or if it lasts for only a few seconds, it is almost certainly not of ischaemic origin. Angina is seldom associated with tenderness of the chest wall, although it may occasionally be so. It is usually, but not always, relieved by glyceryl trinitrate. Angina pectoris is unlikely if walking is not a provoking factor, but some patients take so little exercise that the symptom arises only on emotion or at night.

Fig. 8.2 Horizontal ST depression in myocardial ischaemia.

Physical examination is of comparatively little value except for the exclusion of such causes as aortic stenosis and cardiomyopathy. However, because angina pectoris is often associated with hypertension, with diabetes and with aortic valve disease, the characteristic findings of these conditions may be observed.

Evidence of myocardial ischaemia is provided by the presence of characteristic ST segment changes during an attack. As spontaneous attacks are seldom witnessed, it may be necessary to carry out an exercise test. The patient may be made to exercise on a bicycle ergometer or a treadmill, preferably until the chest discomfort is provoked. Standard and chest lead ECGs should be obtained during exercise and during the first 10 minutes of rest. A positive exercise test is one which shows a horizontal downward sloping ST depression of 1 mm or more (Fig. 8.2). ST segments which slope upwards from the J point should not be regarded as evidence of ischaemia as they are often seen in normal individuals with tachycardia (see Fig. 3.13).

Unfortunately, even after careful history-taking and ECG examination, one may remain uncertain as to whether or not a patient has angina pectoris. Radionuclide studies with thallium-201 may be helpful, but in some cases it is necessary to resort to coronary arteriography to establish the presence of coronary arterial disease. The use of this potentially hazardous procedure is seldom justified for diagnostic purposes alone, but it is essential in patients being considered for coronary artery surgery or angioplasty. It involves the introduction of specially designed catheters into the brachial or femoral arteries. The left and right coronary arteries are entered and radio-opaque medium is injected. Cineangiographic records are obtained in various positions to ensure a good visualization of all the major vessels. Left ventriculography is also undertaken to assess myocardial function.

Deaths from coronary angiography may result from coronary occlusion and dissection. Ventricular fibrillation may occur also, but is usually corrected without difficulty. The mortality of this investigation is between 0.1 and 0.5%.

Differential diagnosis

Although the diagnosis of angina can usually be established on the basis of the history and ECG, there are a number of other conditions which have to be considered in the differential diagnosis. Perhaps the most common difficulty arises with musculoskeletal pains in the chest wall. Frequently no cause is found for such pains which are often associated with tenderness and usually located on one side of the chest rather than centrally. These pains are most likely to be provoked by such actions as lifting and pulling, which produce tension of the muscles attached to the ribs. Amongst identifiable musculoskeletal conditions may be included Tietze's syndrome (in which there is an inflammation of one or more costochondral junctions), a slipping rib cartilage, fractured ribs, or metastatic lesions in ribs. In these conditions, unlike angina, there is tenderness and the symptoms may be aggravated by inspiration. The pain of cervical spondylosis is sometimes most severe in the upper chest region and accompanied by discomfort in the shoulders and arms.

Stabbing pains under the left breast and persistent aches in the same region are common and are most unlikely to be due to ischaemic heart disease. It is often not possible to establish their cause, but these symptoms are very common in those with anxiety neurosis.

Disorders of the gastrointestinal tract may be difficult to differentiate from angina pectoris. Oesophageal reflux, often associated with hiatus hernia, gives rise to a central chest pain, but this seldom radiates to the arms, is of a more burning or bursting character, and is more readily provoked by stooping or lying flat, although it may be produced by exercise. The pain of peptic ulcer is usually situated in the epigastric region, and is associated with tenderness. It is related to food rather than to exertion and is usually relieved by alkalis or milk and not by glyceryl trinitrate. Cholecystitis and cholelithiasis may give rise to pain in the lower sternal region, but there is usually tenderness either in the epigastrium or in the right subcostal area; there is frequently associated nausea, and the pain is not related to exertion. It is important to recognize that these gastrointestinal conditions, particularly hiatus hernia and cholecystitis, are common in patients with ischaemic heart disease, and the presence of one of these disorders does not preclude the coexistence of angina pectoris.

Prognosis

Most patients who develop angina pectoris live a normal or nearly normal life for many years. Symptoms are liable to vary from time to time, becoming worse in winter and improving the subsequent summer. They may disappear altogether for months or years.

It is difficult to give an accurate prognosis for any individual, but the outlook is relatively unfavourable if there is associated hypertension, advanced age, cardiac failure or preceding myocardial infarction. Coronary angiographic studies have shown that the prognosis is good if disease is confined to one artery. By contrast, severe narrowing of the left main coronary artery and diffuse lesions of all three arteries are associated with a high risk of early death.

Most patients live for 5 years and about one-third live for 10 years or more. The risk of sudden death or acute myocardial infarction is always present; before such events occur, there is frequently an exacerbation of the angina.

Treatment

The general management of the patient with angina pectoris is of paramount importance. The anxiety that the diagnosis arouses may cause incapacity, and it is important to emphasize the relatively good prognosis. The patient should be advised to avoid intense cold, walking into a wind or unnecessarily uphill, and taking large meals. He should be told to think about his daily programme in advance so that, for example, he does not have to hurry for a bus or train. Usually, the patient can continue his occupation, but should attempt to avoid unnecessary stresses, and learn to relax. Physical exercise should be encouraged provided it does not induce discomfort, but sudden strenuous effort should be avoided. There is no convincing evidence that low fat diets are of any value in the treatment of ischaemic heart disease, but a reduction in saturated fats with some substitution by polyunsaturated fats is advisable, especially for the younger patient. Obesity must be corrected. Cigarette smoking should be discouraged because it may provoke angina and increase the risk of acute myocardial infarction.

Drug therapy

Nitrates. Nitrates have been in use in the management of angina for more than 100 years, but their mode of action remains uncertain and their place in therapy controversial.

The major pharmacological effect of nitrates is the relaxation of smooth muscle, which seems to result from an increase in intracellular cyclic guanosine monophosphate (cGMP). Dilatation occurs in the coronary arteries, and in the peripheral arteries and veins. The former action leads directly to an increase in coronary blood flow, arterial dilatation leads to a fall in afterload, and a reduction in venous tone causes pooling, with a diminished venous return and preload. The relative importance of these different effects is not clear, and probably varies from one patient to another. Thus, the coronary vasodilator action is of particular value when an increase in coronary artery tone is an important component of angina, whereas it may have little influence in an artery with a fixed stenosis. In the latter situation, it is probably the venodilator action that is most relevant.

Most nitrates undergo extensive first pass metabolism in the liver; this may be overcome by administering large doses, but the effects are rather unpredictable. Alternatives are to use *isosorbide mononitrate* which does not undergo first pass metabolism, or to bypass the gut by sublingual, transdermal, or intravenous administration.

Nitrates have relatively minor side-effects, but headache is very common. This tends to diminish with continued use, but some patients find it even more distressing than the angina. Nitrates (particularly glyceryl trinitrate) may cause hypotension and syncope; patients should be advised to take at least their first dose sitting down.

A problem with continuous nitrate therapy is the development of tolerance. This does not seem to occur if there is a nitrate-free period each day, but is likely to do so if there is not.

Glyceryl trinitrate (nitroglycerin, trinitrin) is standard therapy in angina pectoris. It is given sublingually in a dose of $0.2-0.5$ mg. It will stop an attack of angina in about 2 minutes, but is particularly effective if given prophylactically. Patients should, therefore, be encouraged to take a tablet when they anticipate an attack; they should also be advised that the drug is not addictive, as many fear that they will become drug dependent.

Long-acting oral nitrates are effective if given in sufficient dosage, but headache is a common problem, and the regimen should ensure a nitrate-free period. The same considerations apply to transdermal patches.

Intravenous nitrates are of considerable value in unstable angina and in cardiac failure. Nitrates should be diluted before use. Glass bottles are preferable; with nitroglycerin, intravenous tubing that minimally absorbs the drug is necessary. Nitroglycerin should be given initially in a dosage of 5 µg per minute; the dose may be increased each 5 minutes by 5 µg, and later, 10 µg per minute, as necessary, with very careful observation of the blood pressure. Isosorbide dinitrate therapy may be started at 20 µg a minute, and increased by steps of 20 µg.

Beta-adrenoceptor blocking drugs. These are now given routinely to all but the mildest case, unless there are contraindications to their use. They block the action of catecholamines in increasing heart rate, blood pressure and cardiac contractility and thereby limit the myocardial oxygen needs on exercise or psychological stress. Unfortunately, they can exacerbate cardiac failure and may cause bronchospasm in those with obstructive airways disease. When given to patients free of heart failure or a history of asthma or bronchitis, beta-blocking drugs seldom give rise to serious side-effects but minor ones are quite common. These include fatigue, unpleasant dreams and nausea.

In general, the choice of a particular beta-blocker is not of importance, but it is preferable to use a cardioselective drug for patients with suspected obstructive airways disease or insulin-dependent diabetes. Compliance is more likely to be achieved if one uses a preparation which need be given only once or twice a day, such as atenolol, sotalol or nadolol or the long-acting formulations of propranolol and metoprolol. A lower dosage of a beta-blocker may be effective when it is combined with a long-acting nitrate or calcium antagonist.

Calcium antagonists. Calcium has an essential role in both the electrical and mechanical functions of the heart. It is also involved in the contraction of coronary and peripheral arteries. As described on p. 31, the entry of calcium ions into the cell is an important component in the generation of the action potential, being partially responsible for depolarization and for the plateau phase. The slow calcium current is largely responsible for depolarization of the atrioventricular node. Calcium in the cell blocks the action of troponin, which itself inhibits the actin–myosin reaction. In the resting phase, calcium is bound to a number of structures within the cell including the nucleus, mitochondria, sarcolemma, the T system and the sarcoplasmic reticulum. The small quantity of calcium that enters the cell during depolarization is not sufficient by itself to initiate contraction but appears to stimulate the release of the ion from the sarcoplasmic reticulum and this in turn inhibits troponin and stimulates the actin–myosin contraction. The process is reversed during relaxation. The rate of development of tension in the myocardium and the total tension developed depends on the rate at which calcium becomes available and the amount which becomes available, respectively.

The four main calcium antagonists currently available are verapamil, diltiazem, nicardipine and nifedipine. Verapamil and diltiazem have potent electrophysiological effects, depressing the action potential in the atrioventricular node specifically. They may lead to bradycardia. They are used for the treatment of supraventricular tachycardias involving the atrioventricular node. Their value in angina pectoris is probably due to a combination of peripheral and coronary vasodilatation and a reduction of the tachycardia which occurs on exertion. A dosage of 120 mg verapamil three times daily is usually required to control angina; the commonest side-effect is constipation. Diltiazem is relatively free from side-effects; the customary dosage is 60 mg three times daily. Nifedipine has little effect on the atrioventricular node; it exerts its main pharmacological effect on the peripheral and coronary arteries. The peripheral vasodilatation it induces leads to a reflex tachycardia and may also lead to hypotension. Although effective in exercise-induced angina, it may aggravate it because of tachycardia. It has been found particularly helpful in the management of coronary artery spasm but when used in exercise-induced angina is better combined with a beta-blocking drug. It is also being used in the management of hypertension in association with other antihypertensive drugs. 10−20 mg thrice daily is the usual dosage. Many patients suffer from side-effects with nifedipine but they are seldom serious. Some 20−30% have peripheral oedema as a result of vasodilatation. Others complain of headaches, gastrointestinal disturbances, flushing, dizziness and syncope. Nicardipine is similar to nifedipine. The dosage is 5−30 mg three times a day.

Coronary artery bypass surgery

The narrowed segments of coronary arteries can be bypassed by using a saphenous vein or internal mammary artery. In the former case, one end of the vein is attached to the ascending aorta and the other to the affected artery beyond the most distal obstruction as demonstrated by coronary arteriography. If an arterial graft is used, the proximal end of the vessel is not detached, but the distal end is sectioned and inserted into the coronary artery.

Grafts may, if necessary, be inserted into all the three major arteries, and into their larger branches. Provided left ventricular function is not severely impaired, the mortality of the operation is less than 2% in most centres. A small proportion of vein grafts close shortly after insertion, but most stay open for at least 5 years; following this, there is an increasing tendency to closure, particularly in patients with hyperlipidaemia. It has been found that antiplatelet therapy (e.g. aspirin 300 mg daily) is helpful in maintaining patency, and a lipid-lowering diet should be given to those with hyperlipidaemia.

The results of surgery are usually very satisfactory, at least for 5−10 years. Angina is abolished in at least 50% of cases, and greatly improved in a further 30−40%. As well as relieving angina, coronary artery surgery benefits the prognosis of patients with disease of the left main coronary artery, and also those who have disease of the three major vessels, together with left ventricular dysfunction, provided this is not too severe. Late deterioration may be due to graft closure, or to progression of the disease in the ungrafted vessels.

Surgery is indicated for those whose angina is not adequately relieved by full medical treatment, but it should also be considered as a measure to improve prognosis, even in the absence of severe symptoms, in the younger patient with advanced coronary disease.

Percutaneous transluminal coronary angioplasty (PTCA)

A non-elastic balloon mounted close to the tip of a specially designed catheter can be passed to the site of a coronary stenosis and inflated there. This process produces clefts in the atheromatous lesion, compression and redistribution of its contents, endothelial desquamation, and stretching of the media. In most cases, this results in a substantial increase in the arterial lumen. Initially, angioplasty was used for proximal lesions occurring in patients with disease of only one coronary artery. With greater experience and with improved apparatus, experts in the technique can now successfully dilate lesions in several arteries, even if these are relatively distal. Angioplasty should not be attempted if the left main coronary artery is involved, and it is not likely to be successful if the lesion is long or if the vessel is occluded (although recently occluded vessels may sometimes be reopened). Some 80–90% of apparently suitable stenoses can be dilated, but the procedure may be complicated by acute coronary occlusion due to dissection, spasm or thrombosis. This may require emergency coronary bypass surgery. Angioplasty has a mortality of about 1% and a risk of myocardial infarction of approximately 3%. Restenosis occurs within six months in about 25% of cases, but repeat angioplasty is usually successful.

The main indication for the procedure is angina unresponsive to medical treatment, whether this is stable or unstable. It is also used to supplement thrombolytic therapy in myocardial infarction.

Angioplasty is carried out under local anaesthesia. Patients can usually be mobilized the following day and be discharged one or two days thereafter. If the affected lesions can be dilated, symptoms are relieved, although they may return with restenosis. Because of the risks of thrombosis and coronary artery spasm after angioplasty, patients are often kept on calcium antagonists and antiplatelet agents (such as aspirin) for weeks or months after the procedure.

Unstable angina

Angina is regarded as being unstable if it has developed for the first time recently, or if pre-existing angina has worsened for no apparent reason. Several mechanisms may be involved, which include rupture of an atheromatous plaque, with or without super-imposed thrombosis, and coronary spasm. The clinical picture is very variable, ranging from relatively mild attacks of pain on exertion to recurrent attacks of severe pain at rest which are unresponsive to full medical treatment. During the episodes of pain, there are usually transient ECG changes, such as ST depression or elevation, or T wave abnormalities. The chief concern in unstable angina is the substantial risk of progression to myocardial infarction in the ensuing days or weeks. This outcome affects 10–20% of the patients, but particularly those who do not respond promptly to medical treatment.

It is difficult to be sure of the mechanisms involved in any particular case, and it is probably best to combine beta-blockers and calcium antagonists, if neither are contraindicated. Nitrates should be taken orally as necessary, and if other forms of drug therapy have failed, the addition of intravenous nitrates is often effective (see p. 150). Aspirin in a dosage of about 300 mg a day has been shown to reduce the risk of a myocardial infarction.

If a prompt response to rest and medical treatment is not achieved, it is best to proceed without delay to coronary arteriography, and then to angioplasty or coronary artery bypass surgery if these seem indicated.

Myocardial infarction

Myocardial infarcton is usually due to plaque rupture with super-imposed thrombus.

If death occurs soon after the onset of acute myocardial infarction there are sometimes no gross or microscopic changes in the myocardium, although enzyme-staining reactions and electron microscopy may reveal evidence of damage. Later, the infarction area appears pale and is surrounded by a reddish area due to hyperaemia. Microscopically, the muscle cells lose their nuclei and, subsequently, necrotic changes take place in adjacent connective tissue and blood vessel walls. Leucocytic infiltration occurs at the edges of the infarction. The removal of necrotic muscle fibres starts about the third day and continues for about 2 weeks. At the same time granulation tissue containing blood vessels and fibroblasts invades the necrotic area. Finally, the infarcted area is replaced by fibrous scar tissue over a period lasting between 2 and 8 weeks. If the infarction reaches the endocardial surface, a mural thrombus may develop. If it impinges on the pericardium, pericarditis occurs.

The location and size of a myocardial infarction depend upon the artery that is occluded and the collateral blood supply. In some cases the infarct extends from endocardium to epicardium (transmural infarction); in others, only subendocardial territory is involved. If the left anterior descending artery is occluded, the infarction affects the anterior wall of the left ventricle and may involve the septum. If the left circumflex artery is occluded, the infarction affects the lateral or posterior walls of the left ventricle. If the right coronary artery is occluded, the infarction chiefly affects the inferior (diaphragmmatic) surface of the left ventricle, but also the septum and the right ventricle. Coronary occlusion may not lead to myocardial infarction if the area supplied by the occluded vessel has a collateral supply from adjacent arteries.

The major presenting symptom is chest discomfort. This is predominantly in the sternal region, but may radiate to both sides of the chest, to the jaw, to the shoulders and to one or both arms. It is usually described as tight, pressing, heavy or constricting. Sometimes the patient may deny 'pain' and describe a discomfort, not amounting to pain, in the centre of the chest. Although it can be brief, the pain usually lasts for more than half an hour and may continue for several hours. Unlike the pain of angina, it is seldom associated with exertion and it is not relieved by rest or glyceryl trinitrate. The pain may be maximal at the onset, but often increases in intensity for a period of minutes or hours and then remains constant until it gradually recedes. Frequently, the patient gives a history of the recent onset of angina or the exacerbation of pre-existing angina in the preceding days or weeks.

In some patients, pain is overshadowed by other symptoms, such as breathlessness or syncope. Occasionally, the pain is obscured because the infarction develops during anaesthesia or at the time of a cerebrovascular accident. Rarely, infarction may be truly pain-free.

Once the pain has been controlled, the patient may remain free of symptoms and make an uninterrupted recovery. However, in a substantial proportion of cases, there develop one or more of a number of complications, of which the most important are arrhythmias, cardiogenic shock and left ventricular failure. These complications, which will be considered in detail later, are the common causes of death and are responsible for many of the abnormal physical signs which may be observed.

Physical signs

During the earliest stages of the attack, the patient is obviously distressed, and may be sweaty and cold. The general appearance improves when the pain is controlled and often, within a few hours, the patient looks well.

The pulse may be normal in volume and rate, but in severe attacks it is small and fast. Arrhythmias or bradycardia are also common.

The blood pressure usually falls progressively over a period of hours and days, reaching its minimum some time during the first week, and returning towards normal slowly over the next two or three weeks. There may be, however, a sharp fall in blood pressure at the onset of the infarction, which may progress to the severe hypotension of cardiogenic shock, or may resolve. Transient hypertension, perhaps resulting from intense pain, is sometimes observed.

The jugular venous pressure is usually normal or slightly elevated early in the course of acute myocardial infarction; it is seldom markedly elevated due to right-sided heart failure.

The apex beat, which is often difficult to feel, may be displaced outwards. Between the apex and the left sternal edge a systolic pulsation may be detectable, due to a protrusion of the infarcted anterior wall of the heart.

The first and second heart sounds are often soft. A fourth (or atrial) sound can be heard in most cases; a third heart sound is common when there is heart failure or shock.

A soft pansystolic murmur at the apex is not uncommon and is caused by mitral regurgitation either as a result of papillary muscle malfunction or secondary to dilatation of the left ventricle. Rarely, a loud systolic murmur may develop at the left sternal edge, due to a rupture of the ventricular septum, or at the apex, due to rupture of a papillary muscle. A transient pericardial rub occurs in perhaps 20% of patients, usually on the second or third day.

Pulmonary crepitations are common but of little importance unless they are widespread and numerous because of pulmonary oedema.

Most of the abnormal physical signs described disappear within a few days of the onset of infarction, except in the most severely affected patients.

A fever, seldom exceeding 38°C (101°F), usually commences within the first 24 hours and subsides in under a week. There is often a slight leucocytosis and an increase in the erythrocyte sedimentation rate. The pyrexia, leucocytosis and raised ESR represent a reaction to myocardial necrosis.

Early complications

Disturbances of rate, rhythm and conduction

These occur in 95% of patients with acute myocardial infarction.

In about half of these, they are severe enough to be of clinical importance.

Sinus tachycardia is common and is an index of severity. Sinus bradycardia frequently occurs at the onset of infarction, being sometimes part of the vasovagal syndrome. It is particularly associated with inferior myocardial infarction, but may be provoked by morphine and digitalis. It is usually benign, but can cause hypotension or encourage the development of ectopic rhythms.

The atrial tachycardias, including atrial fibrillation, which occur in about 15% of patients, may precipitate cardiac failure or shock. Atrial fibrillation is usually transient and seldom lasts for more than a few days.

Ventricular ectopic beats are almost invariable; they are usually of no consequence, but those of the R-on-T variety (Fig. 8.3) may be precursors of ventricular fibrillation.

Ventricular tachycardia is dangerous both because it can cause shock and cardiac failure and because it may progress to ventricular fibrillation.

Ventricular fibrillation is the most important single cause of death in acute myocardial infarction and occurs in 8–10% of hospitalized patients. In about half of these cases, there has been no preceding shock or cardiac failure and the ventricular fibrillation is 'primary'. In the remainder, it can be regarded as being secondary to these complications.

Heart block occurs in about 5% of patients with acute myocardial infarction. It is particularly common when the inferior surface of the heart is affected because the right coronary artery supplies both this aspect of the myocardium and the junctional tissues. First degree block (prolonged PR interval) is of little significance except as a precursor of more advanced block. Second degree block, usually of the Wenckebach type, is potentially dangerous because bradycardia may be poorly tolerated and because of the risk of progression to complete heart block and ventricular asystole. In spite of the risk, most patients tolerate

Fig. 8.3 The ventricular ectopic beat interrupting the T wave of a preceding beat. The second R-on-T beat initiates ventricular fibrillation.

these conduction defects well but need to be observed closely for the development of hypotension, cardiac failure or asystole. Normal AV conduction is almost always restored if the patient survives the acute attack.

When heart block complicates anterior infarction, it carries a very high mortality. The block results from damage to both bundle branches and is almost invariably accompanied by widespread myocardial damage. The patients usually have cardiac failure and have a bad prognosis even if their heart block is successfully treated.

Cardiogenic shock

As mentioned, the patient at the onset of infarction is often pale, distressed and hypotensive. This situation, which is often transient, may be attributed to pain and should not be described as cardiogenic shock. This term should be restricted to those patients who have the clinical picture of hypotension, with cold cyanosed extremities, sweating, and mental torpor, which lasts at least half an hour, or who deteriorate rapidly until the blood pressure can no longer be recorded. There is a low cardiac output and a peripheral resistance insufficient to compensate for this, together with oliguria, hypoxia, and acidosis. Arrhythmias and cardiac failure are frequently associated and the mortality is 80–90% irrespective of treatment. Shock is largely the result of severe myocardial damage with more than 40% of the ventricular wall being infarcted. Occasionally, the shock picture is accounted for by arrhythmias such as ventricular tachycardia or complete heart block, in which case correction of the arrhythmia may result in recovery. In a few patients, particularly those who have been receiving diuretics, hypovolaemia may be a factor. Rarely, a surgically correctable disorder, such as a ruptured papillary muscle or a ventricular septal defect may be responsible.

Left ventricular failure

This is seldom present at the onset, but develops within 48 hours in perhaps two-thirds of patients with acute myocardial infarction. It can be suspected from tachycardia, a third heart sound, widespread pulmonary crepitations and pulmonary venous congestion or oedema on the chest radiograph. Catheterization using a Swan–Ganz or similar catheter, will show a pulmonary wedge pressure in excess of 20 mmHg.

Right ventricular failure

A slight elevation of the jugular venous pressure is common in the first days after acute infarction. Infarction of the right ventricle, which is almost always associated with inferior wall infarction, may cause a high venous pressure and, rarely, the shock syndrome, even in the presence of good left ventricular function. The classical features of failure of the right side of heart — peripheral oedema and hepatomegaly — are rare and take several days to develop even in the patient with severe myocardial damage.

Pulmonary embolism and infarction

Twenty or more years ago, pulmonary embolism caused death in about 3% of all patients admitted to hospital with acute myocardial infarction. It has become relatively rare, presumably because patients are now mobilized as soon as possible. It is usually preceded by deep vein thrombosis in the legs, but this may not be clinically evident. Pulmonary embolism should be suspected when there is the sudden development of hypotension or right heart failure some days after the onset of myocardial infarction, and also when there is a pleural type of chest pain with or without haemoptysis.

Systemic arterial embolism

Embolism may occur from mural thrombi situated in the left ventricle or left atrium. Hemiplegia is the most common result, but there may be occlusion of any artery.

Cerebrovascular accidents

Cerebrovascular accidents may precede, accompany or follow acute myocardial infarction. As mentioned, cerebral embolism is one cause, but cerebral infarction may develop as a result of the fall in blood flow in those with cerebral vascular disease.

Cardiac rupture

Rupture through the wall of the left ventricle is responsible for about 10% of all deaths and particularly affects the elderly and the hypertensive. It is most likely to occur during the first few days and usually causes sudden death. Occasionally, the picture may be that of cardiac tamponade.

Rupture through the interventricular septum occurs in about one in every 200 patients with acute myocardial infarction. This produces the sudden onset of severe heart failure, accompanied by a systolic thrill and murmur at the left sternal edge. The patient deteriorates rapidly over a period of a few days; survival for more than a few weeks is unusual.

Papillary muscle rupture and malfunction

When a papillary muscle ruptures, a loud apical pansystolic murmur appears in association with the sudden development of left ventricular failure. Death usually occurs within a few hours or days. Partial rupture may produce the features of mitral regurgitation with or without left-sided heart failure.

The electrocardiogram

The ECG is virtually always transiently or permanently abnormal after acute myocardial infarction. Because the ECG diagnosis of infarction depends upon the observation of a sequence of changes with time, serial records are vital.

The characteristic abnormalities are: the appearance of abnormally large Q waves, the development of ST segment elevation and the development of T wave inversion (Fig. 8.4). Although the precise mechanisms responsible for these ECG changes are not yet determined, it is probable that the Q wave changes are the result of muscle death, that the ST abnormalities are due to muscle injury, and that the T wave abnormalities are due to ischaemia.

Dead tissue, which is unpolarized, takes no part in electrical activation, but can transmit changes in the electrical potential in other tissues. In Fig. 8.5 can be seen the effect of infarcted tissue on depolarization of the heart. With the electrode situated facing

Fig. 8.4   a, b, c, d, e and f, showing the progression of changes recorded by an electrode facing the area of infarction (upper series) and from an electrode placed distant from the infarction (lower series). Note the early development of ST elevation and broad Q wave in the record obtained from the electrode facing the infarction. Subsequently the ST segment becomes iso-electric and the T wave inverted. Finally, the T wave becomes upright, but the pathological Q wave persists. In the lower series, so-called 'reciprocal' ST depression can be seen in b and c.

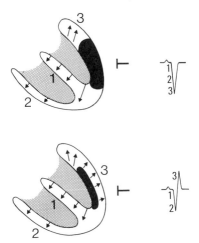

Fig. 8.5 (A) The appearances recorded from an electrode over the left ventricle in extensive left ventricular infarction. The initial vector is directed, as usual, away from the left ventricle due to depolarization of the septum, and is followed by that of depolarization of the right ventricle and non-infarcted areas of the left ventricle in a direction away from the infarction. A totally negative deflection (QS) is obtained. (B) The appearances obtained from an electrode placed over the left ventricle when the infarction is less extensive. The initial vector is, as usual, directed from left to right across the septum, and provides the first component of the Q wave. Subsequently, the right ventricle and the non-infarcted areas of the endocardium of the left ventricle are depolarized, continuing the Q wave. Finally, depolarization reaches the epicardium superficial to the infarcted area, producing a terminal R wave.

the left ventricle, depolarization commences, as usual, from the left side of the septum to the right (vector 1). Subsequently depolarization spreads to affect the right ventricle and those parts of the left ventricle away from the infarct. Vector 2 is therefore directed away from the electrode and produces a deepening of the Q wave. Finally, the muscle around the area of the infarct may become activated and produce a terminal R wave (vector 3). Sometimes, Q wave infarctions are described as 'transmural'; this is an undesirable term, as they do not necessarily involve the full thickness of the myocardium.

In the injured zone, the cells remain polarized, but the transmembrane potential is less than normal, because of loss of cellular potassium. Repolarization of the injured tissue occurs more quickly than normal and a voltage gradient develops between the normal and injured tissue. This is reflected in ST elevation over the area of injury.

The T wave abnormalities are believed to be due to changes in the direction of repolarization in ischaemic tissue.

Q waves may take several hours to develop after the onset of infarction. They usually persist indefinitely because the scar tissue which replaces the infarcted muscle is similarly uninvolved in electrical activation. Normally, Q waves in leads facing the left ventricle do not exceed 2 mm in depth or 0.03 sec in width. Q waves and QS waves are normal in aVR, and are commonly found in V1 and V2. Deep Q waves are often also seen normally in lead III. The Q wave in lead III should only be considered definitely abnormal if it exceeds 0.03 sec in duration, and if it is accompanied by Q waves in either lead II or aVF. The 'normal' Q wave in lead III usually diminishes or disappears on deep inspiration, whereas the 'pathological' Q wave persists.

ST segment elevation often commences within minutes of the onset of myocardial infarction but may be delayed for many hours. In the earliest stage, the elevated ST segment may retain the normal upward concavity, but before long it becomes convex and 'coves' downwards to the T wave. ST elevation is confined to those leads facing the infarct. In leads distant from the infarct, so-called 'reciprocal' ST depression is often seen. The ST segment usually returns to the iso-electric line within 48−72 hours. Persistent elevation suggests a ventricular aneurysm.

T wave inversion occurs slightly later than ST elevation during the course of myocardial infarction; there is a stage when this ST segment is returning towards the iso-electric line whilst the T wave is becoming inverted. Later, the ST segment becomes iso-electric and the T wave becomes symmetrically, often deeply, inverted. As healing takes place, the T wave usually becomes less inverted and eventually upright and normal, but the inversion sometimes persists.

Q waves are often absent in small myocardial infarctions, but ST and T wave changes are almost invariable. The recognition of myocardial infarction on the ECG can be difficult if there has been previous infarction which has resulted in persistent Q waves, ST elevation or T wave inversion.

Left bundle branch block may also obscure the changes of infarction, because in this disorder the septum is depolarized from right to left; this produces an initial R wave in left ventricular leads, preventing the appearance of a Q wave. The diagnosis can sometimes be made from ST and T wave changes.

The leads in which the infarct patterns are seen depend upon its location.

1   Anteroseptal infarction produces changes in one or more of the leads V1 to V4.

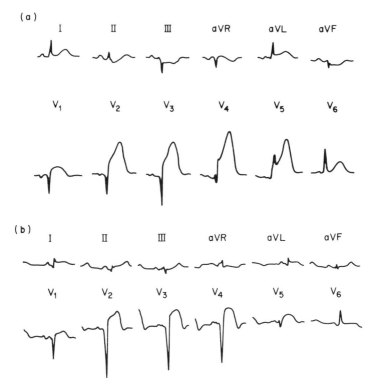

Fig. 8.6 Anterior myocardial infarction. (a) Recent infarction with ST elevation in aVL and V1 to V5; reciprocal ST depression in III and aVF. Large Q waves in V1 to V3. (b) One day later ST elevation in I, II, aVL, Q waves V1–V4. ST segments lower with change in shape V1–V5; T waves are inverted in I, aVL and V2 to V6.

2 Anterolateral infarction produces changes from V4 to V6, and lead I and aVL (Fig. 8.6).
3 Anterior infarction is indicated by more widespread changes including most of the leads from V1 to V6, as well as leads I and II and aVL.
4 Inferior (or diaphragmmatic) infarction is registered by changes in leads II, III and aVF (Fig. 8.7).
5 Strictly posterior myocardial infarction does not produce Q waves in the standard 12 leads. However, the loss of electrical activity from the posterior part of the left ventricle, leads to a tall R in V1, because the forces depolarizing the right ventricle are unopposed.

Fig. 8.7 Inferior myocardial infarction. (a) Recent infarction with ST elevation in II, III and aVF; reciprocal ST depression in I, aVL, V1 and V2. (b) Q waves have become more prominent in II, III and aVF. ST elevation less; T waves inverting.

6 Right ventricular infarction (which is almost always associated with inferior infarction) produces transient ST elevation in V4R.

Further leads may be required for infarcts in unusual sites, V7 and V8 being helpful in lateral infarcts, and leads in the second or third intercostal spaces for high anterior and lateral infarcts.

Serum enzymes (Fig. 8.8)

Certain enzymes, present in high concentration in cardiac tissue, are released by necrosis of the myocardium. Their activity in the serum, therefore, rises and falls after myocardial infarction. The amount of enzyme released roughly parallels the severity of myocardial damage.

Serum creatine phosphokinase (SCK) Creatine phosphokinase, which occurs in heart, skeletal muscle and brain, rises within

Fig. 8.8 Changes in serum enzyme activity following myocardial infarction. Serum creatine phosphokinase (SCK) increases earlier and to a relatively greater extent than SGOT and SLDH (see text).

6 hours of the onset of infarction, reaching a peak in 18 to 24 hours. It may become normal after 72 hours. Apart from myocardial infarction, abnormally high levels occur in muscle diseases, in cerebrovascular damage, after muscular exercise exercise and with intramuscular injections.

The MB isoenzyme of CK is virtually specific for cardiac muscle and is now widely used in the diagnosis of myocardial infarction.

Serum glutamic oxalo-acetic transaminase (SGOT) This enzyme, also called aspartate transaminase (ASAT), is found particularly in the heart, skeletal muscle, brain, liver and kidney. After infarction, the SGOT rises in about 12 hours and reaches its peak in 24 to 36 hours, returning to normal from the third to the fifth day.

Serum lactate dehydrogenase (SLDH) This enzyme is found in the heart, but also in red cells. It rises relatively late after infarction, reach its peak 24 to 48 hours afterwards, and may remain abnormal from 1 to 3 weeks. Unfortunately, even slight haemolysis raises its level. Isoenzymes are more specific.

Diagnostic levels for these enzymes have not been quoted as they vary considerably from one laboratory to another.

Radionuclide and echocardiographic investigations

Perfusion defects can be demonstrated using thallium-201 in most patients within the first few hours, but may disappear later.

Technetium pyrophosphate concentrates in the infarcted area producing a 'hot spot', several hours after the onset; this is not, however, a very specific or sensitive test.

Echocardiography shows loss of the normal systolic thinning of the ventricular wall in the region of the infarction.

Diagnosis of myocardial infarction

In most cases, the diagnosis is suspected from the character, location and duration of the chest pain. The persistence of the pain beyond 15 minutes, its lack of relationship to exercise and the failure of glyceryl trinitrate to relieve it usually serve to differentiate it from angina pectoris. The development of abnormal physical signs, and more particularly, the appearance of arrhythmias, shock and failure also suggest that infarction has occurred. Fever, leucocytosis and raised ESR indicate necrosis rather than ischaemia. The definitive diagnosis depends upon the recognition of the ECG changes, supported by abnormal serum enzyme levels. Infarction is virtually certain if Q waves appear during the course of the illness, or if sequential ST and T wave changes are accompanied by transient but significant elevations of serum enzyme levels. Difficulties in diagnosis arise when the ECG or enzyme level changes are equivocal, or if serial ECG records or enzyme estimations are not made at appropriate times.

It is exceedingly difficult to differentiate some cases of acute myocardial infarction from unstable angina ('acute coronary insufficiency'). This is an ill-defined syndrome, in which there are attacks of ischaemic cardiac pain which are more prolonged and less related to exertion than are those of typical effort-induced angina pectoris, but in which the ECG changes do not indicate infarction, although persisting ST depression may suggest continuing ischaemia. By definition, enzyme changes are absent, and there is no fever, leucocytosis or rise in ESR.

The differentiation of myocardial infarction from massive pulmonary embolism may be difficult, but the chest pain of myocardial infarction is usually more severe and the breathlessness less marked. In pulmonary embolism, the ECG may be normal, or there may be characteristic abnormalities (see p. 286) and although there may be changes in SLDH and SGOT, SCK (and, more specifically MB−CK) is usually not raised. In cases of doubt, pulmonary angiography or radio-isotope scanning of the chest are helpful. Pulmonary infarction can be recognized by the location and pleural character of the pain and the radiographic appearances.

Acute pericarditis may produce symptoms and signs very similar to those of an acute myocardial infarction (see p. 179). In many cases, the pericarditis is preceded by an upper respiratory infection and cough. The chest pain is more aching or stabbing in character, and is made worse by deep inspiration, movement or lying flat. Pyrexia often precedes the pain, whereas the temperature rise of myocardial infarction usually takes at least 12 hours to develop. Although pericarditis may produce ST elevation and T wave inversion, the ST elevation is concave upwards and is widespread rather than focal. Abnormal Q waves do not occur and enzyme changes occur only if there is accompanying myocarditis.

Dissecting aneurysm can cause severe central chest pain similar to that of acute myocardial infarction (see p. 279). The pain usually has a tearing quality, and tends to move into the upper dorsal spinal region and into the abdomen. The ECG does not show the changes of myocardial infarction, except when the dissection involves the origin of a coronary artery. In cases of doubt, the arterial pulses should be repeatedly checked, and a chest radiograph obtained to determine whether there is mediastinal widening. Echocardiography and computed tomography are of diagnostic value.

Prognosis

In about one-quarter of all episodes of acute myocardial infarction, death occurs suddenly within minutes of the onset. Such cases are seldom seen by a physician. The remainder of this discussion is concerned with the prognosis of those who survive this immediate period.

The overall mortality, excluding the very early deaths, is approximately 15−30%. The risk of death depends upon many factors, including the age of the patient, the previous history of coronary disease and the presence of other diseases, as well as the extent of the infarction.

The mortality of the acute attack rises sharply with age. Death occurs in about 10−20% in those under 50 years of age, 20% in those under 60, near 30% in those over 60, and 40−50% in the elderly. Mortality is higher in women than in men, but this is largely accounted for by the fact that infarction occurs relatively uncommonly in the younger female. The mortality is greater in recurrent compared with first infarction, particularly when there has been preceding cardiac failure.

The risk of dying is highest in the first few hours and decreases rapidly thereafter. Some 60% or more of all deaths within 4 weeks occur within the first 2 days. During this time, prognostication is difficult because dangerous arrhythmias may develop unpredictably. At the end of 48 hours, the assessment of the prognosis for the rest of the 4-week period is reasonably accurate if the blood pressure, the signs of cardiac failure and the occurrence of serious arrhythmias are taken into account. Cardiogenic shock carries a mortality of 80–90%. Persistent tachycardia, continuing gallop rhythm and the development of right-sided heart failure are unfavourable features. Ventricular tachycardia, bundle branch block and atrial fibrillation are associated with a high mortality. Death may occur unexpectedly, late in the course of acute myocardial infarction, from further myocardial infarction, rupture and pulmonary embolism.

The ECG provides little information of prognostic value, except that, in general, patients with Q waves do worse than those without. High serum enzyme levels, indicating extensive necrosis, are unfavourable.

In those patients who have survived acute myocardial infarction, the outlook is better than is often appreciated. The prognosis is best in those who are free of hypertension, angina and cardiac failure. Overall, between 80 and 90% of patients survive at least one year, approximately 75% survive 5 years, 50% 10 years and 25% 20 years. The risk of further infarction and sudden death persists but diminishes as time elapses.

Many patients can go back to work within 2 months; nearly all should have returned within 3 months. Failure to do so should call for a careful reappraisal of physical, psychological and social factors.

Treatment

Usually, the most urgent measure is the relief of pain. When this is severe, opiates such as intravenous morphine sulphate (10 mg) or diamorphine (5 mg) are required and may have to be repeated. Unfortunately, these drugs may produce bradycardia, hypotension and respiratory depression, and it is advisable to combine them with atropine 0.5 mg, if there is bradycardia, or a drug such as perchlorperazine if there is not. The inhalation of nitrous oxide 50% and oxygen 50% is useful if other analgesic measures are unavailable or have failed.

General management

In recent years, it has become usual to admit all those with suspected myocardial infarction to hospital. The main purpose of this is to ensure that intensive care is available in the first few unpredictable hours. There is, however, a case for leaving at home those patients whose circumstances are good if the clinical state is satisfactory several hours after the onset, particularly if they are elderly or live a long distance from the nearest coronary care unit.

The patient must be confined to bed immediately, but the degree of restriction depends upon the severity of the infarction. If this has been mild and there is no evidence of cardiogenic shock or cardiac failure, the patient should be allowed to feed himself, use a commode and gently exercise his legs from the outset. Within 1–2 days it may be possible for him to sit out of bed. The mildest cases may be permitted to walk a few steps shortly after this and may be ready for discharge from hospital after 5–10 days, at which time they should be able to walk up a few stairs. The patient with a small infarction should have returned to reasonably normal activity within a period of 1–2 months and can then resume light work. If, however, during the first days there is evidence of a severe infarction, or if there have been dangerous arrhythmias, the patient requires strict bed rest which may have to be continued until the complication has been brought satisfactorily under control. The subsequent progress of patients with more severe infarction is necessarily slow, but in most cases discharge from hospital is possible in 3–4 weeks.

The programme of rest and rehabilitation depends upon the severity of the cardiac disability. Increase in activity should be gradual but progressive. One of the greatest dangers is the development of an unwarranted anxiety. This can be prevented by encouragement and explanation from the onset of the illness, and the patient must understand that he has a good chance of recovery, and of return to near normal activity. At every stage an optimistic attitude should prevail, and it should be apparent that the physician expects his patient to recover. Intensive care units should reduce anxiety; the patient should initially be reassured by the constant observation and the excellence of the medical and nursing care. Subsequently, when the most acute stage is over, he should be encouraged that close supervision is no longer necessary. Finally, on discharge from hospital it should be made clear that the patient is expected to return to a nearly normal life within 8 weeks or so.

Patients usually have little appetite initially; those who are overweight should be given a low calorie diet.

Intensive care

For the first few days after the onset of acute myocardial infarction, the risk of sudden and unexpected death is high. This is largely due to arrhythmias, which can be treated or prevented by appropriate therapy. Because of the close observation required at this time, and the need to have appropriate equipment and skills immediately available, intensive care of a special kind is required.

Intensive care of patients with myocardial infarction has three essential components: the concentration of patients at maximal risk in special areas, their care by nurses and doctors with specialized training, and apparatus for monitoring the ECG and for resuscitation.

Pre-hospital care

The early phase of those with heart attacks is critical; resuscitation from cardiac arrest is most often required at this time and interventions to limit infarct size should be administered as soon as possible. It is, therefore, of great importance that resuscitation and other relevant facilities should be available outside hospital. Depending upon local circumstances, these can be provided by suitably trained and equipped doctors or by paramedical personnel (such as ambulance men).

Anticoagulant therapy

Anticoagulants may be used for several different purposes in myocardial infarction.

1 To prevent the progression or recurrence of thrombosis in the coronary arteries. Their effectiveness in this regard remains to be established.
2 To prevent or treat deep vein thrombosis and pulmonary embolism. Early mobilization has made these complications less common than they used to be; however, they remain a substantial risk in those with large infarctions, particularly if complicated by heart failure.
3 To prevent or treat thrombo-embolism from the left side of the heart; this complication is most likely to occur in those with large anterior infarctions, atrial fibrillation or ventricular aneurysms.

There is little agreement amongst cardiologists about the indications for anticoagulant therapy in myocardial infarction but few would question their value in the high-risk patients mentioned above.

Low-dose heparin (e.g. 5000 units 8-hourly subcutaneously) can prevent the development of deep vein thrombosis, but is inadequate once thrombosis has occurred. Intravenous heparin is then required. Preferably this should be given continuously in a dosage which maintains the partial thromboplastin time (PTT) between 1.5 and 2 times the pre-heparin control value. Alternatively, if PTT monitoring is not available, heparin may be given intravenously, 5000 units every 4 hours.

In general, heparin should be administered for at least 5–7 days, even if warfarin is being given concurrently. The only common unwanted effect is haemorrhage, which can be rapidly counteracted by protamine sulphate. Rarely, there may be thrombocytopenia or anaphylaxis.

When longer-term treatment is needed, oral anticoagulant drugs should be given. Warfarin is the most commonly used of the drugs. It may be administered initially as 10 mg daily for 3 days, and the dosage subsequently adjusted depending upon the prothrombin ratio. Prothrombin ratios should now be expressed in terms of the International Normalized Ratio (INR) which is essentially the same as the British Corrected Ratio (BCR). This should be kept between 2.0 and 4.5, the higher end of the range being aimed for in higher risk patients (e.g. those with recurrent thrombosis and pulmonary embolism).

If warfarin therapy is undertaken, the possibility of interactions with other drugs must be borne in mind. Antagonists include barbiturates and cholestyramine; potentiators include amiodarone, aspirin, cimetidine and phenylbutazone.

Bleeding is quite common with warfarin. If it is mild, all that is required is an adjustment in dosage. Severe bleeding calls for the use of vitamin K, or concentrated factor replacement (the former should not be used if clotting would be particularly hazardous, e.g. in the presence of a prosthetic valve).

There is some evidence that anticoagulant therapy prevents further myocardial infarction. Long-term treatment should be undertaken only if the patient is known to be cooperative, if the doctor is prepared to supervise the patient and his anticoagulant control carefully, and if a reliable laboratory is available.

Management of rhythm and conduction disorders

Ventricular fibrillation is best treated by immediate dc shock of 200 joules, without prior closed-chest cardiac massage or artificial ventilation. If this is given quickly enough, sinus rhythm, blood pressure and consciousness are nearly always restored. If a defibrillator is not immediately available, external resuscitation must be initiated and continued until the apparatus arrives. The prognosis of patients with ventricular fibrillation depends upon their condition prior to the onset of this arrhythmia. If free of shock or cardiac failure, and if dc shock is immediately available, 90% have a chance of being alive 1 month later. If either of these complications has been present, the chances are approximately 25%.

Ventricular fibrillation is frequently preceded by other ventricular arrhythmias, notably ventricular tachycardia and ventricular ectopic beats of the R-on-T variety. When these arrhythmias appear, lignocaine should be given (p. 83). An alternative drug is procainamide, which may be given intravenously under electro-cardiographic and blood pressure control at 50 mg per minute until the arrhythmia is suppressed. Other antiarrhythmic drugs including disopyramide and mexiletine may also be of value.

Atrial flutter and fibrillation, should be treated with digitalis glycosides if the ventricular rate is high. Digoxin or ouabain may be given in a dosage of 0.5 mg intravenously (if digitalis has not been administered during the preceding week). Subsequently, digoxin may be given orally. If the heart rate is not brought under control quickly, sinus rhythm should be restored by syn-chronized dc shock. Supraventricular tachycardias may be treated similarly, if carotid sinus pressure is ineffective.

Asystole responds poorly to therapy, but an attempt should be made to restore electrical activity by a blow on the chest, closed-chest cardiac resuscitation or electrical pacemaking. First-degree heart block requires no treatment but should be closely observed for progression. Bradycardia due to more advanced block is common during the early hours and can often be corrected by atropine. If the bradycardia is persistent, especially if associated with hypotension, an endocardial electrode should be placed in the right ventricle and attached to an external pacemaker. If pacemaking facilities are not available, a slow intravenous in-fusion of isoprenaline may be given (1 to 5 mg in 500 ml 5% laevulose) taking care to avoid sinus tachycardia and ventricular arrhythmias.

Sinus bradycardia is usually relatively harmless, but if it is producing hypotension or is associated with ventricular ectopic activity, atropine in a dosage of 0.3 mg should be given intra-venously, and repeated if necessary, taking care not to induce tachycardia.

Management of cardiac failure and shock

More than 60% of patients with myocardial infarction have some evidence of cardiac failure, as shown by chest radiography, but in many of these it is transient and asymptomatic and requires no treatment. If, on the other hand, there is dyspnoea, or pul-monary oedema, or a gallop rhythm, or prolonged or profound hypotension, the prognosis is poor. In such cases, every effort must be made to determine the factors that have led to cardiac failure, to evaluate carefully the haemodynamic status, and to institute appropriate treatment.

The most important single factor is the extent of myocardial damage sustained in the current and previous myocardial infarc-tions. Others, which are more amenable to correction, are:

1 Arrhythmias and conduction disorders;
2 Hypovolaemia, sometimes the consequence of previous treatment with diuretics, antihypertensives and pressor drugs;
3 Right ventricular infarction, which may produce a clinical picture
   of high venous pressure, with low systemic arterial and pulmonary wedge pressures;
4 Previous treatment with beta-adrenoceptor drugs;
5 Lesions such as a ventricular septal defect which are surgically
   correctable.

If possible patients with cardiac failure or shock should be
categorized using the data available from intravascular monitoring with a Swan–Ganz catheter. Three major groups can be
identified.

1 Those with 'backward' failure, i.e. with a cardiac index >2.2 l
   min^{-1} m^{-2} and pulmonary wedge pressure >18 mmHg. Such
   patients maintain their blood pressure but have pulmonary
   oedema. Appropriate treatment includes diuretics and vasodilators (e.g. nitrates) and, possibly, digitalis.
2 Those with 'forward' failure, i.e. with a cardiac index <2.2 l
   min^{-1} m^{-2} and pulmonary artery wedge pressure <12 mmHg.
   Such patients usually respond to the administration of plasma
   expanders.
3 Those with both pulmonary oedema and hypotension (cardiac
   output <2.2 l min^{-1} m^{-2} and pulmonary artery wedge pressure
   >18 mmHg). The mortality in this group is very high, but an
   attempt should be made to improve left ventricular function
   by reducing afterload (with vasodilators) and increasing contractility with inotropic drugs. (See also Chapter 2).

It is important neither to overload the circulation nor to lower
the filling pressure of the left ventricle excessively. One should
aim to keep the pulmonary artery wedge pressure between 15
and 20 mmHg.

The intra-aortic balloon pump (see p. 322) can cause considerable temporary clinical improvement, but this is not maintained
unless some major factor can be corrected, e.g. the surgical
closure of a ventricular septal defect.

Surgical treatment

Surgery has little part to play in the acute phase of myocardial
infarction except for the few patients who develop a ventricular
septal defect; these require early repair. Other surgically treatable complications include ventricular aneurysm and papillary
muscle rupture; operation is preferably delayed for 6 weeks. If
a patient develops these lesions at a time when corrective

surgery would be inappropriate, an intra-aortic balloon pump
may be invaluable in supporting the circulation for 1–2 weeks.

Late complications in acute myocardial infarction

The major risks of infarction occur during the first few days, but
complications can arise over a period of several weeks. These
include further infarction, the recurrence of serious arrhythmias,
and sudden death. Amongst other complications are ventricular
aneurysm formation, the post-myocardial infarction syndrome
and the shoulder–hand syndrome.

Ventricular aneurysm formation occurs in 10–20% of patients.
Although the prognosis in those affected is reasonably good, the
area of paradoxically moving non-contractile myocardium leads to
extra work for the remaining heart muscle. In some cases this
contributes to cardiac failure, and there is also a risk of embolism
from mural thrombi. The presence of an aneurysm is suggested by
a systolic pulsation of the anterior chest wall lasting more than 3
weeks after the infarction. Other evidence includes persistent QS
waves and ST elevation in the affected leads, an abnormal rounded
protrusion from the left ventricular wall on the chest radiograph
(Fig. 8.9), and paradoxical movement on fluoroscopy. These features
are not always present. The aneurysm may be demonstrated by
echocardiography, radionuclide studies and left ventriculography.

The *post-myocardial infarction syndrome* ('Dressler's') is characterized by pericardial pain, accompanied by pericardial rub, fever,
pleurisy and a leucocytosis. It may occur at any time in the weeks
or months after an infarction, and has been attributed to an
immune reaction to necrotic cardiac muscle.

The *shoulder-hand syndrome* afflicts a small percentage of patients
some weeks after infarction, particularly if there has been prolonged immobilization. There is a limitation of movement of the
shoulder joint, associated with tenderness and pain, and there
may be swelling of the hands and fingers with nodules on the
palms.

Rehabilitation and secondary prevention after myocardial infarction

Although many patients make an initially satisfactory recovery
following myocardial infarction, the longer term outcome in terms
of return to normal activities, including work, and freedom from
recurrences is often disappointing.

Failure to return to a normal life may be due to physical factors,
but is often the result of anxiety or inadequate instruction and

Fig. 8.9 Rounded protrusion on the left border of the heart in ventricular aneurysm.

rehabilitation. It is helpful if, in the milder case, a limited exercise tolerance test is carried out 1 or 2 weeks after the infarction in which the patient exercises until a heart rate of 120 or 130 is achieved. If such a heart rate can be attained without cardiac symptoms or ST depression on the ECG, the outlook is very good and the patient can be encouraged to return quickly to a near-normal life. For example, 4—8 weeks after discharge, the individual should be walking out of doors and up hills and stairs, be able to return to car driving and sexual activity, and should go back to work, provided this is not physically strenuous, shortly thereafter. Patients whose exercise tolerance is less good require slower convalescence and more careful observation. If angina pectoris or dyspnoea are major symptoms, careful attention to drug therapy and consideration for surgery is necessary.

The long-term use of beta-adrenoceptor blocking drugs after myocardial infarction reduces mortality in the succeeding years. They appear to be particularly beneficial in those whose acute episode was complicated by serious arrhythmias or cardiac failure; it is recommended that they are given on a long-term basis to such patients, unless there are contraindications (such as uncontrolled heart failure). They are also indicated for hypertension and angina pectoris.

The stopping of smoking and the control of hypertension and diabetes are all important in the survivor of myocardial infarction.

Drugs, such as mexiletine, disopyramide and amiodarone, are indicated for patients with recurrent serious ventricular arrhythmias, but their effectiveness and safety in the individual patient must be established.

Cardiac failure

In a small proportion of patients with ischaemic heart disease, the initial manifestation is cardiac failure, which may be either left-sided or right-sided. The clinical picture is that of a dilated cardiomyopathy. The ECG may or may not provide conclusive evidence of coronary disease. Echocardiography and radionuclide imaging usually demonstrate regional, as opposed to global, dysfunction and may show an aneurysm. Except in the latter case, surgery (other than transplantation) is not indicated.

Sudden death

Death often occurs suddenly in patients with coronary atherosclerosis. In about 50% of cases, the subject is known to have suffered from angina pectoris, or to have had a previous myocardial infarction. In a proportion of the remainder, it is possible to obtain a history from relatives that an attack of pain had preceded the fatal event, but in quite a substantial number death occurs without any warning whatsoever.

When sudden death occurs under circumstances in which the patient is observed, ventricular fibrillation is nearly always its cause. Occasionally ventricular asystole is responsible; in the elderly ventricular rupture is not uncommon.

Prompt defibrillation is frequently effective in restoring life in those who appear to die suddenly. As most cases occur outside hospital, success depends upon there being someone trained in cardiopulmonary resuscitation at hand and the ready availability of personnel equipped with the necessary apparatus. Those who have been successfully resuscitated require careful observation and evaluation because of the risk of 'recurrent sudden death'. They should be investigated for arrhythmias by dynamic electrocardiography (Holter monitoring) and, probably, by electrophysiological testing to determine whether antiarrhythmic therapy is needed and, if so, which drug is the most suitable.

Further reading

Hjemdahl-Monsen, C.E., Lewis, H.D., Cairns J., Chesebro, J.H. & Fuster, V. (1986) Role of antithrombotic therapy in unstable angina, myocardial infarction, and sudden death. *Journal of the American College of Cardiology* 8: 67B–75B.

Julian, D.G. (Ed.) (1985) *Angina Pectoris*, 2nd edn. Edinburgh: Churchill Livingstone.

Kent, K.M. (1987) Coronary angioplasty. *New England Journal of Medicine* 316: 1148.

Levy, R.I. (1985) Cholesterol and cardiovascular disease. *Circulation 72:* 686.

Norris, R.M. (1982) *Myocardial Infarction.* Edinburgh: Churchill Livingstone.

Oliver, M.F. (1986) Prevention of coronary heart disease. *Circulation 73:* 1.

Parker, J.O. (1987) Nitrate therapy in stable angina pectoris. *New England Journal of Medicine 316:* 1635.

Wenger, N.K. (1986) Rehabilitation of the coronary patient. *Progress in Cardiovascular Diseases. 29:* 181.

Wheatley, D.J. (Ed.) (1986) *Surgery of Coronary Artery Disease.* London: Chapman and Hall.

Diseases of the Pericardium, Myocardium and Endocardium

The pericardium

The pericardium has several functions: it helps to fix the heart and prevent excessive movement, it acts as a barrier against the spread of infection and malignancy from adjacent organs, and it reduces friction between the heart and its neighbouring tissues. It also limits acute cardiac dilatation and plays a part in the distribution and equalization of hydrostatic forces on the heart, being responsible for 'diastolic coupling', such that the diastolic pressures in the two ventricles are closely correlated when the pericardium is intact, but not when it is absent.

Pericardial disease, which may be acute or chronic, is usually associated either with a generalized disorder or with pulmonary disease.

Pathology

Pericarditis may be fibrinous, purulent or constrictive. In acute fibrinous pericarditis, the serous pericardium is inflamed and covered with an adherent layer of fibrin. There may be accompanying effusion. In purulent pericarditis, there is usually a thick fibrinous exudate, containing polymorphonuclear cells and organisms. In pericardial constriction, the pericardium is a dense mass of fibrous tissue which is often heavily calcified. Sometimes a mixed picture of effusion and constriction is seen ('effusive—constrictive pericarditis').

Acute pericarditis

Aetiology

1 Infective; viral, pyrogenic, fungal, parasitic, tuberculous
2 Connective tissue disorders: rheumatic fever (p. 196), rheumatoid arthritis (p. 306), systemic lupus erythematosus (p. 307), polyarteritis (p. 307), scleroderma (p. 307) and sarcoid.

3 Allergic and autoimmune reactions, including the postcardiotomy (p. 216) and post-myocardial infarction syndromes (p. 174).
4 Neoplastic invasion, particularly from carcinoma of the lung.
5 Metabolic and endocrine: uraemia and gout.
6 Myocardial infarction.
7 Trauma.
8 Idiopathic.
9 After cardiac surgery.
10 Drug induced: daunorubicin, hydralazine, isoniazid, methysergide, penicillin, procainamide.

'Idiopathic' pericarditis is common but is probably, in most instances, due either to a viral infection or to allergy or autoimmunity. The viruses most frequently identified have been of the Coxsackie B group, but influenza, measles, mumps and chickenpox may also be responsible. Purulent pericarditis usually results from the spread of infection from adjacent lung.

Tuberculous pericarditis is preceded by infection in contiguous mediastinal lymph nodes.

Clinical features and diagnosis

Chest pain is the commonest symptom but is not invariable. Its distribution simulates that of acute myocardial infarction, being central and sometimes radiating to the shoulder and upper arm. The pain may be most severe in the xiphisternal or epigastric regions. It is often sharp and severe, but may be aching or oppressive. Unlike ischaemic cardiac pain, it is accentuated by inspiration, by movement and by lying flat.

The most definitive sign of pericarditis is a pericardial rub, although this is not always present. A to-and-fro scratchy or grating noise may be heard in systole, mid-diastole and presystole, or in only one of these phases. It is often localized to a small area but varies in position from time to time. It is usually accentuated if the patient leans forward, with the breath held in expiration, but is sometimes heard better towards the end of inspiration. Although the rub may disappear with the development of the pericardial effusion, it does not necessarily do so. Other signs may include those of pericardial effusion and, occasionally, of pericardial tamponade.

In the early stages, the ECG usually shows widespread ST elevation with the ST segment concave upwards (Fig. 9.1). After a few days the ST segment returns to the iso-electric line and the T wave becomes inverted. The ECG may simulate that of myocardial infarction, but Q waves are not seen and the ST segment elevation is of a different configuration.

180 *Cardiology*

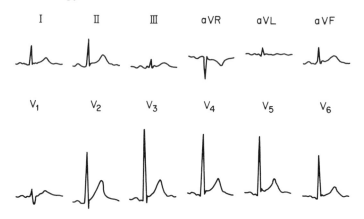

Fig. 9.1 ECG appearances in acute pericarditis. Notice widespread ST elevation, with preservation of the normal upward concavity of the ST segment.

The chest radiograph is not helpful unless there is a large pericardial effusion or there is concomitant pulmonary or pleural disease. Echocardiography is valuable in the detection of pericardial effusion.

Acute pericarditis is most likely to be confused with acute myocardial infarction, spontaneous pneumothorax and pleurisy. In differentiating it from acute myocardial infarction, the following points are of importance: (1) the character of the pain, the absence of pre-existing angina, and the history of an upper respiratory infection or of pyrexia preceding the onset of chest pain, (2) the absence of Q waves and of the characteristic infarction type of ST elevation on the ECG, and (3) the absence of serum enzyme changes. In spontaneous pneumothorax, the diagnosis can usually be made without difficulty by the detection of hyper-resonance and absent breath sounds over the affected lung or by the radiological demonstration of air in the pleural space. There is sometimes a coexistent pneumo-mediastinum which can cause a crunching or crackling sound with each heart beat. Pleurisy can be distinguished by the location and character of the pain, the presence of a pleural rub and, sometimes, by the clinical and radiological evidence of pleural effusion. Pleurisy and pericarditis commonly coexist.

Aetiological diagnosis

Viral pericarditis should be suspected if there is a history of an upper respiratory infection and fever preceding the chest pain, and can be confirmed by the demonstration of changing titres of viral antibodies in the blood, or the culture of viruses from the stools. Tuberculous pericarditis may be difficult to diagnose, because there is often no evidence of either pulmonary or miliary infection. Usually, however, there is a history of malaise and weight loss for some weeks prior to the pericarditis. Tuberculosis is unlikely if tuberculin skin tests are negative. If necessary the diagnosis may be confirmed by pericardial aspiration or biopsy. In pericarditis due to staphylococci, streptococci or pneumococci, there is usually infection in the lung or elsewhere in the body. In rheumatic fever, there is accompanying evidence of the rheumatic process as well of myocarditis and endocarditis. In pericarditis due to hypersensitivity or autoimmunity, there is no preceding respiratory infection but there is often a history of similar episodes in the past.

Treatment

This consists of the symptomatic relief of pain by salicylates (600 mg orally every 3—4 hours) or indomethacin (25—75 mg orally four times daily), the removal of fluid when this is causing pericardial tamponade, and the treatment of the underlying cause when this is possible. No specific therapy is usually necessary for viral or allergic pericarditis, although corticosteroids may be used to abbreviate their course if this is protracted. Tuberculous pericarditis requires prolonged treatment with antituberculous drugs and corticosteroids. Pericardial resection may be necessary even during the acute phase if pericardial constriction develops. Bacterial pericarditis should be treated with the appropriate antibiotics; surgical removal of pericardial pus may be necessary.

Pericardial effusion

Pericardial effusion may result from transudation (in cardiac failure), exudation of serous fluid or pus (in pericarditis) or blood (from trauma or malignant disease). It is also a feature of myxoedema. The hydropericardium of cardiac failure causes few if any symptoms, although it may cause compression of the lungs and reduce the vital capacity. Pericardial effusion due to other causes may produce pain and pericardial tamponade.

Large effusions may be detected by percussion. With the patient lying flat, increased dullness may be noted in the second left interspace, as well as in the fourth and fifth right interspaces, and to the left of the apex beat.

Auscultation may reveal pericardial friction and heart sounds which are often, but not always, soft.

The chest radiograph is valuable in diagnosis, particularly if several films are taken over a period of days — a sudden increase in the cardiothoracic ratio being very suggestive of pericardial effusion. When there is a considerable effusion, the cardiac silhouette is enlarged and the normal demarcation between the chambers is obliterated (Fig. 9.2). The heart shadow takes on a pear or waterbottle shape, and on fluoroscopy little pulsation can be observed. Similar abnormalities may be seen in some cases of cardiac failure, but the presence of a very large heart shadow in the absence of pulmonary vascular congestion makes the diagnosis of pericardial effusion likely. Pericardial effusion produces low-voltage ECG complexes which may vary considerably in amplitude from cycle to cycle, sometimes alternating in height ('electrical alternans').

Echocardiography has proved to be a useful diagnostic method. When fluid separates the contracting and relaxing posterior wall of the heart from the stationary posterior pericardium, an echo-free space is produced (Fig. 9.3). Similarly, the anterior wall of the heart is separated from the chest wall.

The diagnosis may be most certainly established by pericardial aspiration, but this is best avoided because of its potential danger. Fortunately, echocardiography can establish the diagnosis in most cases but paracentesis may be required for diagnostic purposes, e.g. to identify a causative organism. No specific treatment is required for a pericardial effusion unless there is tamponade.

Pericardial tamponade

The pericardium does not normally impede ventricular distension during diastole. An accumulation of pericardial fluid, or pericardial fibrosis or calcification may prevent adequate filling. This may develop acutely, as when the pericardium fills with fluid, or slowly, as in chronic pericardial constriction. Probably the commonest causes are neoplasm and idiopathic or viral pericarditis, but it may develop in such conditions as uraemia, myocardial infarction, and after a traumatic cardiac catheterization, cardiac surgery and chest injury.

Fig. 9.2 Radiographic appearances in pericardial effusion.

Fig. 9.3 Cross-sectional echocardiogram in the long axis parasternal view of a patient with a large pericardial effusion. An echo-free space is seen behind the posterior left ventricular wall. No anterior effusion is seen. LV = left ventricle. MV = mitral valve. E = pericardial effusion. The arrows point to a thickened aortic valve and a calcified mitral valve.

The inability of the ventricles to fill during diastole leads to raised diastolic pressures in right and left ventricles, an increase in systemic and pulmonary venous pressures, and a fall in cardiac output and in systemic blood pressure. There is a compensatory sinus tachycardia and the pulse is small and often of the paradoxical type. If the cardiac compression is acute and severe the picture is one of shock, whose cause may not be obvious. The recognition of raised venous pressure is of crucial importance. The echocardiogram is particularly valuable in diagnosis.

Tamponade can be rapidly fatal; relief by paracentesis or surgery is urgent.

Pericardial constriction ('constrictive pericarditis')

Constriction of the heart by a fibrosed or calcified pericardium is relatively uncommon. In most patients, no identifiable cause can be found, although in some communities a tuberculous infection is responsible for the majority of cases. Constriction can also be a late complication of other types of infection, neoplastic invasion and intrapericardial haemorrhage.

Adequate filling of the ventricles during diastole is prevented by thick, fibrous and, often, calcified pericardium. Although extension of the disease process may affect the superficial areas of the myocardium, the rest of the heart is usually normal.

The inability of the ventricles to distend during diastole leads to an increase in diastolic pressure and to a consequent rise in pressure in the left and right atria and in both pulmonary and systemic veins. The stroke volume is low and there is a compensatory tachycardia.

The onset may be subacute or chronic. Symptoms resemble those of right-sided cardiac failure. The presenting complaint is often that of abdominal swelling due to ascites, but dyspnoea and ankle swelling are also common.

The pulse is of small volume and may exhibit paradox. Sinus tachycardia is usually present, but atrial fibrillation develops in the advanced case. The neck veins are grossly engorged and show two characteristic features: a rapid 'y' descent and an increase in pressure on inspiration. The first and second heart sounds are soft, and there is nearly always an early diastolic sound heard best at the lower end of the sternum. This is an unusually early third heart sound associated with rapid but abbreviated ventricular filling.

The liver is enlarged and often tender, although it may be difficult to feel because of gross ascites. In contrast with the severity of the ascites, peripheral oedema is comparatively slight.

One of the most characteristic features of pericardial constriction is the shell-like rim of calcified pericardium, which is particularly well seen in lateral radiographs of the heart (Fig. 9.4). However, calcification is not invariable, nor does its presence necessarily imply constriction. The heart is usually small or of normal size, but is occasionally large. Reduced cardiac pulsation is observed on fluoroscopy. The ECG is not diagnostic, but usually shows low-voltage QRS complexes associated with flattened or slightly inverted T waves. If atrial fibrillation is not present, the P waves are often broad and bifid.

Cardiac catheterization reveals raised left ventricular diastolic, left atrial, pulmonary arterial, right ventricular diastolic and right atrial pressures. In the right ventricular pressure pulse, there is an early diastolic dip followed by a plateau (Fig. 9.5). This appearance is not specific to pericardial constriction and may be seen in cardiomyopathy.

Pericardial constriction is suggested by a small and paradoxical pulse, a high venous pressure, a quiet heart with an early third heart sound and pericardial calcification, although not all these features are necessarily present. An important clue to the diagnosis is the combination of advanced right-sided failure with a normal-sized heart.

Fig. 9.4 Calcification of the pericardium, outlining the ventricles, in the lateral view.

Fig. 9.5 Characteristic right ventricular pressure pulse in pericardial constriction. Note early diastolic dip, followed by a plateau.

Pericardial constriction is most likely to be confused with cirrhosis of the liver, but the characteristic arterial and venous pulses in pericardial constriction should permit differentiation. In other forms of right-sided heart failure, cardiac valve lesions or pulmonary disease are usually evident. Differentiation of pericardial constriction from cardiomyopathy may be difficult or impossible without thoracotomy if there is no pericardial calcification and no evidence of concomitant disease elsewhere. However, in most cases of cardiomyopathy, even of the so-called restrictive type, there is cardiac enlargement.

The medical treatment of the failure associated with pericardial constriction is seldom successful, although some improvement may follow the use of diuretics. Digoxin is of value only if atrial fibrillation supervenes.

The only effective treatment is surgical removal of the thickened pericardium. However, pericardial constriction sometimes occurs during the acute or subacute phase of tuberculous pericarditis, and preliminary treatment should then be undertaken with antituberculous drugs and corticosteroids.

Progress following pericardiectomy is usually satisfactory but may not be so if there has been extensive myocardial involvement or severe liver damage.

Pericardial paracentesis

Fluid may have to be removed from the pericardium either for diagnostic purposes or to relieve tamponade. It is a potentially dangerous procedure and should be undertaken only if essential. The patient should be sitting nearly upright, with his back supported. The needle may be inserted in the angle between the left costal margin and the xiphisternum and advanced sharply upwards. If the aspiration is being carried out for diagnostic purposes only, a 20-gauge needle attached to a plastic 3-way tap and a 10 ml syringe may be used, but for aspiration of larger quantities or of blood or pus, an 18- or 16-gauge needle some 10 cm long should be used. The site of insertion should be anaesthetized with 2% lignocaine. The ECG should be monitored during the procedure. If possible, this should be done using the needle as an electrode; a sterile insulated wire with a clip at each end is attached both to the needle and to the V lead terminal. If the atrium is entered, a large P wave is seen. ST segment elevation is observed if the needle is in contact with a ventricle. The needle should be advanced slowly while gentle suction is applied. A sudden 'give' will usually be felt when the pericardial space is entered. If blood is withdrawn, it should be observed for clotting to determine whether the specimen has been obtained from a cardiac chamber. Fluid from a haemopericardium will not clot.

Myocardial disease

The myocardium is involved in most types of heart disease. The terms *myocarditis* and *cardiomyopathy* are reserved for those relatively uncommon types of myocardial disease which cannot be attributed to coronary atherosclerosis, congenital or valvar heart disease, thyrotoxicosis or hypertension.

Myocarditis is used to describe inflammatory disorders of the myocardium due to infection and toxins. Cardiomyopathy is used for chronic disorders of heart muscle; the term may be restricted to those disorders whose cause is unknown, and the term 'specific heart muscle disease' for those of identified aetiology.

Myocarditis

Myocarditis usually forms part of a generalized infection (particularly viral) but can also be due to physical and chemical agents (see Table 9.1). It is often associated with pericarditis. Occasionally, septicaemia may lead to focal suppurative lesions. Myocarditis is

Table 9.1 Causes of myocarditis.

Infections	Other
Viruses	Hypersensitivity states
Mycoplasma	Radiation
Bacteria	Drugs, e.g. sulphonamides, doxorubicin, lithium, emetine, cyclophosphamide
Spirochaetes	Heavy metals
Rickettsiae	Insect stings
Fungi	
Parasites and protozoa	

an important component of acute rheumatic fever (see Chapter 10).

Mild forms of myocarditis occur in a large number of infectious diseases but often cause only sinus tachycardia and non-specific ECG changes. They may, however, give rise to arrhythmias such as atrial fibrillation or supraventricular tachycardia without producing other overt cardiac effects.

In severe cases, tachycardia may be considerable, or, particularly in diphtheria, there may be a bradycardia due to heart block. The symptoms and signs of left and right cardiac failure may develop, with dyspnoea, gallop rhythm, cardiac enlargement and murmurs due to dilatation of the ventricles. Chest pain is common, but usually attributable to associated pericarditis. There is a risk of acute circulatory failure (shock) and of sudden death. Minor ECG abnormalities are common, but such changes may occur in infections even in the absence of myocarditis. Occasionally, there is ST elevation (due to pericarditis) or depression, or inversion of T waves, or disturbances of conduction and rhythm. There may be enzyme evidence of myocardial necrosis. Echocardiography and radionuclide imaging may be useful in demonstrating ventricular dysfunction. Endomyocardial biopsy is of limited value in diagnosis.

The diagnosis may be supported by the isolation of a virus from tissue or fluid specimens, or by increases in the titre of virus-neutralizing, complement fixing, or haemagglutination-inhibiting antibodies.

There is no specific treatment. Rest and the usual therapy for cardiac failure are required, but digitalis is usually ineffective.

Cardiomyopathy and specific heart muscle diseases

Aetiologically, cardiomyopathies fall into two groups: those in which the heart disease is the major or only abnormal feature, and those in which the myocardial disease is a complication of a generalized disorder which may be described as 'specific heart muscle diseases'. Cardiomyopathy may be secondary to connective tissue disorders (systemic lupus erythematosus, scleroderma and polyarteritis), to amyloidosis, sarcoidosis, neuromuscular diseases (Friedreich's ataxia, progressive muscular dystrophy and myotonia atrophica) to haemochromatosis, and to glycogen storage disease.

There are three distinctive clinical patterns, dilated, hypertrophic and restrictive.

Dilated cardiomyopathy

Dilated (congestive) cardiomyopathy is the commonest type of heart muscle disease. In many patients no aetiological agent can be identified, but it is likely that a substantial proportion follow a viral infection. Alcohol abuse seems to be an important factor in some cases.

The major physiological defect is the decreased contractile force of the left ventricle, with slow and inadequate systolic emptying. The ventricle dilates and the pressure rises in the left atrium. Subsequently, pulmonary hypertension and right ventricular failure occur.

Patients usually present with dyspnoea and oedema whose onset may be abrupt or insidious. Tachycardia is common as are ventricular ectopic beats and atrial fibrillation. The venous pressure is raised and there may be systolic venous pulsation from tricuspid regurgitation. Cardiac enlargement affects both left and right ventricles. Third and fourth heart sounds are common. There may be the pansystolic murmurs of mitral or tricuspid regurgitation.

The ECG frequently demonstrates arrhythmias, as well as abnormalities of the ST segment and T waves. The chest radiograph confirms cardiac enlargement affecting all chambers. Echocardiography and radionuclide imaging reveal dilated, poorly contracting ventricles. Cardiac catheterization and angiocardiography are of little value in diagnosis as they demonstrate only evidence of ventricular failure and, occasionally, tricuspid and mitral regurgitation.

The diagnosis requires the exclusion of coronary artery disease, thyrotoxicosis, hypertension, rheumatic heart disease and congenital heart disease as aetiological factors: it is supported by evidence of one of those generalized disorders which is associated with cardiomyopathy.

Treatment depends on the stage of disease. Alcohol should be forbidden. Bed rest may be necessary in severe cases; diuretics are first-line drug treatment. Digitalis is valuable in controlling atrial fibrillation; vasodilators, especially the angiotensin converting enzyme (ACE) inhibitors, are usually effective in helping to combat the features of congestive failure, at least temporarily. The prognosis is poor, 50% dying within 2 years of diagnosis and nearly all in 5 years. Cardiac transplantation is indicated if disability is severe and life expectancy short.

Hypertrophic cardiomyopathy

In this condition there is massive hypertrophy of the ventricles. The rigid non-compliant chambers impede diastolic filling. The ventricular septum is often the site of the most conspicuous hypertrophy, which may obstruct the left ventricular outflow tract (obstructive cardiomyopathy or idiopathic hypertrophic subaortic stenosis). The obstruction increases as systole progresses, and the more vigorously the ventricle contracts the more severe is the obstruction.

Hypertrophic cardiomyopathy is sometimes a familial condition and one may obtain a history of heart disease or sudden death in relatives.

The symptoms are often those which occur in aortic stenosis, including dyspnoea, angina and syncope. Arrhythmias are common and there is a high risk of sudden death. The pulse has a steep upstroke due to the rapid ejection of blood by the hypertrophied ventricle during early systole. The venous pulse may show a large 'a' wave, and there may be evidence of both left and right ventricular hypertrophy. Left ventricular outflow obstruction causes the systolic murmur and thrill of subaortic stenosis, maximal at the lower left sternal edge or apex. The pansystolic murmur of mitral regurgitation is frequent; less often there may be the signs of tricuspid regurgitation or of pulmonary stenosis. A fourth heart sound is usual. Both the 'a' wave and fourth heart sound are due to forceful atrial contraction against the non-compliant hypertrophied ventricle.

The ECG shows left ventricular hypertrophy and, sometimes, conduction defects. The echocardiogram is of great value. Characteristic features are asymmetrical hypertrophy of the septum (ASH), systolic anterior movement of the mitral valve (SAM) and mid-systolic closure of the aortic valve (Fig. 9.6). Cross-sectional echocardiography demonstrates the asymmetric hypertrophy and the obliteration of the ventricular cavity during systole. The chest

Fig. 9.6 M-mode echocardiogram in hypertrophic cardiomyopathy. The arrow indicates a systolic anterior movement of the mitral valve (SAM). The interventricular septum is grossly thickened.

radiograph may show left ventricular hypertrophy. On cardiac catheterization, a systolic pressure difference can be demonstrated between the body and the outflow tract of the left ventricle if there is obstruction. This difference is increased by drugs such as isoprenaline, which increase myocardial contractility, and may be abolished by drugs such as propranolol, which decrease myocardial contractility. Angiocardiography demonstrates a small left ventricular cavity with narrowing of the outflow tract and, often, mitral regurgitation. Obstructive cardiomyopathy has usually to be differentiated from other types of aortic stenosis. In valvar aortic stenosis, the pulse is usually small and flat and there is either an early systolic click or calcification of the aortic valve. In congenital subaortic stenosis, the pulse is small and flat and there is frequently aortic regurgitation, which is not a feature of obstructive cardiomyopathy.

The prognosis is very variable. Minor forms of the disease are quite common and patients with severe hypertrophy may remain alive and well for many years. The main concern is sudden death; often this is preceded by ventricular arrhythmias.

Beta-blockers and calcium antagonists are both helpful in relieving chest pain (especially the combination of beta-blocker and nifedipine). Resection of part of the septum relieves the symptoms in some patients. Amiodarone appears particularly beneficial in those with severe ventricular arrhythmias and may prevent sudden death.

Restrictive cardiomyopathy

This resembles constrictive pericarditis because the rigid myocardium impedes filling. In the Western world, the main causes are amyloidosis, polyarteritis, leukaemic infiltration and haemochromatosis. Elsewhere, the commonest cause is endomyocardial fibrosis, with or without eosinophilia. The clinical differentiation from pericardial constriction may be impossible but helpful clues are the absence of pericardial calcification and the presence of cardiac enlargement; cardiac biopsy may be diagnostic. Treatment is seldom effective, but if eosinophilia is present steroids and cytotoxic drugs are helpful. Surgical resection of the endocardium may be life-saving.

Endocardial disease

Endocarditis is an inflammation of the inner lining of the heart, affecting predominantly the valve structures. It may be infective or non-infective. The non-infective processes, which include rheumatic fever and systemic lupus erythematosus, are considered in more detail elsewhere.

Infective endocarditis

Infective endocarditis may be due to bacteria, fungi, *Coxiella* or *Chlamydia* and may be acute or subacute. The commonest variety is bacterial in origin and subacute in its course. Infective subacute endocarditis seldom affects a previously normal heart. The process is most frequently superimposed upon pre-existing mitral or aortic valve disease, a ventricular septal defect or persistent ductus arteriosus. Prosthetic valves may also become infected and an increasing number of cases are being seen in intravenous drug abusers. Acute endocarditis (most frequently *Staphylococcus aureus*) may occur on previously normal hearts.

Infective endocarditis used predominantly to affect the young female with rheumatic heart disease. It is now seen quite as frequently in the elderly male with calcific aortic disease.

Pathology

Streptococcus viridans An oral commensal of several varieties, this is the organism most frequently responsible for endocarditis. Other organisms include *Streptococcus faecalis*, *Staphylococcus aureus*, fungi, *Coxiella burnetii*, and *Chlamydia psittaci* (psittacosis).

The infection leads to the formation of friable vegetations which have necrotic tissue, platelets, fibrin, white cells and red cells in their base, with superficial layers of fibrin and micro-organisms. Ulceration may lead to erosion or perforation of the valve cusps or of a sinus of Valsalva. The location of the endocarditis depends upon the underlying lesion. In aortic regurgitation, endocarditis affects the ventricular surface of the valve; in mitral regurgitation it involves the atrial surface of the mitral valve. In a ventricular septal defect, the vegetations may form around the defect itself but are often located either on the tricuspid valve or where the jet impinges on the right ventricular wall. Invasion of the adjacent myocardium is common and may proceed to abscess formation, and to pericardial involvement.

Embolization from the vegetations is frequent and is responsible for many of the clinical features of the disease. Large emboli may cause occlusion of the cerebral, renal or splenic arteries. Micro-emboli affect nearly all parts of the body and, in particular, lead to skin lesions and a glomerulonephritis. Pulmonary emboli develop when the right side of the heart is involved, as it is when there is a ventricular septal defect or persistent ductus arteriosus.

Several of the manifestations of the disease, including arthritis and glomerulitis, are thought to be due to immune complex deposition.

Clinical features

A history of dental treatment or infection is present in some patients, and in a small proportion there has been preceding urethral, pelvic or cardiac surgery.

The onset is often insidious with malaise and feverishness being the earliest complaints. The symptoms often mimic those of influenza. If left untreated, a characteristic clinical picture develops which was common in the days before antibiotic therapy. The complete syndrome of fever, anaemia, petechiae in the skin, clubbing, splenomegaly, a cardiac murmur and microscopic haematuria is seldom seen nowadays.

Fever is usual but not invariable. Non-specific symptoms, such as backache and malaise are common, and pallor characteristic. Petechiae may develop in any part of the body, but should be looked for particularly in the conjunctivae, in the ocular fundi and under the nails (splinter haemorrhages). They may have pale centres and tend to occur in crops. Other superficial lesions include tender, palpable nodules in the tips of the fingers and toes (Osler's nodes). Clubbing of the fingers takes 1−2 months to develop.

In nearly all patients there are signs of organic heart disease, but the infection sometimes obscures them. The cardiac signs may become more obvious either because of the anaemia or because of further damage to valves. Murmurs may, therefore, appear or disappear during the course of the disease. Heart failure is not common in the earlier stages, but frequently complicates the recovery process.

Most patients with infective endocarditis are anaemic, but the anaemia is not of a specific type. The spleen is often enlarged and occasionally tender. Proteinuria and microscopic haematuria are usual.

Neurological complications are common and are due to embolic occlusion of cerebral vessels or to mycotic aneurysms. Coma, convulsions and hemiplegia may occur and meningitis, encephalitis and subarachnoid haemorrhage may be mimicked.

The chest x-ray and ECG are of little value except in the diagnosis and assessment of the underlying cardiac abnormality. Echocardiography is now an essential investigation in this disorder, both because of its ability to demonstrate vegetations, and because it can help in the assessment of the severity of valvar involvement. Vegetations can be seen in some 75% of cases by the cross-sectional technique.

Diagnosis

The diagnosis should be suspected in all patients with valve disorders or congenital heart disease in whom unexplained pyrexia develops. Confirmation of the diagnosis depends on obtaining a positive blood culture, which is possible in some 90% of cases. At least six specimens of blood should be obtained over a period of 1 or 2 days. The blood should be incubated aerobically and anaerobically, and special cultures should be set up for fungi. If the patient has received penicillin previously, penicillinase should be incorporated in the culture medium. Complement fixation tests must be undertaken for the diagnosis of *Coxiella* and *Chlamydia* infection.

Prognosis

Recovery from infective endocarditis is rare unless effective and prolonged antibiotic therapy is given. Death, which may be due to heart failure, emboli or renal failure, often does not occur until several months after the onset. Even if the infection is cured, damage to the valves may be so serious as to lead to intractable heart failure. However, the mortality is probably now in the region of 15–30%.

Treatment

It is important that the responsible organism should be identified without delay, so that the appropriate antibiotics can be given. However, the start of therapy should not be postponed beyond 2 to 3 days in spite of negative blood cultures. Bactericidal agents should be employed, because bacteriostatic drugs produce only temporary suppression of the infection.

When the organism is penicillin-sensitive, a penicillin (penicillin G or ampicillin) is given. Administration is usually intravenous, at least for the first 2 weeks and adequate dosage (e.g. penicillin G, 8 million units/day), preferably confirmed by laboratory testing, is essential. Change to oral therapy may be possible later, given a good response. In penicillin-resistant infection (e.g. *Streptococcus faecalis*) a combination of a penicillin (penicillin G or ampicillin) and an aminoglycoside (streptomycin, or increasingly, gentamicin) will be necessary. Infections due to penicillin-sensitive staphylococci will respond to penicillin, but the more common penicillin-resistant strains demand large doses of penicillinase-resistant drugs, e.g. flucloxacillin 2 g intravenously every 4 hours. Blood culture-negative endocarditis should be treated as for *Streptococcus faecalis* infections, infection with *Coxiella* and *Chlamydia* having first been excluded. A minimum of 4 weeks therapy is thought necessary in all cases. Antibiotic therapy is constantly changing as new drugs become available and as organisms become resistant to those in current use.

The temperature usually falls to normal within 3 days of the start of effective antibiotic therapy. The recurrence of pyrexia suggests the emergence of resistance organisms, superinfection by another organism or, perhaps most commonly, the development of a reaction to the antibiotic. Further blood cultures should be obtained and a change of antibiotic considered.

Surgery may be necessary for the correction of congenital heart disease or for the replacement of damaged valves, but should, if possible, be deferred until the infection is under control.

Prophylaxis

Although endocarditis may occur in the absence of any obvious cause and in patients without known heart disease, many cases are probably preventable. All patients known to be at risk should pay great attention to oral hygiene, and should be aware of the need to have antibiotic cover for dental extractions, genito-urinary surgery and other procedures in which infection is likely. For dental extractions, it is recommended that oral amoxycillin 3 g is given prior to the procedure. Prophylaxis for genital or urinary operations, and for patients with prosthetic valves should also include an aminoglycoside, e.g. gentamicin.

Non-bacterial thrombotic endocarditis

This term is used to describe verrucous lesions on the endocardium which are found in a variety of chronic wasting conditions, infectious diseases and neoplasms. These vegetations consist of platelet thrombi containing fibrin. There is no infection primarily involved; their importance lies in their liability to superimposed infective endocarditis and to embolisation to the brain and elsewhere.

Further reading

Fowler, N.O. (1981) Pericardial diseases. Key references *Circulation 63:* 1429.

Goodwin, J.F. (Ed.) (1985) *Heart Muscle Disease.* Lancaster: MTP Press.

Hirschmann, J.V. (1978) Pericardial constriction. *American Heart Journal 96:* 110.

Krikorian, J.G. & Hancock, E.W. (1978) Pericardiocentesis. *American Heart Journal of Medicine 65:* 808.

Maron B.J. *et al.* (1987) Hypertrophic cardiomyopathy *New England Journal of Medicine 316:* 780, 844.

Perloff, J.K. (1981) The cardiomyopathies: dilated and restrictive. Key references. *Circulation 63:* 1189.

Rahimtoola, S.H. (1978) *Infective Endocarditis.* New York: Grune and Stratton.

Shabetai, R. (1978) The pericardium: an essay on some recent developments. *American Journal of Cardiology 42:* 1036.

Shulman, S.T. et al (1984) Prevention of bacterial endocarditis. *Circulation 70:* 1123A.

Working Party of the British Society for Antimicrobial Chemotherapy (1982) The antibiotic prophylaxis of infective endocarditis. *Lancet i:* 1323.

Rheumatic Heart Disease

Rheumatic fever and its sequel, chronic rheumatic heart disease, is a major cardiac cause of disability and death.

Rheumatic fever

Acute rheumatic fever is a disease which follows infection by group A haemolytic streptococci and produces manifestations in many tissues and organs. Arthritis is often the most conspicuous feature, but cardiac involvement is of much greater importance. The duration of rheumatic activity is very variable; it may cease in 2 weeks or persist for many months. Recurrences are common. Death is rare in the acute phase but chronic rheumatic heart disease is responsible for a considerable morbidity and mortality.

Aetiology

Rheumatic fever seems to occur only after a group A streptococcal infection. It is complication of less than 1% of episodes of streptococcal pharyngitis, developing some 10−20 days after the onset of the sore throat. No history of sore throat, however, can be obtained in some 30−50% of cases; nonetheless virtually all patients with acute rheumatic fever have a streptococcal antibody response.

It is still far from clear how the infection leads to rheumatic fever. It seems probable that rheumatic fever is a result of a hyper-immune reaction either to bacterial allergy or to autoimmunity.

Over the last 50 years, rheumatic fever has been becoming progressively less frequent and less severe in many countries, including the United Kingdom, the United States and Scandinavia. However, in Asia and South America, there seems to have been little or no reduction in its incidence and severity. The decline of rheumatic fever in Western countries cannot be solely the result of the use of antibiotics for it preceded their discovery. It may be attributed both to a change in the virulence of streptococci and to improving social conditions, for poverty is associated with a relatively high risk of the disease. Overcrowding is an important factor, probably because it encourages cross-infection.

Rheumatic fever most commonly occurs between the ages of 5

and 15, with the peak about the age of 8. It is rare under the age of 4 and becomes progressively less common after the age of 15, although occasional cases are seen even after the age of 30. Rheumatic fever affects males and females equally often, but females are more susceptible to chorea. Rheumatic fever or its sequelae are often seen in more than one member of the same family. Although this may in part be due to the sharing of unfavourable social circumstances, there is good evidence of a genetic predisposition to the disease.

Pathology

Microscopic evidence of acute rheumatic fever is widespread, but particularly affects tissues lined by endothelium such as blood vessels, the endocardium, the pericardium and synovial membranes. The earliest lesion is one of swelling in and around collagen fibres, accompanied by oedema and lymphocytic infiltration. Later, and more specifically, granulomatous Aschoff nodules appear. These are formed by collections of round cells, fibroblasts and multinucleated giant cells, and are usually surrounded by an area of polymorphonuclear cells, lymphocytes and plasma cells. The Aschoff nodules occur throughout the heart and are common in the interstitial tissue close to small blood vessels situated beneath the endocardium of the left ventricle.

Macroscopically, the lesions of rheumatic fever are most obvious in relation to the heart valves and the pericardium. The valve cusps become thickened by oedema and by the infiltration of capillaries. Grey or yellow warty vegetations ('verrucae') form along the lines of closure. These are common on the mitral and aortic valve cusps, and seldom affect the tricuspid or pulmonary valves. When the pericardium is involved, it becomes thickened and may contain a fibrinous straw-coloured effusion.

Chronic rheumatic heart disease is a sequel to acute rheumatic carditis, and many of its features are the result of fibrosis occurring during the healing of the acute lesion. Its pathology will be discussed in more detail later in this chapter.

Clinical features

In most cases, some 2–3 weeks after the onset of acute pharyngitis, the child begins to feel unwell, loses his appetite and complains of pains in the limbs. Fever is present, but it is not usually high. The major clinical features are carditis, polyarthritis, subcutaneous nodules, erythema marginatum and chorea.

Carditis. This occurs in about half of the first attacks of rheumatic fever. *Endocarditis*, with valvar involvement, is suggested by the appearance of cardiac murmurs; of all patients who develop carditis, three-quarters have murmurs in the first week. An apical pansystolic murmur indicates either mitral valve damage or functional mitral regurgitation associated with myocarditis. Rheumatic involvement of the mitral valve is also strongly suggested by the appearance of a low-pitched and short mid-diastolic apical murmur (Carey Coombs). This murmur is usually transient, but may persist for months or years until the characteristic features of mitral stenosis develop. However, the presence of a short mid-diastolic murmur at the apex in rheumatic fever cannot be taken as evidence of mitral stenosis or of its subsequent development. Midsystolic murmurs in the aortic or pulmonary area are less certain evidence of cardiac involvement, as they are common in febrile children without heart disease and usually disappear as recovery takes place. The diastolic murmur of aortic regurgitation is not uncommon, and usually persists after the acute rheumatic process has subsided.

Myocarditis is an important and common feature of acute rheumatic fever, but is difficult to diagnose with confidence. It is suggested by a tachycardia which is greater than would be expected from the height of the fever or which persists after the temperature falls, and by cardiac enlargement. More diagnostic is the appearance of left-sided or right-sided heart failure when this cannot be attributed to valve damage. The symptoms include dyspnoea, orthopnoea and oedema. Gallop rhythm is common but does not necessarily imply myocarditis, as it may occur in any child with fever and tachycardia.

When clinical evidence of *pericarditis* is present, the carditis is usually severe and involves the myocardium and endocardium as well (pancarditis). Retrosternal pain and pericardial friction occur and there may be a pericardial effusion.

When rheumatic activity has subsided, there are often residual signs of valve damage. Because of this, abnormal cardiac signs cannot be taken as evidence of continuing activity.

Polyarthritis. This is common but its severity is variable. Characteristically, the joints become swollen, painful and hot, but in the younger child there may be only vague aches. The arthritis usually affects one joint after another, giving the impression of 'flitting', but it may involve several joints simultaneously. The knees, ankles, shoulders, wrists and elbows are most commonly involved, but the smaller joints of the hand and feet may be affected, particularly in the older patient. The inflammation in each joint usually develops within a few hours and may take up to a week to subside. Salicylates and corticosteroids produce relief of symptoms and signs promptly and are of some diagnostic value in this respect. Even in the absence of treatment, the polyarthritis usually disappears within 3 weeks and leaves no residual abnormality.

Subcutaneous nodules. These seldom give rise to symptoms but are of diagnostic importance. They are firm painless structures which are attached to tendon sheaths, joint capsules and fascia, and the skin is movable over them. They occur mainly over the extensor surfaces of the wrists, elbows, knuckles, knees and Achilles tendon and also over the scalp. They usually last about a week.

Erythema marginatum. This consists of lesions which develop rapidly from small macules or papules into large circles with pink, slightly raised, sharply circumscribed edges and pale centres. As these circles intersect, a pattern of segments develops. These appear and disappear within a period of hours. Erythema marginatum affects the trunk and limbs, but never involves the face. It is neither painful nor itchy; recurrences may ensue after all other features of rheumatic fever have disappeared.

Chorea (St Vitus' dance). This is a neurological manifestation of the acute rheumatic process. It often occurs without the other features, but cardiac involvement is common. It can affect children of either gender, but after puberty, it is confined to females. The onset is usually insidious with the development of an apparent clumsiness in an otherwise healthy child. Jerky and non-repetitive movements occur and muscle tone is reduced. When the arms are extended the wrist is flexed and the fingers hyperextended, giving rise to a 'dinner fork' configuration. Chorea must be differentiated from tics, which are also jerky but are repetitive, and from athetosis, in which the movements may not be repetitive but are of a more writhing character.

Laboratory investigations

In most cases there is a moderate leucocytosis of $12\,000-15\,000$ white blood cells per mm^3 and an increased erythrocyte sedimentation rate (ESR). These features suggest rheumatic activity, but they are not reliable indices when steroids are given as the leucocytosis may persist or rise, and the ESR fall as a result of the therapy itself. However, a persistently raised ESR suggests, but does not prove, continuing activity.

In only about one-quarter of patients can a group A streptococcus be grown from the throat. The presence of a high antistreptolysin 'O' (ASO) titre provides good evidence of recent infection, particularly if it rises and falls. Other antibody tests, such as those for anti-DNase B and anti-streptozyme (ASTZ) are also of value.

A number of electrocardiographic abnormalities occur in acute rheumatic fever. Amongst these are a prolonged PR interval and, more rarely, more advanced degrees of atrioventricular block. Non-specific T wave changes are common and the ST and T wave changes characteristic of pericarditis may be seen.

The diagnosis of rheumatic fever

There is no certain way of establishing the presence of rheumatic fever, but the combination of certain clinical features and laboratory findings is highly suggestive. It may be diagnosed with some confidence if evidence of a recent streptococcal infection is present together with two or more of the following: carditis, polyarthritis, chorea, erythema marginatum and subcutaneous nodules. The diagnosis is also probable if evidence of streptococcal infection is combined with *one* of the clinical features mentioned together with two or more of the following: previous evidence of rheumatic fever or rheumatic heart disease, arthralgia, fever, raised ESR or white cell count, or prolonged PR interval. (Revised Jones Criteria, American Heart Association, 1984.)

Differential diagnosis

The diagnosis of rheumatic fever is often difficult because the complete picture is seldom present. Furthermore, although the criteria described are valuable, they depend upon accurate observation and the correct timing and performance of laboratory tests. A history of sore throat may be misleading, as this is often due to organisms other than streptococci. Likewise, polyarthritis may be wrongly diagnosed when only the vague limb pains so common in childhood have occurred. Cardiac signs can also be deceptive, as functional systolic murmurs often come and go in the child with pyrexia from any cause. Another problem is posed by the patient with chronic rheumatic heart disease who develops a sore throat. Nevertheless, if the above-mentioned criteria are adhered to, the correct diagnosis will usually be made.

Diseases which are particularly important to differentiate from rheumatic fever are bacterial arthritis, rheumatoid arthritis and subacute infective endocarditis. In most cases of acute septic arthritis, the disease process is confined to a single joint and the inflammation is liable to extend into adjacent soft tissue. The diagnosis can be confirmed by bacteriological examination of fluid from the joint. Staphylococcal and meningococcal septicaemias can be diagnosed from blood cultures. Rheumatoid arthritis tends to involve smaller joints than rheumatic fever, but observation over a long period may be necessary in order to be certain of the diagnosis. Subacute infective endocarditis may be difficult to differentiate from rheumatic fever if blood cultures are negative, but a polyarthritis is rare, and some of the characteristic features such as microscopic haematuria and anaemia, which are seldom found in rheumatic fever, are usually present.

Course and prognosis

The course of rheumatic fever is variable and unpredictable. In some apparently severely ill patients, complete recovery takes place within a few days, whereas in others the disease drags on for months. In either case, the liability to recurrences of rheumatic activity following further streptococcal infection remains and it is common for the victim of one attack to experience one or more further episodes over the succeeding years.

The first attack is seldom fatal, but recurrences may lead to increasing cardiac damage and heart failure. By contrast, if the patient has escaped cardiac damage in the first attack, it is unlikely to develop subsequently. It has been estimated that more than two-thirds of patients who have experienced rheumatic fever eventually develop chronic rheumatic valve disease.

It is rare for the young child with rheumatic fever to escape cardiac damage. The risk of developing valve disease after an acute episode diminishes with age and it is not unusual for those first affected in adult life to have no sequelae. There can be no doubt that many cases of rheumatic fever escape diagnosis because about half of the patients with proven chronic rheumatic disease give no history of an acute episode.

Treatment

During the acute phase of the disease the subject wants and needs bed rest. When the temperature, pulse rate and ESR have returned to normal and the evidence of acute arthritis and carditis has disappeared, the patient may be gradually mobilized and rehabilitated. Active carditis requires complete rest, and this may have to be continued for several weeks. Subsequent increases in activity must depend upon the individual response, and a full resumption of normal physical activity usually has to be delayed to 6 months from the time when the last signs of active carditis have resolved.

Both salicylates and corticosteroids have a dramatic effect on the fever and polyarthritis of rheumatic fever. Although contro-versy continues as to the relative merits of the two forms of drug therapy, it is now common practice to use salicylates for rheumatic fever without carditis, and to add or substitute corticosteroids if there is undoubted evidence of cardiac involvement. However, it does not seem that any drug prevents the development of chronic valve damage. It is important not to give large doses of salicylate which can lead to salicylate intoxication; it is particularly undesirable to administer large doses of sodium salicylate as the sodium may precipitate cardiac failure. For children, 50 mg of acetylsalicylic acid per kg body weight may be given daily, and the dose subsequently adjusted to control symptoms. For adults, 4—8 g a day may be appropriate, in divided doses, given every 4 hours. Salicylates should be continued until signs of rheumatic activity have ceased. There is great variation in the dosage of corticosteroids necessary to control activity. An initial dose of 40 mg of prednisone daily may be given and subsequently reduced to 20 mg daily, continued for 6 weeks and gradually withdrawn. Some patients have a rebound of rheumatic activity subsequently, and it is best to try to control this with salicylates.

The manifestations of cardiac failure are often suppressed by corticosteroids but diuretics and digitalis should be administered if necessary.

Prevention of rheumatic fever

Rheumatic fever may be prevented by the prophylaxis and treatment of acute streptococcal infections.

Acute streptococcal infections are probably most effectively treated by a single injection of 0.6—1.2 mega-units of benzathine penicillin, but this is painful. Alternatively, phenoxymethylpenicillin may be given for 10 days.

All patients who have experienced acute rheumatic fever should receive long-term prophylactic therapy. For this purpose, benzathine penicillin may be injected monthly in a dosage of 0.6—1.2 mega-units, or oral therapy given as 125 mg phenoxymethylpenicillin twice daily or sulphadiazine 0.5 g twice daily. It is not known how long prophylaxis should be continued, but it is common practice to recommend this up to the age of 25.

The healing of rheumatic carditis and the development of chronic rheumatic heart disease

Chronic rheumatic heart disease is the result of damage produced by recurrent attacks of acute rheumatic carditis and the subsequent healing process. These changes are largely confined to the valve structures, although in some instances myocardial damage may also be severe. Rheumatic pericarditis heals without residual effects. It is difficult to know to what extent the chronic lesions are the result of continuing and smouldering rheumatic activity. It is unusual for adult patients with chronic rheumatic heart disease to exhibit clinical evidence of acute rheumatic infection, but laboratory investigations may reveal evidence of repeated subclinical streptococcal infections, and biopsy of myocardial muscle in the adult frequently shows Aschoff bodies.

Because valve damage predominates in patients with chronic rheumatic heart disease, this condition will be considered in detail under the individual valve lesions. Nevertheless it is important to recognize that myocardial damage coexists and that correction of a valve abnormality will not necessarily restore normal cardiac function.

The pathological processes that cause valve deformity include thickening and distortion of the cusps at the time of rheumatic fever, contracture of the valve structures, fusion of the commissures, shortening of the chordae tendineae and, finally, calcification during the phase of healing. The nature of the valve lesion depends upon the relative importance of these factors in the individual case. Stenosis occurs if fusion of the cusps predominates; regurgitation is produced by shortening of the chordae tendineae and contracture of the valve leaflets.

The valve deformities may take many years to develop and, in particular, narrowing is not critical until the affected orifice is reduced to less than a quarter of its normal size. Regurgitation may be important from the time of the attack of acute rheumatic fever but its appearance as a symptomatic disorder, also, is likely to be delayed. Therefore, although the signs of mitral and aortic regurgitation may be present in childhood or early adult life, symptoms due to these lesions seldom develop until the third or fourth decade. The same is true for mitral stenosis; in aortic stenosis symptoms are often postponed even longer.

Further reading

Ad Hoc Committee to Revise the Jones Criteria (modified) of the Council on Rheumatic Fever and Congenital Heart Disease of the American Heart Association (1984) Jones Criteria (revised) for guidance in the diagnosis of rheumatic fever. *Circulation 69:* 203A.

Committee on Rheumatic Fever and Infective Endocarditis of the Council on Cardiovascular Disease in the Young (1984) Prevention of rheumatic fever. 70, 1118A.

Disciasco, G. & Taranta, A. (1980) Rheumatic fever in children. *American Heart Journal 99:* 63.

Disorders of the Cardiac Valves

Mitral valve disease

The normal mitral valve (Fig. 11.1) consists of the valve ring, two unequal cusps (leaflets), chordae tendineae and papillary muscles. The larger antero-medial (or aortic) cusp is interposed between the mitral and aortic orifices, and forms part of the outflow tract of the left ventricle (Fig. 11.2). The papillary muscles arise from the ventricular wall opposite the commissures and are attached to the cusps on either side of the commissures by the chordae tendineae (Fig. 11.3). The chordae are collagenous strands, which, when tensed by the contracting papillary muscles, prevent the cusps from prolapsing into the left atrium during ventricular systole.

Chronic mitral valve disease is frequently due to rheumatic endocarditis. This may take the form of pure mitral stenosis but some degree of regurgitation is often associated. Pure mitral regurgitation is usually non-rheumatic in origin; mitral valve prolapse is a common abnormality. Regurgitation may also be due to ruptured or defective chordae tendineae, papillary muscles or valve cusps, or to dilatation of the valve ring following left ventricular enlargement from a variety of causes.

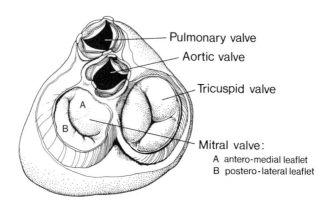

Fig. 11.1 Appearances of the heart valves during systole, with the atria and great vessels removed. The heart is viewed from behind, with the left ventricle and mitral valve on the left.

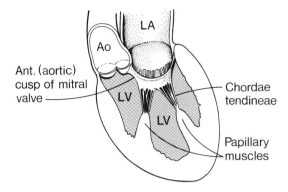

Fig. 11.2 Diagrammatic representation of relationships of left atrium (LA), left ventricle (LV) and aorta (AO). Note that the aortic cusp of the mitral valve separates the mitral valve orifice from the outflow tract of the left ventricle.

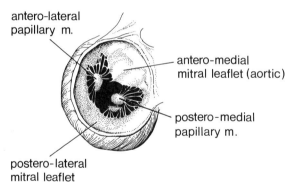

Fig. 11.3 Open mitral valve viewed from the left atrium. Note that the papillary muscles arise opposite the commissures and are attached to the cusps on either side of the commissures by the chordae tendineae.

Mitral stenosis

Pathology

Mitral stenosis is usually the result of recurrent rheumatic inflammation followed by healing. The leaflets adhere at their commissures, leaving a central orifice. In some instances the valve cusps remain pliant and mobile; in others fibrosis and calcification make them rigid. In about 10% of cases severe shortening of the chordae tendineae produces a funnel-shaped orifice.

Pathophysiology

Serious haemodynamic consequences develop only when the mitral valve orifice is reduced from the normal size of approximately 5 cm^2 to about 1 cm^2. In severe mitral stenosis, the orifice is a slit less than 1 cm long and 0.5 cm across.

In the normal heart there is little pressure difference across the mitral valve between its opening in early ventricular diastole and its closure. In mitral stenosis, a pressure difference develops which depends upon the area of the mitral valve orifice and the volume of blood flowing through it (Fig. 11.4).

When the stenosis is relatively mild, the mean pressure in the left atrium may be normal at rest (i.e. less than 12 mmHg) but increases on exercise as the cardiac output rises. In more severe stenosis, the pressure is raised even at rest, and in the most severe grades is persistently elevated to 25 mmHg or more. The left ventricular pressure is normal, provided there is no disease affecting this chamber.

When the stenosis is slight, the cardiac output may be normal, but as the narrowing increases, the cardiac output diminishes to about half the normal value, and may not rise in response to exercise.

The pressure in the pulmonary veins and capillaries parallels that in the left atrium. If the pulmonary capillary pressure rises rapidly to 30 mmHg, pulmonary oedema develops as the hydrostatic pressure exceeds plasma osmotic pressure. If the process takes place slowly, fluid exudes into the alveolar wall and a physical barrier eventually develops between capillaries and alveoli consisting of a thickened capillary basement membrane, increased collagen and oedema. These changes increase the tissue tension of the alveolar wall and limit the exudation of fluid. As a consequence, patients with mitral stenosis can sometimes tolerate high pulmonary capillary pressures without developing severe pulmonary oedema. Because of the increased fluid in the interstitial tissues, the lymphatics become engorged.

As the pulmonary capillary pressure increases, there is a concomitant rise in pulmonary arterial pressure. Thus, as left atrial and pulmonary capillary pressures increase from about 10 to 30 mmHg, the pulmonary mean arterial pressure rises from 20 to 40 mmHg. However, in many cases of severe mitral stenosis, pulmonary arterial hypertension is much more severe than can be accounted for by this passive rise. This disproportionate elevation of pulmonary arterial pressure does not occur until there is a persistently high left atrial pressure. It is largely due to an increase in tone in the pulmonary arterioles and small pulmonary arteries, which is largely reversible when the mitral valve disease is cor-

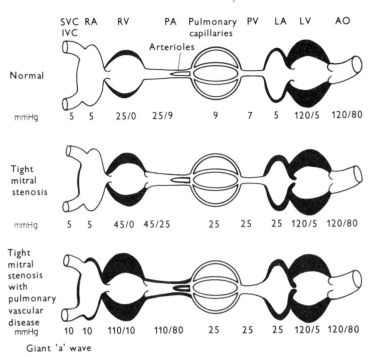

	SVC RA IVC	RV	PA	Pulmonary capillaries	PV	LA	LV	AO

Fig. 11.4 The haemodynamic effects of mitral stenosis. In the normal heart, the pressure in the left atrium is similar to that of the left ventricle during ventricular diastole. With the development of mitral stenosis, the pressure in the left atrium rises, and this rise is transmitted to the pulmonary veins, capillaries and arteries. When pulmonary vascular disease develops, there is a narrowing of the pulmonary arterioles which leads to a disproportionate rise in the pulmonary arterial and right ventricular systolic pressures. With right ventricular failure, both the right ventricular end-diastolic pressure and the mean right atrial pressure may rise to 10 mmHg.

rected. Sometimes pulmonary arterial hypertrophy and secondary atheroma develop; these changes may be irreversible. Severe pulmonary arterial hypertension is disadvantageous in that it leads to right ventricular hypertrophy and failure. However, the increased resistance of the pulmonary arterial vessels prevents an abrupt rise in right ventricular output on exercise and therefore protects the lungs from a sudden increase in pulmonary capillary pressure.

The pulmonary vascular congestion typical of mitral stenosis leads to increased rigidity (decreased compliance) in the lungs.

As a consequence, patients with severe mitral stenosis may have to double or treble the work of breathing.

Complications

Atrial fibrillation develops sooner or later in most cases of mitral stenosis. At first this may be paroxysmal, but it is usual for it to become permanent. At its onset the ventricular rate is often more than 140 per minute and the patient may be rapidly precipitated into acute pulmonary oedema. It is an important complication, both because it contributes to the development of cardiac failure and because it is responsible for atrial stasis and the consequent risk of thrombosis and embolism.

Pulmonary embolism and infarction frequently occur, especially when the disease is far advanced, as thrombosis is encouraged by atrial fibrillation, cardiac failure and bed rest.

Systemic embolism is common and often follows the onset of atrial fibrillation. The embolism is cerebral in a high proportion of cases but may involve the mesenteric, renal or other arteries.

The congested respiratory tract makes the patient liable to attacks of acute bronchitis and to the development of chronic bronchitis. Infective endocarditis is rare in pure mitral stenosis but is commoner as a complication of mixed mitral stenosis and regurgitation.

Symptoms

The patient with mitral stenosis, who is often symptom-free for many years, eventually develops features of left-sided cardiac failure and, later, those of right-sided failure. Various factors, such as pregnancy and the onset of atrial fibrillation, may suddenly precipitate the patient from one of these stages into the next.

The major symptom of mitral stenosis is shortness of breath. This occurs at first only on strenuous exercise, but as time passes less and less exertion is required to evoke it. Eventually, orthopnoea develops and the patient is liable to attacks of paroxysmal dyspnoea and acute pulmonary oedema. Acute pulmonary oedema is less likely when severe pulmonary arterial hypertension has developed.

Haemoptysis occurs in some 10–20% of patients with mitral stenosis but is seldom severe. In some cases, the sputum is frothy and pink due to acute pulmonary oedema, but frankly bloody sputum may be expectorated by a patient who is almost free of breathlessness. This is probably due to the rupture of dilated pulmonary or bronchial veins. Another important cause of haemoptysis is pulmonary infarction.

Patients may also complain of palpitation, cough and angina

pectoris. Severe breathlessness and orthopnoea have usually been present for years before right-sided heart failure develops. The earliest symptom of this is oedema of the legs, but abdominal discomfort due to engorgement of the liver or to ascites also occurs.

Physical signs

Patients with long-standing mitral stenosis often have a characteristic facies — a dusky malar discoloration. This may be attributed to peripheral cyanosis associated wth a low cardiac output and vasoconstriction.

The arterial pulse is usually normal in volume but may be small, and is often irregular due to atrial fibrillation. In the earlier stages, the venous pressure is normal, but rises with the onset of right-sided heart failure. When there is severe pulmonary hypertension, there may be a large venous 'a' wave due to forceful right atrial contraction against the hypertrophied non-compliant right ventricle.

The apex beat is usually in the normal place but may be deviated to the left by right ventricular hypertrophy. It often has a tapping quality, which is associated with the characteristic loud first heart sound. In more advanced cases, right ventricular hypertrophy produces a heaving impulse to the left of the lower sternum. Mid-diastolic and presystolic thrills may be present at, or internal to, the apex beat.

There are four cardinal auscultatory features of mitral stenosis: a loud first sound, an opening snap, a mid-diastolic murmur, and a presystolic murmur (Fig. 11.5). The first sound is accentuated and the opening snap loud when the cusps are mobile; these signs may disappear with the development of rigidity and calcification of the valves (see p. 108). A mid-diastolic murmur is usually present, and its length, but not its intensity, gives an indication of the severity of the lesion. The presystolic murmur is often an early sign but may not be heard unless the patient is exercised and then turned into the left lateral position. A mitral systolic murmur signifies concomitant mitral regurgitation.

The second sound splits normally, but the pulmonary component is often accentuated because of pulmonary hypertension. An apical third heart sound is impossible in significant mitral stenosis because the rapid filling of the left ventricle necessary for its production cannot occur.

The ECG

If sinus rhythm is present, there is usually P mitrale (Fig. 11.6). Atrial fibrillation is common; other atrial and ventricular ar-

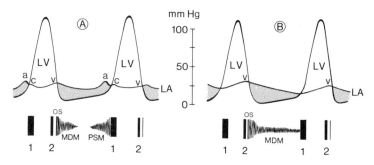

Fig. 11.5   (A) The pressure pulses in left ventricle and left atrium and the phonocardiographic appearances in mitral stenosis. A pressure difference is present throughout diastole (shaded area), and is accentuated by atrial contraction ('a' wave). Mid-diastolic and presystolic murmurs result. (B) Atrial fibrillation has developed with loss of the 'a' wave and of the presystolic accentuation of the murmur.

Fig. 11.6   Broad and notched P wave in mitral stenosis (P mitrale).

rhythmias occur occasionally. Evidence of right ventricular hypertrophy develops in cases with severe pulmonary hypertension.

Radiological appearances

The most characteristic radiological feature of mitral stenosis is the selective enlargement of the left atrium, which, in the posteroanterior view, produces a bulge below the pulmonary artery on the left border of the heart, and a rounded dense shadow within or outside the middle part of the right border of the heart (Fig. 11.7). Left atrial enlargement can be confirmed by observing the displacement of the barium-filled oesophagus in the lateral view. Other radiological features may include calcification of the mitral valve, a normal or small left ventricle, and a normal or small aorta. The upper pulmonary veins are usually prominent. When the pulmonary capillary pressure is high, horizontal septal lines (Kerley's B lines) appear in the costophrenic angles, and the radiological features of pulmonary oedema may be seen. Haemosiderosis may produce mottling of the lungs. Pulmonary

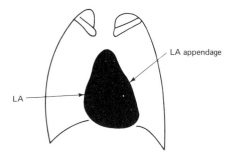

LA appendage

LA

Fig. 11.7 The bulge produced by the left atrial appendage is seen on the left border of the heart between the pulmonary artery and the left ventricle. The left atrium may also bulge out on the right side of the heart, but more commonly forms a dense shadow behind the right atrium.

artery, right ventricular and, occasionally, right atrial enlargement may also be present when there is pulmonary arterial hypertension.

Echocardiography

In mitral stenosis, the M shape normally seen in diastole is lost, and the diastolic (EF) slope is reduced (Fig. 11.8A). Echoes from the valve are increased if it is fibrotic or calcified, and make the leaflets appear thickened. Separation of the leaflets is diminished, and the two leaflets may move in the same direction. Cross-sectional echocardiography allows visualization of the stenotic mitral valve orifice (Fig. 11.8B), and estimation of the rate of filling of the left ventricle. Doppler ultrasound permits quantification of the rate of flow through the valve.

Cardiac catheterization

Cardiac catheterization reveals the haemodynamic changes previously described. This investigation is seldom required for diagnostic purposes, but may be helpful in assessing the severity of the lesion. This is most accurately done by simultaneously measuring the pressure on either side of the mitral valve and estimating the cardiac output. Angiocardiography is mainly of value in assessing the severity of any associated mitral or aortic regurgitation.

Combined valve disease

Mitral stenosis is frequently complicated by disease of the other cardiac valves. The combination of rheumatic aortic regurgitation with mitral stenosis is a common one; in most cases the aortic regurgitation is the less important defect. The severity of the aortic regurgitation can be judged with reasonable assurance by the pulse volume, and by the diastolic pressure, which in severe

Fig. 11.8A   Severe mitral stenosis — an M-mode parasternal echocardiogram. The left atrium is hugely enlarged and the mitral valve shows the characteristic slow diastolic closure rate. RVOT = right ventricular outflow tract. MV = mitral valve. LA = left atrium.

cases is usually less than 60 mmHg. The combination of severe mitral stenosis and aortic stenosis is unusual but important, because one may mask the presence of the other.

Severe tricuspid stenosis complicates about 3% of cases of mitral stenosis and often obscures its signs.

Tricuspid regurgitation is common in advanced mitral stenosis because the tricuspid valve ring dilates with right ventricular enlargement. The associated pansystolic murmur may be heard not only at the left sternal edge but as far out as the apex. This may lead to the erroneous diagnosis of mitral regurgitation. Systolic venous pulsation in the neck, the increase in the murmur on inspiration, and the lack of transmission of the murmur to the axilla serve to identify its tricuspid origin.

Diagnosis

The presence of mitral stenosis can often be suspected from a history of rheumatic fever combined with progressive dyspnoea, a small and irregular pulse, and a mitral facies. In the milder case, these features may be absent, and palpation and auscultation first

Fig. 11.8B Cross-sectional echocardiogram in mitral stenosis. The upper panel shows a short axis parasternal view. The mitral valve orifice is small and there is considerable thickening particularly on the left hand side of the orifice. The lower panel shows the long axis parasternal view with the hammocking appearance of the anterior cusp as it comes to the end of its opening movement.

reveal the diagnosis. A high proportion of patients have a tapping apex beat, right ventricular heave, loud first sound, opening snap, and mid-diastolic and presystolic murmurs. The experienced auscultator is usually first struck by the loud first sound and the opening snap rather than by the diastolic murmurs, which may be audible only if they are specifically sought with the patient lying in the left lateral position. The diagnosis is supported by P mitrale in the ECG, by the demonstration of left atrial enlargement in the radiograph and by the characteristic echocardiographic and catheterization features.

Probably the commonest cause for the mistaken diagnosis of mitral stenosis is the misinterpretation of normal splitting of the first sound for a presystolic murmur (a presystolic murmur is seldom the only auscultatory abnormality in mitral stenosis). A third heart sound may be wrongly interpreted as being an opening snap or a mid-diastolic murmur, and differentiation may be impossible without a phonocardiogram. One should hesitate to diagnose mitral stenosis on the basis of either a presystolic murmur or a short 'mid-diastolic murmur' alone without collateral evidence.

When an apical pansystolic murmur complicates the physical signs in mitral stenosis, it may be difficult to establish whether there is a significant degree of mitral regurgitation. This is unlikely if there is a loud first sound and an opening snap, or if there is evidence of advanced pulmonary hypertension. Important mitral regurgitation is probable if the systolic murmur is loud and radiates to the axilla, or if there is left ventricular hypertrophy, a soft first heart sound or a third sound rather than an opening snap. Doppler ultrasound and angiography are valuable in the diagnosis and assessment of regurgitation.

Mitral stenosis may be simulated by the mid-diastolic murmurs encountered in conditions leading to high flow through the mitral valve, such as ventricular septal defect and persistent ductus arteriosus, and by the Austin Flint murmur associated with severe aortic regurgitation as well as by the mid-diastolic murmur of left atrial myxoma. The possibility that a mid-diastolic murmur is not due to mitral stenosis should be considered particularly if there is neither a loud first sound nor an opening snap. In left atrial myxoma, the signs may entirely mimic those of mitral stenosis, but tend to vary from time to time (see also p. 308). Echocardiography is particularly valuable in differentiating the mid-diastolic murmur of mitral stenosis from that due to other causes.

Course and prognosis

The characteristic physical signs of mitral stenosis, which can be present within a year of acute rheumatic fever, may precede the development of symptoms by 10 or 20 years. Breathlessness, usually the first complaint, is most likely to start between the ages of 20 or 30 but may be delayed much longer. In those in whom complications do not develop, the course is slowly but steadily downhill over a number of years. However, in Western countries, patients with signs of rheumatic mitral valve disease are now mainly seen in middle or old age, whereas in parts of Asia and Africa, it is predominantly found in adolescents and young adults.

Sooner or later, some complication usually arises which leads to temporary or permanent deterioration. In young women, pregnancy is often responsible for the onset or aggravation of breathlessness; in the patient with severe stenosis, parturition may lead to pulmonary oedema and death. Rapid deterioration may also occur as a result of pulmonary infection or infarction and at the onset of atrial fibrillation. Although these complications are often serious and even fatal, one or more pregnancies may be well tolerated, and patients may return to normal activity after infection or infarction has been treated, or atrial fibrillation controlled.

Once right-sided heart failure has developed, the prognosis without surgical treatment is poor.

Medical treatment

Surgery is eventually required in most cases, but it is usually necessary to prepare the patient for it by appropriate medical therapy. Even after successful surgery, treatment is often needed for the control of arrhythmias and the prevention of emboli.

Patients with mitral stenosis should be encouraged to live reasonably normal lives, but to avoid excessive exertion. They should be advised against being overweight, and discouraged from smoking. Infections should be promptly treated with appropriate antibiotics, and anticoagulants used if there is evidence of venous thrombosis or of pulmonary or systemic embolism and should be considered in all patients with atrial fibrillation. Careful supervision is required during pregnancy (see p. 311).

Digitalis is required for atrial fibrillation, but is of no value in pure stenosis in sinus rhythm. Cardiac failure is best treated by diuretics. An attempt to restore sinus rhythm should be made after mitral valve surgery in patients with atrial fibrillation, if this is known to be of fairly recent onset.

Surgical treatment

Two types of surgery are available: mitral valvotomy and mitral replacement. Mitral valvotomy can be performed as a closed operation (i.e. without direct vision of the valve and without cardiopulmonary bypass) or under the conditions of open heart surgery. When the valve cusps are pliant and mobile, this procedure leads to relief of the stenosis for many years, but restenosis of the valve frequently takes place after 5–10 years. When the valve is rigid or calcified, valvotomy is seldom successful for more than a few years, if at all. The mortality of mitral valvotomy depends upon the severity of the disease and the presence of complications. If the patient is in reasonably good health prior to the operation, and free of severe pulmonary hypertension and mitral regurgitation, the mortality should be less than 5% and, in the most favourable cases, less than 1%. Where there is advanced pulmonary hypertension or right-sided failure, the mortality may rise to 10% or more. In reaching a decision as to whether valvotomy should be undertaken, one must take into account the mortality even in relatively mild cases, the possibility of producing mitral regurgitation, the relatively high incidence of re-stenosis and the risk of causing cerebral embolism. Operation should be avoided in the presence of rheumatic activity. Surgery should also be deferred until cardiac failure has been brought under control or if there has been recent pulmonary or systemic embolism.

Mitral valvotomy is indicated when there are symptoms attributable to pure or almost pure mitral stenosis. It should be considered when there are signs indicating severe stenosis, particularly if there is advanced pulmonary arterial hypertension, even in the absence of symptoms. 'Prophylactic' valvotomy should be undertaken in young women with moderate or severe stenosis to avoid operating during pregnancy.

Atrial fibrillation develops shortly after the operation in about one-quarter of cases but often resolves spontaneously within 3 weeks. If it fails to do so, correction with dc shock should be undertaken.

The postcardiotomy syndrome, which is characterized by pericarditis, pleurisy, pyrexia and malaise, may arise 1–8 weeks after surgery. It has been attributed to an autoimmune reaction to heart muscle, or to the presence of blood in the pericardium. Corticosteroids relieve the symptoms but are usually unnecessary.

Successful valvotomy is effective in reducing symptoms, but signs of residual stenosis usually persist. The loud first heart sound and opening snap remain, but the diastolic murmurs are shortened or abolished.

When there is marked rigidity or severe calcification of the valve cusps. mitral valve replacement must be undertaken. This requires cardiopulmonary bypass, with its increased risks, and involves the complications associated with the use of prosthetic materials (see also Chapter 18).

Because of an operative mortality of about 5%, and the risks of subsequent morbidity, mitral valve replacement should only be undertaken in patients in whom symptoms are severe or whose prognosis is clearly limited to a few years.

Mitral regurgitation

Mitral regurgitation can be caused by a number of different disease processes:

It is frequently the end-result of *rheumatic endocarditis* and may predominate over mitral stenosis. The valve cusps are usually rigid and deformed and the chordae tendineae fused and shortened. Calcification is common. In a small proportion of cases, however, the valve cusps are preserved, but the orifice enlarges as a consequence of scarring and dilatation of the mitral valve ring. Regurgitation may develop at the time of rheumatic fever, especially if this is severe, but does not usually produce major haemodynamic effects for several years because the progression of valve damage is slow.

Infective endocarditis may produce destruction or perforation of the cusps, or rupture of chordae tendineae.

Congenital mitral regurgitation occurs with or without other congenital abnormalities (see 'atrial septal defect', p. 241).

Papillary muscle malfunction or rupture may result from myocardial infarction.

Tearing of cusps may occur at *mitral valvotomy*.

Left ventricular dilatation from any cause, such as hypertension, coronary artery disease and aortic valve disease may lead to dilatation of the valve ring. The mitral regurgitation so produced leads to further enlargement of the left ventricle, and therefore further dilatation of the valve ring, with the development of a vicious circle.

Spontaneous rupture of chordae tendineae of unknown aetiology may occur.

Mitral valve prolapse (billowing or ballooning of the posterior mitral valve leaflet) is a common condition which may be associated with rheumatic and ischaemic heart disease and with the Marfan syndrome. Usually, however, there is no other disease process; in such cases, there is a myxomatous change of the valve leaflets, which are voluminous and redundant. The usual auscultatory finding is a midsystolic click and/or a late apical systolic murmur, but the click and murmur may occur at other times during systole. In any individual, the auscultatory features may vary considerably from time to time, and can be made to do so by standing, sitting, and straining in the Valsalva manoeuvre. Most patients are asymptomatic, but chest pain and arrhythmias affect some patients. The ECG may show minor ST abnormalities. Echocardiography (Fig. 7.15), which has demonstrated this abnormality in some 5% of normal young people, characteristically reveals a midsystolic 'buckling' of one or both leaflets into the left atrium. Some cases have a posterior 'hammocking' of the leaflets throughout systole. Although there is a slight risk of infective endocarditis and of serious arrhythmias, the prognosis is usually excellent. Patients with definitive evidence of mitral regurgitation should receive prophylaxis against infective endocarditis. Reassurance is an essential part of management; an anxiety state is the commonest complication of this lesion.

Pathophysiology

The severity of mitral regurgitation depends on a number of factors.

1   The size of the mitral valve orifice during ventricular systole. Although this can be of fixed size, as it is when the valve is calcified, it may be variable, depending on the degree of left ventricular dilatation.
2   The pressure relationships between the left ventricle, aorta and left atrium.
3   The left ventricular output.

Any factor which augments left ventricular output or raises aortic impedance increases mitral regurgitation. The degree of mitral regurgitation is limited by the distensibility of the left atrium and pulmonary veins. However, the pressure in the left atrium is much lower than that in the aorta, so that with a large valve orifice, as much blood may regurgitate into the left atrium during systole as is ejected into the aorta. A feature of chronic severe mitral regurgitation is that the left atrium is much larger than is usual in mitral stenosis.

During systole, the pressure in the left atrium may rise to a high 'v' peak, but will not do so if the regurgitated blood is readily accommodated in a voluminous left atrium. When mitral regurgitation develps abruptly, as with the rupture of papillary muscles or chordae tendineae, the left atrium is often small and the 'v' wave tall.

In diastole, there is a large flow from left atrium to left ventricle, consisting of the blood received from the pulmonary circulation combined with that which regurgitated during the preceding systole. At this time the pressure in the left atrium falls rapidly to the ventricular level. Therefore, although there may be a high 'v' wave the mean left atrial pressure is often not greatly raised, and the pulmonary capillary pressure is seldom as high as that encountered in mitral stenosis. Eventually, however, with the development of left ventricular failure, the pulmonary capillary pressure rises and, with it, the pulmonary arterial pressure. Severe pulmonary hypertension and right-sided cardiac failure are unusual unless there is also an appreciable degree of mitral stenosis.

Complications

The complications are similar to those of mitral stenosis. Atrial fibrillation is frequent when mitral regurgitation is of rheumatic origin but less so when other disease processes are responsible. Infective endocarditis is relatively common.

Symptoms

In cases of rheumatic origin, the physical signs precede symptoms by many years. When symptoms do occur, they usually increase slowly. Fatigue, perhaps attributable to the low cardiac output, may be the first complaint, but eventually dyspnoea on exertion, orthopnoea and, rarely, paroxysmal nocturnal dyspnoea develop.

When mitral regurgitation is due to perforation of a cusp, or to rupture of chordae tendineae or papillary muscles, the onset of symptoms is abrupt; the patient may present with acute pulmonary oedema.

Physical signs

The pulse is usually of normal volume; irregularity due to atrial fibrillation is common. The venous pressure is normal except when there is right-sided cardiac failure. The apex beat, which may be displaced downwards and outwards, often has the vigorous thrusting character of left ventricular hypertrophy and dilatation, and there is sometimes a systolic thrill.

The first sound is usually soft and introduces an apical pansystolic murmur which radiates to the axilla. The murmur may be of the same intensity throughout systole, but often increases towards the end of this period. When the regurgitation is due to papillary muscle malfunction or ballooning of a mitral cusp, the murmur may be exclusively in late systole. Rarely, it may radiate to the left sternal edge rather than to the axilla and may be mistaken for aortic stenosis. The intensity of the murmur bears some relation to the severity of the regurgitation, but is not a reliable guide. In most severe cases there is a third heart sound, followed by a short mid-diastolic murmur due to rapid filling of the left ventricle.

The ECG

The ECG may be normal but P mitrale is often present if atrial fibrillation has not supervened. Left ventricular hypertrophy occurs in severe mitral regurgitation, but if there is significant stenosis there may be evidence of biventricular hypertrophy or no abnormality.

Radiography and echocardiography

Radiologically, the most conspicuous feature is the marked enlargement of the left atrium, but there may also be left ventricular enlargement. Calcification of the mitral valve is often visible in rheumatic cases. Evidence of pulmonary dilatation and pulmonary oedema develops when there is left ventricular failure.

When mitral regurgitation is of acute onset due to malfunction or rupture of valve cusps, papillary muscles or chordae tendineae, there may be little left atrial or left ventricular enlargement in spite of high left atrial pressure and pulmonary oedema.

Echocardiography may not reveal any abnormality in mitral regurgitation, but if the reflux is large, there is dilatation of the left atrium and left ventricle. Calcification or thickening of the cusps may be seen. Other possible findings include mitral valve prolapse or a flail valve due to ruptured chordae or papillary muscles. Doppler ultrasound is a good technique for demonstrating mitral regurgitation, but does not allow accurate estimation of its severity.

Cardiac catheterization and angiocardiography

The confirmation and quantitation of mitral regurgitation is best made by injecting radio-opaque contrast medium into the left ventricle. Left ventriculography is of particular value in assessing the severity of mitral regurgitation complicating mitral stenosis. The presence of left ventricular failure may be confirmed by finding a high left ventricular end-diastolic pressure. A tall 'v' wave in the left atrial or pulmonary arterial wedge pressure tracing is suggestive of, but not diagnostic of, mitral regurgitation.

Diagnosis

The diagnosis is usually based on the finding of an apical pansystolic murmur radiating to the axilla. The pansystolic murmur of tricuspid regurgitation may reach the apex, but does not radiate further and is usually increased on inspiration. The systolic murmur of aortic stenosis may be heard best at the apex, but is midsystolic and does not radiate to the axilla. The murmur of ventricular septal defect is heard best at the lower left sternal edge.

It may be difficult to differentiate mitral regurgitation from a benign systolic murmur, but benign murmurs are never pansystolic, are seldom of grade 3 or greater intensity and tend to vary with posture and respiration.

Suggestive evidence of mitral regurgitation is provided by left atrial and left ventricular enlargement on the chest radiograph, and by P mitrale and left ventricular hypertrophy on the ECG. Echocardiography is valuable in prolapse of the mitral cusps and in ruptured chordae and papillary muscles. The definitive diagnosis is made by left ventriculography.

In mitral regurgitation of non-rheumatic origin, the diagnosis may be suggested by the sudden appearance of a loud apical systolic murmur accompanied by left ventricular failure.

Course and prognosis

The course of patients with mitral regurgitation is very variable. Those with mild regurgitation and without cardiomegaly may live a normal life span, although exposed to the risk of infective endocarditis. In rheumatic mitral regurgitation of moderate severity, the course is one of slow deterioration over 10–20 years with gradually increasing heart size until left ventricular failure develops. Unless this has been precipitated by a complication that can be corrected, the prognosis is then poor and death is likely to occur within a few years. When mitral regurgitation has been due to ruptured chordae tendineae, papillary muscles or cusps, the prognosis is generally poor, although the regurgitation is occasionally slight and well tolerated.

Medical treatment

Medical treatment does not differ from that for mitral stenosis, except that inotropic drugs, such as digitalis, may be of value even in sinus rhythm. Reduction in afterload, by vasodilator therapy, is helpful, particularly in acute mitral regurgitation.

Surgical treatment

Mitral regurgitation can be successfully treated surgically only under direct vision, with cardiopulmonary bypass. In some instances, it is possible to restore valve function by plicating the ring or ruptured chordae. In many cases, however, it is necessary to insert a mitral valve prosthesis. The problems associated with this are discussed on p. 321.

Because of the risks of open-heart surgery and of prosthetic valves, patients with mitral regurgitation should be considered for surgery only if they are becoming increasingly disabled and it is likely that they will succumb to their disease within a few years. The long-term outlook of mitral valve replacements is, as yet, inadequately known, although there are many patients who have received benefit from such valves for a period of more than 10 years.

Aortic valve disease

The normal aortic valve consists of three semi-lunar cusps attached to a fibrous valve ring. Immediately above the insertion of the valve cusps are the sinuses of Valsalva, from two of which the coronary arteries arise. In about 1% of individuals the aortic valve has only two cusps.

The aortic valve and adjacent structures may be involved in congenital, rheumatic, bacterial, syphilitic and atherosclerotic changes. Both stenosis and regurgitation may occur as isolated lesions but are often combined. Calcification of the cusps is an important factor in the development of aortic valve disease and is often responsible for the stenosis that occurs in those with congenitally bicuspid valves.

Aortic stenosis

Aortic stenosis is most commonly the result of disease of the aortic valve cusps, but may also be due to narrowing in the outflow tract of the left ventricle below the cusps (subvalvar) and, very rarely, a constriction in the first part of the aorta (supravalvar stenosis).

Aetiology and pathology

Aortic valve stenosis may be congenital, rheumatic or sclerotic. Most instances of aortic stenosis occur in late middle or old age, in whom there is no evidence of involvement of other valves. In these patients, calcification of the valve is severe and is largely responsible for the stenosis. Even at necropsy it is seldom possible to determine the aetiology, but many have congenitally bicuspid valves. Rheumatic aortic stenosis results from adherence of adjacent cusps with thickening, fibrosis and subsequent calcification.

Subvalvar aortic stenosis may result from a congenital membrane or from fibrous tissue situated in the outflow tract of the left ventricle. This may be combined with valve stenosis, and thus form a tunnel in the outflow tract. A distinctive form of subvalvar stenosis is caused by hypertrophy of the muscle of the outflow tract of the left ventricle, particularly affecting the interventricular septum. This disorder has received a large variety of names including 'idiopathic hypertrophic subvalvular aortic stenosis' and 'hypertrophic obstructive cardiomyopathy' (see also p. 189).

Supravalvar aortic stenosis is congenital and may be associated with a distinctive facial appearance and mental deficiency.

Aortic stenosis is commonly associated with regurgitation. This is especially so in rheumatic and congenital valve stenosis and in congenital subvalvar stenosis. It is seldom severe in the calcific stenosis of the elderly and almost unknown in hypertrophic subaortic stenosis. Mitral valve disease usually predominates over aortic stenosis in rheumatic valve disease.

The left ventricle hypertrophies in response to the pressure load imposed upon it. The weight of the heart is often doubled in severe cases. There is usually little ventricular dilatation unless there is associated aortic regurgitation. Coronary artery disease may coexist with aortic stenosis, but commonly the coronary arteries are larger than normal. In aortic valve stenosis, there is a dilatation of the ascending aorta (an effect of the jet of blood which is propelled through the valve).

Pathophysiology

A minor degree of stenosis has little or no effect upon the function of the heart; only when the area of the valve orifice is reduced to a quarter of the normal are there serious consequences. The left ventricle responds to the pressure load by contracting more forcibly, and the left ventricular systolic pressure increases (see Fig. 11.9). A systolic pressure difference develops between the left ventricle and aorta (Fig. 11.10). The magnitude of this difference in pressure depends on the size of the orifice and the flow of blood through it. The obstruction delays emptying of the left ventricle, so that the phase of ejection becomes prolonged. The cardiac output is usually maintained within the normal range but at the expense of a considerable increase in left ventricular work. In consequence, left ventricular hypertrophy increases progressively as the valve orifice narrows. Although the hypertrophy is a compensatory phenomenon, it eventually contributes to the burden on the heart. The thickened ventricle is less compliant and is therefore less easily filled during diastole; atrial contraction contributes more and more to the filling process. The hypertrophied muscle increasingly outstrips the ability of the coronary arteries to supply it with blood.

Symptoms

There is a characteristic triad of symptoms: breathlessness, syncope on exertion, and angina pectoris. To this may be added the liability to sudden death.

Breathlessness is the earliest symptom in most cases. Later orthopnoea and paroxysmal nocturnal dyspnoea may occur. Eventually, right-sided heart failure with peripheral oedema may develop.

Fig. 11.9 Relationships between left ventricular volume and pressure in the normal heart, in aortic stenosis and in aortic regurgitation. M_1 = mitral valve closure. A_2 = aortic valve closure. Note high pressure generated in aortic stenosis and large end-diastolic volume (at M_1), with increased stroke volume in aortic regurgitation.

Syncope is much commoner in aortic stenosis than in other types of valvar heart disease and its relationship to exertion is of diagnostic value. Its mechanism is uncertain, but it may be due to the inability of the heart to increase its output sufficiently, or to reflex vasodilatation, or to arrhythmias.

Like syncope, anginal pain is much commoner in aortic stenosis than in other valve lesions. It does not differ in character from that seen in coronary artery disease.

Death is often sudden and may not be preceded by any symptoms. However, it is particularly likely to occur in those who have experienced syncope or angina pectoris. It is believed that ventricular fibrillation is usually responsible.

Physical signs

An aortic systolic murmur is the first abnormality to appear and may be present for decades before evidence of severe stenosis develops.

The pulse is abnormal in most severe cases (Fig. 11.11). Characteristically it is small in volume, rises slowly to its peak, and takes an unusually long time to pass the finger. The pulse pressure is correspondingly small. When there is an appreciable degree

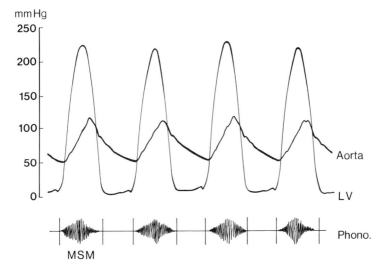

Fig. 11.10 Simultaneous pressure recordings and phonocardiographic appearances in aortic stenosis. Note the systolic pressure difference ('gradient') between the left ventricle and aorta, and the corresponding midsystolic murmur (MSM).

Fig. 11.11 Small, flat pulse in aortic stenosis.

of aortic regurgitation as well, the pulse pressure may be normal or large, and the pulse may take on a 'bisferiens' quality in which a double pulse is felt.

The apex beat may be in the normal position or displaced downwards and to the left. It has a slow heaving quality. A systolic thrill can often be felt in the second right intercostal space, and also in the carotid arteries and along the left edge of the sternum.

There is a midsystolic murmur, which is usually loud and harsh. This may be best heard in the second right interspace, along the left sternal edge, or even at the apex. It is often audible over the carotid arteries. It is accompanied by an early systolic ('ejection') click in those cases in which there is aortic valve stenosis without heavy calcification. This sign is probably due to sudden tension of the valve cusps at the time of opening. Other signs may include a fourth (atrial) heart sound over the left ventricle and reversed splitting of the second heart sound. This latter sign is due to delay in left ventricular emptying and aortic valve closure. The aortic component of the second heart sound may not be audible if there is calcification.

ECG, chest radiography, echocardiography and Doppler ultrasound

The ECG usually shows left ventricular hypertrophy, the extent of which roughly parallels the severity of the stenosis. Other abnormalities which sometimes occur include asymmetrical inversion of T waves and left bundle branch block. The chest radiograph may be normal, but the ascending aorta is usually dilated in aortic valve stenosis. Left ventricular enlargement may be evident. Calcification of the valve when present is best visualized by fluoroscopy. Apex cardiography is of value in demonstrating large 'a' waves which provide an index of severity.

Echocardiography may reveal thickening and calcification of the cusps; bicuspid valves are seen to open eccentrically. The supravalvar or subvalvar location of the obstruction may be apparent. Doppler ultrasound (Fig. 11.12) can be used to estimate the severity of aortic stenosis, and may obviate the need for cardiac catheterization. It is of particular value in allowing the non-invasive follow-up of patients who do not have a critical stenosis when first seen.

Cardiac catheterization

The systolic pressure difference across the stenosis is measured with catheters in left ventricle and aorta or by the withdrawal of a catheter from left ventricle to aorta (Fig. 11.13). If the stenosis is severe, the left ventricular systolic pressure exceeds that in the aorta by more than 50 mmHg. In advanced cases the cardiac output falls, and the gradient may be less than this in spite of extreme narrowing.

Complications

The most frequent cause of death is cardiac failure, but there is considerable risk of sudden death. Infective endocarditis may occur and, by eroding the cusps, cause severe aortic regurgitation.

(Facing Page)

Fig. 11.12 Continuous wave Doppler recording in a patient with aortic stenosis and atrial fibrillation. The height of the signal varies with the velocity of the jet and in this case varies from cycle to cycle depending on the preceding cycle length. The maximum velocity is 6 metres per second which calculates out at a gradient of 144 mmHg.

ECG

CW
DOPPLER

Fig. 11.13   (A) Pressure tracing recorded as catheter is withdrawn from left ventricle to aorta in aortic valve stenosis. Note sudden fall in systolic pressure as the catheter tip enters the aorta. (B) Pressure tracing from the left ventricular body (LV), subvalvar area of left ventricle, and aorta, when catheter is withdrawn from left ventricle to aorta in subaortic stenosis. Note the fall in systolic pressure as the catheter is withdrawn past the subvalvar stenotic area, with preservation of the left ventricular diastolic pressure. No further systolic fall is observed as the catheter is withdrawn into the aorta, but the diastolic pressure rises.

Diagnosis and differential diagnosis

The diagnosis is often suggested by the triad of symptoms (dyspnoea, angina, syncope on exertion), or by the finding of the typical murmur associated with a thrill and a small pulse. Calcification of the valve seen on fluoroscopy provides confirmatory evidence. Hypertrophic subaortic stenosis can be differentiated from other varieties by the pulse, which rises rapidly rather than slowly, and by the absence of an ejection click, valve calcification and aortic regurgitation; the diagnosis is established by echocardiography.

Systolic murmurs in the aortic area occur not only in aortic stenosis, but also when the aortic valve is sclerosed, and when the aorta is dilated by hypertension, atherosclerosis or syphilis. These conditions are not associated with the small pulse and massive left ventricular hypertrophy characteristic of aortic stenosis.

Prognosis

Cases of mild aortic stenosis have a good prognosis; if there is no appreciable degree of left ventricular hypertrophy, the patient is likely to survive for many years. Once the symptoms of breathlessness, angina or syncope have developed, death is likely to occur suddenly at any time, or within 5 years from heart failure.

Treatment

Little or no benefit can be expected from medical treatment. When symptoms have developed, strenuous activity should be avoided and the conventional treatment of heart failure and angina pectoris employed. Surgery is indicated for nearly all patients; this necessitates open-heart techniques. In some cases of non-calcific aortic valve stenosis and in subvalvar stenosis, corrective operations to widen the stenosed orifice may be successful. When there is calcification of the aortic valve, it must be replaced. For this purpose, either prosthetic valves, homograft or heterograft valves can be inserted (see p. 321). The mortality of aortic valve replacement varies greatly from centre to centre, but averages about 5%. This risk must be weighed against the grave prognosis in those with advanced symptoms.

Aortic regurgitation (Synonyms: aortic incompetence, insufficiency)

Aetiology

Aortic regurgitation is commonly due to rheumatic heart disease. It can also be of congenital origin, in which case it is usually of less importance than the lesions which accompany it, such as aortic and subaortic stenosis and ventricular septal defect. Other causes include bicuspid valves, hypertension, infective endocarditis, the Marfan syndrome, dissecting aneurysm, syphilitic aortitis, ankylosing spondylitis and Reiter's disease. In a substantial proportion of cases no cause can be found, i.e. they are 'idiopathic'.

Pathology

Aortic regurgitation can result either from damage to the cusps or from dilatation of the aorta and the valve ring. In rheumatic heart disease, the cusps are thickened and shortened and there may be some fusion of commissures. Varying degrees of stenosis and regurgitation occur. Calcification of the valve, which is usually severe in aortic stenosis, is seldom of importance in pure aortic regurgitation.

Syphilitic aortitis leads to aortic regurgitation as a result of dilatation of the aorta and the valve ring; stenosis is not a feature.

Infective endocarditis can cause erosion or perforation of the cusps, which have usually had some pre-existing abnormality.

Pathophysiology

In aortic regurgitation, a large volume of blood is regurgitated into the left ventricle in each diastole. The left ventricular output may be more than doubled. The increased stroke volume necessary to achieve this is associated with dilatation of the left ventricle (see Fig. 11.10). The regurgitant flow is greatest in early diastole when the difference in pressure between the aorta and left ventricle is maximal. The amount of blood that regurgitates is largely determined by the severity of the aortic valve disease but is also influenced by the compliance of the left ventricle and the systemic vascular resistance.

The dilated left ventricle contracts more powerfully in accordance with Starling's law, but there is an increased tension in the myocardium and increased oxygen consumption. The initial dilatation thus leads eventually to hypertrophy.

The diastolic pressure in the aorta is abnormally low, partly due to the leak and partly to peripheral vasodilatation. The left ventricular end-diastolic pressure is normal in the milder case but rises when cardiac failure supervenes.

Clinical features

Rheumatic aortic regurgitation usually develops at the time of acute rheumatic carditis and persists subsequently. Many years elapse between the appearance of the murmur and the onset of symptoms.

Almost invariably the first complaint is that of dyspnoea on exertion, although fatigue is also frequent. Other minor symptoms include dizziness and an awareness of the vigorous heart action.

The dyspnoea progresses slowly; eventually orthopnoea and paroxysmal dyspnoea may develop. Typical angina pectoris is infrequent except when the regurgitation is severe. In the advanced case, signs of right-sided failure complicate those of left-sided failure.

The arterial pulse in aortic regurgitation, often called 'collapsing' or 'water-hammer', rises rapidly and falls abruptly. This is most easily appreciated by placing the palm of one's hand on the anterior aspect of the patient's forearm (the arm being held vertically upright) because by this means one may accentuate the backflow of blood during diastole. Sometimes the pulse is of bisferiens type, i.e. is felt to have two equally prominent waves, particularly if the regurgitation is accompanied by stenosis. The cardiac rhythm is usually normal unless there is associated mitral valve disease. The systolic pressure is often abnormally high and the diastolic low. In a severe case the systolic pressure may be 250–300 mmHg and the diastolic 30–50 mmHg. Vigorous arterial pulsation is often visible in the neck.

If the regurgitation is substantial, the apex beat is displaced outwards and downwards and is overactive and heaving. The essential feature on auscultation is an early diastolic murmur, usually best heard over the midsternal region or at the lower left sternal edge. In some cases, particularly in syphilitic aortitis, it is loudest in the second right intercostal space. There is often an accompanying systolic murmur; this does not necessarily indicate coexistent aortic stenosis but may be due to the increased stroke volume. The early (or 'immediate') diastolic murmur is often difficult to hear, and is frequently overlooked by the inexperienced. It must be specifically sought, with the stethoscope diaphragm placed at the lower left sternal edge, with the patient sitting up, his breath held in expiration.

In some patients with advanced aortic regurgitation, a mid-diastolic murmur may be heard even in the absence of mitral stenosis. This murmur (known as the Austin Flint murmur) has been attributed to the effect of the regurgitant jet on the aortic leaflet of the mitral valve which is interposed between the mitral and aortic valve orifices (see Fig. 11.2). One should hesitate to diagnose an Austin Flint murmur in rheumatic heart disease because concomitant mitral stenosis is likely, particularly if there is a loud first sound or opening snap.

ECG, chest radiography, echocardiography and Doppler ultrasound

The ECG shows increasing evidence of left ventricular hypertrophy as the disease process advances. On the chest radiograph, there is usually left ventricular enlargement, with an elongated heart shadow and dilatation of the ascending aorta. Echocardiography often shows a vibration of the anterior leaflet of the mitral valve, and, if the regurgitation is severe, the mitral valve is seen to close abnormally early. Doppler ultrasound is a sensitive technique for demonstrating the presence, but not the severity, of aortic regurgitation.

Cardiac catheterization

Gross aortic regurgitation is so readily recognized clinically and by non-invasive methods that cardiac catheterization is seldom required for diagnostic purposes. This investigation is, however, necessary when the degree of severity is in doubt; it is of particular value in evaluating the significance of an aortic diastolic murmur in a patient needing surgery for concomitant mitral valve disease. The cine-angiographic demonstration of the regurgitation of contrast medium injected into the aorta provides a good estimate of severity.

Differential diagnosis

The clinical diagnosis of aortic regurgitation is usually not difficult if it is moderate or severe. A large pulse pressure is also observed in other conditions, such as persistent ductus arteriosus, arteriovenous fistulae, pregnancy, anaemia and thyrotoxicosis. The early diastolic murmur may be confused with that of pulmonary regurgitation, but this rare lesion is seldom found in the absence of severe pulmonary hypertension. Doppler ultrasound is useful in differentiating the two conditions, and echocardiographic demonstration of fluttering of the mitral valve is very suggestive of the aortic origin of the regurgitation.

In determining the aetiology of aortic regurgitation, it is important to look for other valve lesions and for evidence of disease in other systems. The signs of mitral stenosis or regurgitation suggest a rheumatic origin. Syphilis should be suspected particularly when there is aneurysmal dilatation of the aorta or calcification of the ascending aorta. Congenital aortic regurgitation is usually overshadowed by aortic or subaortic stenosis.

Clinical course and prognosis

Minor degrees of aortic regurgitation are compatible with freedom from symptoms and a normal life span although the risk of infective endocarditis is ever present. In the moderate to severe case, symptoms and signs develop slowly, and it is usually not until the fourth or fifth decade that disability sets in. The severity of aortic regurgitation can be judged, to a large extent, by the pulse pressure and the size of the left ventricle. Increasing dyspnoea and an enlarging heart are signs that the patient is unlikely to survive for more than a few years. Sudden death is unusual in asymptomatic patients but may occur when an advanced stage has been reached.

Treatment

In less severe cases, considerable symptomatic improvement can be obtained by conventional treatment of cardiac failure such as the restriction of activity, and the use of digitalis and diuretics. When symptoms or heart size are increasing in spite of medical measures, surgery should be considered. In good hands the results of aortic valve replacement, either by artificial valves or bioprostheses are reasonably satisfactory, but there is an operative mortality of about 5%. Artificial prostheses necessitate anticoagulant therapy; bioprostheses do not. Successful surgery is accompanied by a diminution in heart size, although not necessarily to normal. Symptoms are relieved, but medical measures may still be required.

Combined aortic stenosis and regurgitation

Aortic stenosis and regurgitation are often combined. When the lesion is congenital, atherosclerotic or calcific, the stenosis is usually the more important. In rheumatic heart disease, all gradations between the two can occur. In deciding which is dominant, the character of the pulse and the pulse pressure are of great value. A collapsing pulse is incompatible with severe stenosis; a small pulse makes major regurgitation unlikely. The murmurs can be deceptive as loud aortic systolic murmurs are not uncommon in aortic regurgitation even when stenosis is slight or absent. Likewise, the intensity of an aortic diastolic murmur is an unreliable guide to the severity of regurgitation. Echocardiography and Doppler ultrasound supplemented, if necessary, by cardiac catheterization and angiocardiography permit adequate assessment of the relative contribution of each lesion.

Tricuspid valve disease

The structure of the tricuspid valve is similar to that of the mitral valve, except for the presence of three cusps. It may be affected by either stenosis or regurgitation. Tricuspid stenosis is nearly always rheumatic in origin and is rarely the dominant cardiac lesion. Some degree of tricuspid stenosis occurs in about 10% of cases of rheumatic heart disease, but is of significance in only about 3%. Organic tricuspid regurgitation, which is uncommon, is usually due to rheumatic heart disease. Functional tricuspid regurgitation is a frequent complication of right ventricular failure whatever the cause.

When tricuspid valve lesions are due to rheumatic heart disease, the pathological appearances are similar to those seen in the mitral valve. The valve cusps are thickened and the chordae may be adherent and shortened. Dilatation of the tricuspid valve ring is a major factor in regurgitation and occurs as a result of either dilatation of the right ventricle or the rheumatic process.

Tricuspid stenosis

The narrowed valve obstructs flow from the right atrium to the right ventricle during ventricular diastole. As a consequence, right atrial pressure rises, cardiac output falls, and the right atrium and venae cavae dilate. Atrial contraction becomes increasingly forceful and produces large 'a' waves in the venous pulse if sinus rhythm is preserved as it usually is. Hepatic engorgement follows and ascites and peripheral oedema eventually develop.

In most cases of tricuspid stenosis, mitral stenosis is also present and dominates the clinical picture. For this reason, breathlessness is the commonest symptom, but because tricuspid stenosis restricts right ventricular throughput, pulmonary congestion is often less severe than it is in isolated mitral stenosis. The patient with mitral stenosis may become less breathless as tricuspid stenosis progresses, but at the expense of right-sided cardiac failure.

Large flicking venous 'a' waves may be seen even in early cases. When the lesion is more advanced the venous pressure as a whole is elevated. The 'a' wave disappears when atrial fibrillation develops. The flow of blood from the atrium into the ventricle during diastole is slow and the 'y' descent of the venous pulse is therefore prolonged. The liver is enlarged and may exhibit presystolic pulsation corresponding with the large 'a' waves. On auscultation, mid-diastolic and presystolic murmurs may be heard at the lower left sternal edge which are similar in timing to those of mitral stenosis but of a rather more scratchy quality. The murmurs are accentuated by inspiration, because of increased venous return to the right atrium at this time. It is not uncommon in the patient with tricuspid stenosis for the signs of mitral stenosis to be masked.

On the ECG the only characteristic feature is the presence of the tall P waves of right atrial enlargement. The chest radiograph shows enlargement of the right atrium and superior vena cava; the features of mitral stenosis are also usually present. The lung fields are often relatively clear. Echocardiography may reveal reduced movement or thickening of the cusps.

On cardiac catheterization, a diastolic pressure difference can be demonstrated between right atrium and right ventricle, and there is usually a large 'a' wave in the right atrial pulse.

The prognosis of patients with tricuspid stenosis is often relatively good. However, if the lesion is severe, progressive signs of right-sided cardiac failure develop; ascites, jaundice and cachexia are characteristic.

In the majority of patients with tricuspid stenosis, the lesion is

insufficiently severe to warrant surgery, which should be undertaken only if the stenosis is responsible for major symptoms.
Valvotomy seldom restores normal valve function; replacement
by a prosthesis is usually necessary.

Tricuspid regurgitation

As mentioned, functional tricuspid regurgitation is a common
complication of right ventricular failure and pulmonary hypertension. Since most patients with this condition have evidence of
rheumatic heart disease, it is often difficult to be sure whether or
not there is organic tricuspid disease as well. One can, however,
deduce that the regurgitation is functional if the signs disappear
with the use of digitalis and diuretics or the successful treatment
of mitral valve disease.

The features of tricuspid regurgitation are the consequence of a
large volume of blood being regurgitated through the valve from
the right ventricle. As a result, the forward flow into the pulmonary circuit is reduced and the right ventricle has to cope with a
large volume load. When regurgitation is severe, large systolic
('cv') waves develop in the right atrium, which are transmitted to
the peripheral veins and liver. There is a high flow of blood
through the tricuspid valve during diastole, as both the regurgitated and the forward flow must be transported at this time. Both
diastolic and systolic flow through the valve is increased on
inspiration as an increased volume of blood is drawn into the
heart.

Coexistent mitral valve disease usually dominates the clinical
picture and dyspnoea is the major symptom. Tricuspid regurgitation may reduce the effects of the mitral valve disease on the
lungs at the expense of producing right-sided heart failure. As
the disease progresses, there is an increase in venous pressure,
hepatic enlargement, ascites and peripheral oedema. Large systolic
waves are present in the jugular veins; systolic pulsation of the
liver may be felt. A systolic murmur is heard at the lower left
sternal edge; this is usually increased on inspiration. There may
also be a tricuspid diastolic murmur due either to concomitant
tricuspid stenosis or to high flow through the orifice during this
phase.

There are no specific ECG features of tricuspid regurgitation;
the chest radiograph usually shows right atrial enlargement. If
the tricuspid regurgitation is secondary to mitral valve disease
and pulmonary hypertension, the characteristic radiological features of these lesions will be present.

On cardiac catheterization, the chief feature is the large systolic venous wave of the right atrial pulse. The finding of severe pulmonary hypertension suggests the regurgitation is functional. A near normal pulmonary artery pressure is an indication that the tricuspid disease is organic.

It is often difficult to differentiate mitral regurgitation from tricuspid regurgitation, or to determine whether there is a combination of the two. Mitral regurgitation is suggested by radiation of the murmur to the axilla and by left ventricular enlargement, tricuspid regurgitation by systolic venous pulsation and by inspiratory accentuation of the murmur. Doppler ultrasound is a sensitive technique for detecting tricuspid regurgitation and gives some impression of its severity.

Tricuspid regurgitation is often tolerated for a long time, but sooner or later the features of advanced right-sided cardiac failure become disabling, often with jaundice and cachexia. Severe oedema and ascites develop and are progressively less responsive to treatment.

If the tricuspid regurgitation is functional, there may be striking improvement with digitalis and diuretic therapy. Usually, surgery for associated mitral valve disease is required, and, if successful, leads to the disappearance of the tricuspid leak. When severe tricuspid regurgitation does not diminish in response to these measures, repair or replacement of the valve by a prosthesis becomes necessary.

Pulmonary valve disease

Pulmonary valve disease is relatively uncommon. Pulmonary stenosis is usually of congenital origin and is discussed in Chapter 12. Other causes of pulmonary stenosis include rheumatic heart disease, and malignant carcinoid. Obstruction of the outflow tract of the right ventricle may occur in hypertrophic cardiomyopathy and mediastinal tumours.

Pulmonary regurgitation is usually secondary to pulmonary hypertension, but occasionally occurs as a consequence of infective endocarditis, as a complication of the surgical relief of pulmonary stenosis, and as a congenital anomaly. It is nearly always overshadowed by the heart disease to which it is secondary. In most cases, there are signs of pulmonary hypertension, and the only feature which suggests the diagnosis is an early diastolic murmur (the Graham Steell murmur) in the second or third left intercostal spaces which becomes louder on inspiration. It is often difficult to decide whether a murmur in this position is due to pulmonary or aortic regurgitation. Pulmonary regurgitation is unlikely in the absence of signs of pulmonary hypertension and right ventricular hypertrophy. Aortic regurgitation is suggested by a collapsing pulse and the signs of left ventricular hypertrophy, although these signs may be absent if the regurgitation is slight. The diagnosis may be confirmed by Doppler ultrasound. Pulmonary regurgitation seldom produces serious haemodynamic effects and its prognosis and treatment are those of the associated pulmonary hypertension.

Further reading

Bonchek, L.J. (1981) Current status of cardiac valve replacement: selection of a prosthesis and indications for operation. *American Heart Journal* 101: 96.

Greenberg, B.H. & Murphy, E. (Eds) (1987) *Valvular Heart Disease.* Littleton: PSG.

Hall, R.J.C. & Julian, D.G. (1988) *Diseases of the Cardiac Valves.* Edinburgh: Churchill Livingstone.

Key References (1982) Natural history of valvular heart disease *Circulation* 65: 1283.

Rapaport, E. (1975) Natural history of aortic and mitral valve disease. *American Journal of Cardiology 35:* 221.

Symposium (1987) Clinical and epidemiological issues in mitral valve prolapse. *American Heart Journal 113:* 1265.

Congenital Heart Disease

A congenital abnormality of the heart is present in nearly one in every hundred babies born. About half of the affected babies die either from their heart disease or from some associated congenital anomaly during the first year of life if untreated. The prognosis of those who survive this period is reasonably good; from 5 years of age until early adult life, the prevalence of congenital heart disease remains at about three per thousand. The less severe types of lesion then begin to take their toll and it is unusual for patients with uncorrected congenital heart disease to survive much beyond the age of 40. Most forms of congenital heart disease are amenable to surgery; in some cases this leads to cure, but in others some residual abnormality is left that may require continuing attention.

Embryology

At an early stage, the heart consists of a simple tube of endocardium surrounded by myocardium and epicardium. As it grows, the tube twists into an S shape and by the fourth week of pregnancy it is divided by constrictions into five segments: (1) the sinus venosus, which receives the systemic veins, (2) the common atrium, (3) the common ventricle, (4) the bulbus cordis, and (5) the truncus arteriosus (Fig. 12.1). Between the fifth and eighth week, changes of the greatest importance occur; it is at this time that congenital abnormalities are most likely to arise through arrested or faulty development. Septa develop in the atria and in the ventricles to subdivide each of these chambers into two. Simultaneously, the atria are divided from the ventricles by endocardial cushions from which the mitral and tricuspid valves are formed (Fig. 12.2A). A spiral septum divides the bulbus cordis into the outflow tracts of the left and right ventricles respectively, and the truncus arteriosus into aorta and pulmonary artery (Fig. 12.2B).

By the end of the eighth week, the heart has largely assumed the features which it retains until birth. The right atrium in the fetal circulation then receives blood from the superior vena cava and from the vitello-umbilical veins which later become the inferior vena cava. A proportion of the venous blood, particularly that from the superior vena cava, flows into the right ventricle,

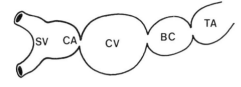

Fig. 12.1 The heart at the fourth week of pregnancy, divided by constrictions into sinus venosus (SV), common atrium (CA), common ventricle (CV), bulbus cordis (BC) and truncus arteriosus (TA).

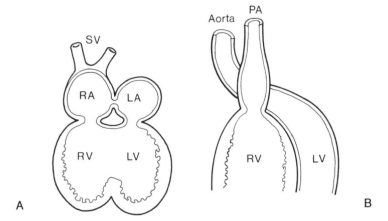

Fig. 12.2 (A) The heart at 8 weeks. The ventricles and atria are each being divided by septa into two chambers. Endocardial cushions develop from which the mitral and tricuspid valves are formed. (B) The spiral septum divides the bulbus cordis into the outflow tracts of the left and right ventricles, and the truncus arteriosus into the aorta and pulmonary arteries.

thence into the pulmonary artery and, by way of the ductus arteriosus, into the descending aorta. Only about 5% of the blood flow traverses the pulmonary circulation. Most of the highly oxygenated inferior vena caval blood is directed through the foramen ovale in the atrial septum into the left atrium and thence, by the left ventricle, into the ascending aorta. Within a few hours or, at most, days of birth the ductus arteriosus closes, and the relatively high pressure in the left atrium keeps the valve of the foramen ovale shut.

Aetiology

No aetiological factor can be found in most cases of congenital heart disease. In a minority there is evidence of either a genetic abnormality or an environmental factor affecting the mother during the early stages of pregnancy.

When congenital malformations are multiple, particularly in Down's syndrome (mongolism or Trisomy 21), Turner's syndrome and Marfan's syndrome, the heart is often involved. Congenital heart disease rarely affects more than one member of a family. If rubella occurs during the first 3 months of pregnancy, there is a considerable risk of cardiac malformation in the fetus. Other virus infections may occasionally be responsible, as may some drugs, including thalidomide, warfarin and alcohol.

The varieties of congenital heart disease

The varieties of congenital heart disease can be divided into three types.

1. Communications between the left (systemic) and right (pulmonary) circulations, e.g. atrial septal defect, ventricular septal defect and persistent ductus arteriosus.

The impedance to flow is normally lower on the right side of the heart and in the pulmonary artery than it is on the left side of the heart and in the aorta. Consequently, the intracardiac pressures are relatively low on the right side. When the two sides of the heart are in communication, provided there is no other abnormality, there is a shunt of blood from left to right through the defect and an increased blood flow through the lungs. In ventricular septal defect and persistent ductus arteriosus, the volume load falls predominantly on the left ventricle, which enlarges accordingly. In atrial septal defect, the load falls on the right ventricle.

The greatly increased pulmonary blood flow frequently leads to a moderate elevation of pulmonary arterial pressure. In most cases, the resistance of the pulmonary arteries is normal but, sometimes, changes take place in the arterial walls which cause a high pulmonary vascular resistance. Severe and irreversible pulmonary hypertension may then ensue and, eventually, lead to reversal of the shunt (Eisenmenger syndrome p. 255).

2. Obstructive lesions, e.g. coarctation of the aorta, aortic stenosis and pulmonary stenosis.

When these lesions are isolated, they impose a burden on the related ventricle and may eventually cause cardiac failure on this account. They may be combined with abnormal communications, the most important anomaly being that of tetralogy of Fallot, in which there is pulmonary stenosis with a ventricular septal defect.

3. *Displacement or absence of chambers, vessels or valves.* These may be associated with abnormal communications or obstructions. Some displacement lesions such as dextrocardia and right-sided aorta may be unimportant. Others, such as transposition of the great arteries, are associated with a high mortality.

Abnormal communications

Atrial septal defect (ASD)

The foramen ovale, which is unsealed in some 25% of adults, does not normally permit the flow of blood from the left atrium to the right atrium because of its valvar construction (Fig. 12.3A).

There are three types of abnormality which permit a flow of oxygenated blood into the right atrium (Fig. 12.3 B, C and D.)

1 The ostium secundum defect, which may be large but does not encroach upon the atrioventricular valves. This is much the commonest variety.
2 The ostium primum defect which is situated close to the atrioventricular valves and is often associated wth abnormalities of these valves and, sometimes, with a partial or complete atrioventricular defect ('endocardial cushion' defect).
3 One or more of the pulmonary veins may be attached to the right atrium or great veins instead of the left atrium. There is usually an atrial septal defect as well.

The right ventricle is normally thinner and more distensible than the left and, at a given pressure level, more easily filled with blood. Therefore when both atria are in communication, blood flows preferentially into the right ventricle from both atria and the shunt through the defect is almost exclusively from left to right. The pulmonary blood flow is usually two or three times the aortic blood flow, but the distensibility of pulmonary arterioles is such that they can readily accommodate this with little or no increase in pulmonary arterial pressure. The increase of pulmonary blood flow maintained over many years, however, sometimes leads to changes in the small pulmonary vessels which increase pulmonary vascular resistance and cause severe pulmonary hypertension.

Defects of the atrial septum seldom give rise to disabling symptoms before the third decade of life, but breathlessness and

Fig. 12.3 (A) Unsealed foramen ovale. The valvar construction of the foramen ovale prevents shunting from left to right. (B) Atrial septal defect of ostium secundum type. The valve cusps are not affected. (C) Anomalous drainage of the right pulmonary veins into the right atrium, associated with an atrial septal defect of the secundum type. (D) Ostium primum defect, associated with abnormalities of the mitral or tricuspid valves.

fatigue are likely to develop before the age of 40. Symptoms are usually progressive and are exacerbated when atrial arrhythmias develop, as they commonly do.

The arterial pulse is relatively small; the venous pressure is usually normal. The right ventricle is strikingly overactive. Splitting of the second sound is wide, and varies little with respiration. This is due to relatively late closure of the pulmonary valve as a consequence of delayed emptying of the overburdened right ventricle. A systolic murmur in the second left interspace due to high flow across the pulmonary valve is almost invariable. Larger defects causes mid-diastolic murmur at the lower left sternal edge, accentuated by inspiration, and produced by increased flow through the tricuspid valve. In the ostium primum type of defect, in which an abnormal mitral valve may permit regurgitation, there may be left ventricular enlargement and an apical systolic murmur.

The ECG nearly always shows the features of partial right bundle branch block ('rsr' complex). In the common ostium secundum type, there is frequently right axis deviation, whilst in the ostium primum type there is usually left axis deviation. This feature is of importance in differentiating the two types of defect (Fig. 12.4).

On the chest radiograph, the heart is usually slightly enlarged, and the pulmonary artery and its branches prominent, as are the right atrium and the right ventricle. The aorta is abnormally small and may not be visible. Expansile pulsation of the pulmonary arteries ('hilar dance') may be a striking feature on fluoroscopy.

Echocardiography, in ostium secundum defect, demonstrates 'paradoxical' septal motion. As a result of right ventricular overloading, the septum moves towards the right ventricle in systole instead of its usual movement towards the posterior left ventricular wall at this time.

In ostium primum, abnormalities of the mitral valve are usual.

Cross-sectional echocardiography reliably demonstrates primum and secundum defects and differentiates easily between them. Doppler ultrasound provides supporting evidence and may permit an assessment of the shunt.

These clinical features are usually sufficiently characteristic for accurate diagnosis. Confirmation by cardiac catheterization is

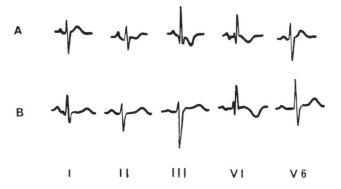

Fig. 12.4 ECG appearances in (A) ostium secundum defect, and (B) ostium primum defect. Note left axis deviation in the latter.

required when the diagnosis is in doubt or surgical treatment is planned. The oxygen saturation in the right atrium is markedly higher than that in the superior vena cava, and the catheter tip may be advanced through the septal defect into the left atrium and thence to the left ventricle. In the ostium primum defect, injection of radio-opaque contrast medium into the left ventricle often reveals mitral regurgitation. When there are anomalies of the pulmonary veins (Fig. 12.3C), the anomalous veins may be entered directly from the right atrium, or, occasionally, from connections to the superior or inferior venae cavae.

Closure of an ostium secundum defect is relatively easy, carries a low mortality and is advisable in all patients with pulmonary blood flow more than twice the systemic blood flow. Correction of the ostium primum type of defect, with its associated anomalies, is more difficult and carries a higher mortality. Surgery is usually undertaken if there are symptoms or when the shunt is large.

Ventricular septal defect (VSD)

The ventricular septum consists of four components: the trabecular or muscular septum extending to the apex, the inlet or posterior septum lying between the atrioventricular valves, the outlet or infundibular septum subtending the great arteries, and the membranous septum which lies under the aortic root and abuts on to the other three components. Defects can arise in any one of these components, but the membranous septum is the most commonly affected.

Defects of the ventricular septum, which may be large in relation to the size of the heart at birth, tend to become smaller or to close in early childhood. If closure is insufficient to prevent a large shunt, the small pulmonary vessels may be damaged by being exposed to the ejectile force and pressure of left ventricular contraction. Irreversible pulmonary hypertension may be produced.

The effect of a ventricular septal defect depends upon its size and upon the impedance to blood flow imposed by the pulmonary arterial vessels. If the defect is small, the jet of blood from the high-pressure left ventricle to the low-pressure right ventricle has little haemodynamic effect. If the defect is large and the impedance of the pulmonary vessels low, a large shunt develops and the pulmonary blood flow becomes more than twice the systemic flow. If, on the other hand, there is a high pulmonary vascular resistance, the pulmonary blood flow is little or no more than the systemic and the pressure in both circuits is similar. If the pulmonary vascular resistance is very high, the shunt reverses.

In the patient with a small defect ('maladie de Roger'), there are no symptoms, but there is a loud 'tearing' pansystolic murmur accompanied by a thrill, maximal to the left side of the lower sternum.

A large left-to-right shunt at ventricular level is liable to produce cardiac failure in the second or third month after birth. The special problems associated with this type of abnormality are discussed under the section 'The diagnosis and management of the infant with heart failure and cyanosis' (p. 259). If a large shunt does not produce symptoms during infancy, there is usually little disturbance until late adolescence or early adult life. Breathlessness and fatigue may then develop and cardiac failure subsequently ensue. In the presence of a large left-to-right shunt with pulmonary blood flow greater than twice systemic, the pulse is usually small and the venous pressure normal, unless there is right heart failure. Both left and right ventricles may be hyperdynamic, and there may or may not be a systolic thrill between the apex and the left sternal edge. A pansystolic murmur is heard at this site, usually accompanied by a mid-diastolic murmur at the apex due to high flow through the mitral valve.

In patients with a high pulmonary vascular resistance, breathlessness, fatigue and cyanosis are likely to develop during the second or third decade with progression to effort syncope, recurrent haemoptysis or heart failure. The signs of the ventricular septal defect are then less obvious, although there may still be a systolic murmur between the apex and the left sternal edge. Right ventricular hypertrophy is evident; the pulmonary second sound may be accentuated and followed by the early diastolic murmur of pulmonary regurgitation.

The ECG in small defects is normal. When the left-to-right shunt is large there is usually evidence of biventricular enlargement, manifested by abnormally deep but narrow Q waves and tall R waves in the left chest leads and an rsr pattern in V1. In cases with a high pulmonary vascular resistance, the ECG pattern of isolated right ventricular hypertrophy develops.

The chest radiograph is normal with a small defect, but with a large left-to-right shunt there is some enlargement of the heart and, more specifically, prominence of the pulmonary vessels, left atrium and both ventricles.

With small defects, the cross-sectional echocardiogram is often normal. With larger defects, there is usually a 'drop-out' of septal echoes, and both left atrium and ventricle may be enlarged. Doppler ultrasound can usually provide unequivocal evidence of a ventricular septal defect and, in association with echocardiography, permit an assessment of its size and the flow through it.

Correlation of these features usually provides sufficient evidence for accurate clinical diagnosis in spite of the various forms which defects of the ventricular septum may take. Further investigation may be advisable when the diagnosis is not clear-cut and is necessary if surgical treatment is contemplated. Cardiac catheterization usually demonstrates that the oxygen saturation of right ventricular blood is higher than that in the right atrium. However, if the defect is small or if there are equal pressures in the systemic and pulmonary circulations, no shunt of oxygenated blood may be demonstrable. The injection of radio-opaque material into the left ventricle may then be necessary for the angiocardiographic visualization of the defect.

The prognosis of ventricular septal defect depends upon the age of the patient, the size of the defect, and the pulmonary vascular changes. Large ventricular septal defects are an important cause of death in the infant; in those who survive, the defect usually becomes smaller or closes. After the first year, few affected children die, but death is likely to occur in those with major defects between the ages of 20 and 40. Patients with small defects usually live a normal life span, but are exposed to the risk of infective endocarditis.

In deciding upon the appropriate therapy for a patient with ventricular septal defect, the expected prognosis must be taken into account. In all patients precautions must be taken to avoid infective endocarditis. Because the outlook in small defects is excellent, surgery is not indicated. If there is a large left-to-right shunt, the defect should be closed. When the pulmonary vascular resistance is high, surgery is usually contraindicated as it cannot correct and may, indeed, worsen the pulmonary hypertension.

Persistent ductus arteriosus (Fig. 12.5)

During fetal life, the ductus arteriosus permits blood to flow from the pulmonary artery into the aorta. Within a few hours or days or birth, it narrows and then closes.

In a few infants, the ductus arteriosus remains open and permits a large flow of blood from the high-pressure aorta to the low-pressure pulmonary artery. This may cause heart failure and death in the first few weeks of life. More commonly the ductus arteriosus undergoes partial closure and the shunt from aorta to pulmonary artery is relatively small. This gives rise to no symptoms during the first few years of life and is usually detected at a routine physical examination. A persistent ductus arteriosus of this kind may eventually become harmful for three reasons. First, it may act as a focus for infective endarteritis. Secondly, the leak of blood from the aorta to the pulmonary artery and the consequent high pulmonary blood flow may lead to cardiac failure in adolescence or adult life. Thirdly, but rarely, severe pulmonary hypertension may develop.

Fig. 12.5 Persistent ductus arteriosus. The shunt is from aorta to pulmonary artery because of the low resistance of the pulmonary circuit.

The patient is usually in good general health. The pulse may be of normal volume if the duct is small, but if it is large, the diastolic leak from the aorta causes a collapsing pulse. Correspondingly, the diastolic blood pressure may be low. The heart may be of normal size, or the left ventricle enlarged. The most characteristic feature of the condition is the 'continuous murmur', situated in the second left intercostal space by the sternal edge but often loudest 5–7.5 cm above or to the left of this. This murmur continues from systole into diastole and is maximum about the time of the second sound (Fig. 12.6). It seldom lasts for the whole of systole and diastole and may occupy only the latter part of systole and the earlier part of diastole. In a few instances, particularly in infants, it may occur as a crescendo in late systole only. The murmur is due to flow of blood from the aorta through the persistent ductus arteriosus into the pulmonary artery in both phases of the cardiac cycle. If the shunt is large, the increased venous return from the lungs causes a mid-diastolic murmur at the apex as it crosses the mitral valve.

The ECG is usually normal but may show the deep Q and tall R waves of left ventricular hypertrophy. The chest radiograph may show enlargement of the left ventricle, aorta and pulmonary artery, and the features of increased pulmonary blood flow. The duct can sometimes be visualized by cross-sectional echocardiography. Enlargement of the left atrium and left ventricle on the M-mode echo confirms the presence of left ventricular volume overload.

The clinical diagnosis is usually easy because of the characteristic continuous murmur. Special investigation is seldom required even prior to surgical treatment. Care, however, is necessary to avoid confusion with the venous hum which is common in normal children. The hum is usually maximal to the right of the sternum below the right clavicle, diminishes or disappears when the child lies flat and can usually be abolished by compression of the jugular veins on the right side. Continuous murmurs due to other causes are rare and their maximum intensity is usually

Fig. 12.6 The continuous murmur of a persistent ductus arteriosus.

below and medial to the pulmonary area. When in doubt because of the site or quality of the murmur or the lack of correlation with the electrocardiographic and radiological features, special investigation is necessary. At cardiac catheterization there is a 'step-up' in oxygen saturation in the pulmonary artery. This can be shown to result from a persistent ductus by the passage of the catheter through it into the descending aorta, or by the angiocardiographic delineation of the ductus by the injection of contrast medium into the arch of the aorta.

Surgical treatment of a persistent ductus arteriosus by division and suture carries little risk and is the correct management in almost all patients. Operation should be performed, if possible, before the child starts school.

In symptomatic low birth weight premature infants, the ductus frequently causes life-threatening cardiac decompensation. Although immediate surgery is probably still the most successful mode of treatment, administration of indomethacin, a prostaglandin inhibitor, can induce duct closure medically. This method is, however, less certain of success and associated with side-effects which may preclude its use.

Obstructive lesions

Coarctation of the aorta

Coarctation of the aorta is a narrowing of the lumen, usually just beyond the origin of the left subclavian artery (Fig. 12.7). It is characteristically of severe degree and is commonly associated with a bicuspid aortic valve which may be or may become stenosed or allow regurgitation. The ductus arteriosus may also persist, particularly if the coarctation is proximal to its attachment to the aorta.

The systolic pressure in the aorta and its branches proximal to the coarctation is raised, but this may not be obvious in early childhood; diastolic hypertension is uncommon before adult life and is seldom severe at rest. The hypertension may induce irreversible changes in the arterioles so that the blood pressure may not return to normal even after the removal of the coarctation.

Fig. 12.7 Coarctation of the aorta. The constriction is usually in the descending aorta just below the left subclavian artery. Beyond the constriction, there is post-stenotic dilatation.

Only a small volume of blood flows through the narrowed segment; much of the blood supply of the lower part of the body is by way of collateral vessels which attain great size. The blood pressure in the lower half of the body is lower than that in the upper half and the pulse wave takes longer to arrive.

The hypertension is eventually liable to cause left ventricular failure. Other risks include infection of the coarctation or of a bicuspid aortic valve, rupture or dissection of the ascending aorta, and cerebral haemorrhage. Cystic medial necrosis of the aortic wall, which is present in only a few patients with coarctation, is the deciding factor in rupture. Rupture of an intracranial aneurysm, which occurs in 5–10% of affected individuals, is the usual cause of subarachnoid haemorrhage.

Coarctation may produce no symptoms and is most often suspected during a routine medical examination when a systolic murmur is heard or hypertension detected. However, long segment narrowing in the preductal area of the aorta is associated with heart failure in infancy. In such infants, commonly, the ductus is patent, and pulmonary hypertension is present; a VSD may coexist.

The blood pressure in the upper limbs is raised: that in the legs is normal or low. The femoral arterial pulse is small and delayed in comparison with the radial pulse. In adults, collateral vessels may be seen and felt along the borders of the scapulae and over the posterior chest wall. The left ventricle is occasionally enlarged. A systolic murmur is almost invariably heard over the area of the coarctation at about the level of the fourth intercostal space posteriorly, and tends to be louder than a systolic murmur which is often audible in the second intercostal spaces close to the sternum. A more continuous murmur may be heard over collaterals.

The ECG is usually normal; left ventricular hypertrophy is uncommon before adult years. The chest radiograph is seldom abnormal in childhood, but characteristically shows an abnormal aortic knuckle with an enlarged left subclavian artery and post-stenotic dilatation of the aorta in adults. Another feature is notching of the undersides of the ribs due to the erosion by enlarged intercostal arteries. The left ventricle may also be enlarged.

The diagnosis is usually made without difficulty on clinical grounds. It may be confirmed by intra-aortic pressure tracings above and below the coarctation and the precise anatomy can be outlined by aortography.

The correct treatment is surgical resection of the coarctation and restoration of the aorta by end-to-end anastomosis or, if necessary, by the insertion of a graft. This should be performed electively in childhood. Nonetheless, hypertension may not be completely abolished or may recur later. Follow-up is necessary.

Aortic stenosis

This condition is considered in Chapter 11.

Hypoplastic left heart

This term is used to describe a number of disorders, such as mitral atresia and aortic atresia, in which the characteristic feature is virtual absence of left ventricular outflow. The diagnosis can usually be established by echocardiogram which reveals a small left ventricle and absent aortic valve. Life can be sustained if there is a large persistent ductus which allows blood to flow from the pulmonary artery to the aorta. Affected infants are intensely cyanosed and usually die within hours of birth. There is, as yet, no treatment. The abnormality can be detected at about the 18th week of pregnancy by fetal echocardiography; termination can then be considered.

Pulmonary stenosis

Pulmonary stenosis is almost invariably of congenital origin. Except when it is complicated by a ventricular septal defect (see 'tetralogy of Fallot', p. 252) the stenosis is usually confined to the valve cusps. These may be fused to form a cone-shaped structure with a narrow orifice. Beyond the obstruction the pulmonary artery is dilated; proximal to it the right ventricle is hypertrophied.

The obstruction to right ventricular emptying leads to a high right ventricular systolic pressure and a systolic pressure drop across the pulmonary valve. In the more severe cases, right ventricular failure develops. If the foramen ovale is unsealed, or if there is an atrial septal defect, a right-to-left shunt with central cyanosis may develop as the right atrial pressure rises.

Although pulmonary stenosis may cause cardiac failure in the first few weeks of life, survival into late childhood or adult life is usual. Often the lesion is first detected on routine clinical examination, but some patients present with fatigue, breathlessness or syncope. Frequently, the lesion is so mild that symptoms never occur.

The arterial pulse may be normal or small. The jugular venous pulse is usually normal, but in severe grades it exhibits a large 'a' wave as the right atrium contracts forcibly in the face of the non-compliant hypertrophied right ventricle. On palpation, there is nearly always a systolic thrill in the second left intercostal space; the left parasternal heave of right ventricular hypertrophy can sometimes be felt. The first heart sound is normal, but it is often followed by an early systolic 'ejection' click and a loud midsystolic murmur best heard in the second left intercostal space. The second sound is normal in the mild case, but in the more severe it is split abnormally widely and the second (pulmonary) element is soft.

The electrocardiogram provides useful evidence of the severity of the pulmonary valve stenosis for, in general, the greater the degree of right ventricular hypertrophy seen on the ECG, the tighter the stenosis. The chest radiograph shows the post-stenotic dilatation of the pulmonary artery. In severe cases, right ventricular hypertrophy and diminution in the pulmonary vascular markings may be detected.

An accurate diagnosis can usually be made clinically. Cardiac catheterization provides confirmatory evidence; the systolic pressure difference across the pulmonary valve is a valuable index of severity, a drop of more than 50 mmHg suggesting severe stenosis (Fig. 12.8). Doppler ultrasound provides reliable evidence of the severity of the stenosis, and is particularly valuable as a means of follow-up. Unless the foramen ovale is unsealed or there is an associated atrial septal defect, no intracardiac shunting can be detected.

A minor degree of pulmonary stenosis is compatible with a normal life span. When the stenosis is more severe, death is likely to ensue sooner or later from right ventricular failure; relief of the stenosis should not be delayed too long as irreversible fibrotic changes take place in the hypertrophied right ventricle. Recently, balloon valvoplasty has been shown to be an effective and safe method of enlarging the valve orifice. Its long-term

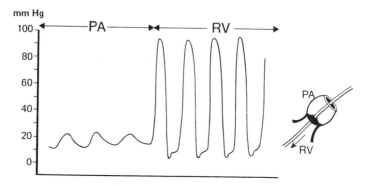

Fig. 12.8 The pressure pulse obtained as the catheter is withdrawn from pulmonary artery to right ventricle in pulmonary valve stenosis.

effects are not yet known, but it seems likely to replace surgical valvotomy in most cases.

Tricuspid atresia

In this relatively uncommon disorder, there is absence of the normal atrioventricular connection on the right side. For life to be sustained in the extra-uterine state, an atrial septal defect and a ventricular septal defect must be present. Frequently there is associated pulmonary stenosis or pulmonary atresia and, more rarely, transposition of the great arteries. The left ventricle is large and the hypoplastic right ventricle receives blood by the VSD. Cyanosis in infancy is the rule. The ECG shows left axis deviation and left ventricular hypertrophy. Cross-sectional echocardiography reveals the absent connection and can also demonstrate the VSD and ASD.

Surgical treatment in infancy by creation of an aortopulmonary shunt is life saving. In later childhood a conduit is inserted between the right atrium and the right ventricular outflow tract or pulmonary artery (Fontan procedure).

Combined obstructive and shunt lesions

Pulmonary stenosis and ventricular septal defect (tetralogy of Fallot)

When pulmonary stenosis coexists with a ventricular septal defect, the stenosis may be slight and shunting exclusively from left-to-right. In most cases, however, pulmonary stenosis is severe and the ventricular septal defect large, and there is a right-to-left shunt. These abnormalities are the major features of the 'tetralogy of Fallot', of which the other components are dextroposition of the aorta (with the aortic root overriding the defect) and right ventricular hypertrophy (Fig. 12.9). The pulmonary stenosis is situated in the infundibulum of the right ventricle and, often, at the pulmonary valve as well. The infundibular stenosis tends to become more severe with advancing age and there is a progressive increase in the proportion of blood shunted from right-to-left.

In the most severe cases, symptoms start soon after birth. More frequently, cyanosis develops in the second half of the first year or not until later in childhood.

With increasing cyanosis, dyspnoea becomes more severe. The child is liable to sudden attacks of intense cyanosis, sometimes associated with syncope, for which spasm of the infundibulum of the right ventricle may be responsible. Children with the tetralogy of Fallot are liable to squat after exercise. It is believed that the squatting position, by compressing the abdominal aorta and the femoral arteries, increases the arterial resistance and therefore diminishes the right-to-left shunt at the ventricular level.

The child is often abnormally small and has central cyanosis with finger clubbing. The arterial pulses are small and venous pulses normal. Clinical evidence of right ventricular hypertrophy is slight. There is a loud systolic murmur accompanied by a thrill in the second or third left intercostal space unless the stenosis is so severe that virtually no blood traverses it. The second heart sound is single because the pulmonary valve component is inaudible. The electrocardiogram shows moderate right ventricular hypertrophy. The chest radiograph is characteristic in showing a 'boot-shaped' heart with a concavity on the left border in the place where the pulmonary artery is normally seen, and a prominent and elevated apex (Fig. 12.10). The pulmonary vascularity is

Fig. 12.9 Tetralogy of Fallot. Note infundibular pulmonary stenosis and ventricular septal defect, with right-to-left shunt at ventricular level.

Fig. 12.10   Radiographic appearances in tetralogy of Fallot. Note prominent and elevated apex.

decreased. Echocardiography shows that the aorta is large and overrides the septum, the normal continuity between the anterior aortic wall and septum being lost. Polycythaemia, secondary to the cyanosis, is usual.

The tetralogy of Fallot is the underlying lesion in 70% of children with central cyanosis over the age of 3. This frequency and the characteristic clinical, electrocardiographic and radiological features usually make the diagnosis easy in childhood. In infancy and also in later life, a confident diagnosis can less often be reached without further investigation.

On cardiac catheterization, a systolic pressure drop can be demonstrated between the body and the outflow tract of the right ventricle. Pressures in the right and left ventricles are identical. The oxygen saturation in the aorta is reduced. Injection of radio-opaque contrast medium into the right ventricle delineates the region of stenosis and demonstrates the shunt through the ventricular septal defect.

Patients with severe pulmonary stenosis and large ventricular septal defects often die in childhood and rarely reach middle age without surgery. Death may result from hypoxic episodes during childhood, from cerebrovascular accidents as a result of thrombosis promoted by polycythaemia, from infective endocarditis and from cerebral abscesses. Virtually all patients require surgery at some stage, but the type of surgery depends upon the severity of the lesion and the age. Ideally, the abnormality should be totally corrected by relief of the pulmonary stenosis and by closure of the ventricular septal defect. In severely affected infants, some surgeons prefer to perform a palliative procedure such as the creation of a shunt between the aorta and pulmonary circulations, either directly (Waterston operation) or by anastomosing the subclavian artery to the pulmonary artery (Blalock—Taussig procedure). This increases the proportion of blood going through the lungs and thus becoming oxygenated. By one or other of these operations the child can be given several years of comparatively good health before the corrective procedure is performed.

Severe hypoxic attacks should be treated with oxygen and morphine (0.1 mg/kg). The baby should be placed in the knee—chest position. Blood $P\text{co}_2$ and pH should be estimated and sodium bicarbonate given intravenously as necessary. Propranolol is possibly of value.

High pulmonary vascular resistance with right-to-left shunt through a septal defect or ductus arteriosus (Eisenmenger syndrome)

Eisenmenger originally described a patient with a ventricular septal defect with central cyanosis in the absence of pulmonary stenosis. It is now known that the reason for the right-to-left shunt in such cases is the presence of a severe pulmonary vascular disease. Because the clinical pictures of pulmonary hypertension with right-to-left shunt are so similar, irrespective of whether the shunt is at atrial, ventricular or aorto-pulmonary level, the term Eisenmenger syndrome is employed to describe all three lesions.

The cause of the pulmonary vascular disease responsible for the pulmonary hypertension is unknown. Factors which may be involved include:

1   lack of regression of the fetal type of pulmonary vasculature (see p. 289);
2   prolonged exposure to high pulmonary blood flow;
3   prolonged exposure to high pulmonary blood pressure;
4   genetic predisposition.

Although irreversible pulmonary arterial changes may develop during early childhood, they more commonly occur during adolescence. Dyspnoea and fatigue, which are usually the first symptoms, are liable to develop in late childhood, adolescence or early adult life. Other complaints include syncope, angina pectoris, oedema and haemoptysis.

On examination the patient is usually cyanosed. When the shunt is through a ductus arteriosus, the venous blood is directed into the descending aorta and only the lower limbs become cyanosed ('differential cyanosis').

The arterial pulse is usually small, due to a low stroke volume; a large 'a' wave may be present in the venous pulse, due to forceful atrial contraction in the face of right ventricular hypertrophy. On palpation, one can detect right ventricular hypertrophy and the shock of pulmonary valve closure. On auscultation, the signs are mainly those of pulmonary hypertension: a loud second heart sound, a right ventricular fourth heart sound, a pulmonary early systolic ('ejection') click and, occasionally, the early diastolic murmur of pulmonary regurgitation and the pansystolic murmur of functional tricuspid regurgitation. In atrial septal defect, the second sound remains split on expiration (because only the right ventricle is overburdened). In ventricular septal defect, there is a single second sound, because the pressure in both ventricles is identical. In persistent ductus arteriosus, there is normal splitting of the second heart sound.

The ECG shows right atrial and right ventricular hypertrophy. On the chest radiograph there are large main pulmonary arteries but small peripheral arteries, together with right ventricular and right atrial enlargement. Cross-sectional echocardiography can reliably demonstrate the ventricular or atrial septal defects in these patients.

The diagnosis is suggested by the combination of central cyanosis and pulmonary hypertension in an adolescent or young adult. The Eisenmenger syndrome differs from the tetralogy of Fallot, (the commonest cardiac cause of central cyanosis in this age group), in there being no pulmonary systolic thrill or loud murmur, in the greater severity of right ventricular hypertrophy, and in the large pulmonary arteries on the chest radiograph. The diagnosis can be confirmed by demonstrating by cardiac catheterization that the pulmonary artery pressure equals the systemic pressure, and by angiocardiographic delineation of the shunt. The progress of the Eisenmenger syndrome is usually slowly downhill, death commonly occurring between the ages of 20 and 40. The main causes of death are pulmonary infarction, right heart failure and arrhythmias and, less often, infective endocarditis. Pregnancy is particularly hazardous in these patients and should be avoided or terminated early.

No surgical treatment, other than heart−lung transplantation, is of value because the major defect is the irreversible change in the small pulmonary arteries. Temporary benefit may result from the conventional treatment of cardiac failure.

Displacement lesions

Transposition of the great arteries (Fig. 12.11)

In transposition of the great arteries, the aorta arises from the right ventricle and the pulmonary artery from the left. As a consequence, there are separate systemic and pulmonary circulations; life cannot be sustained unless there is some communication between them. Usually there is one or more of the following:

a patent foramen ovale, an atrial septal defect, a ventricular septal defect, or a persistent ductus arteriosus.

The infant is characteristically of normal size and well nourished. Cyanosis develops at birth or shortly thereafter. There is difficulty in completing feeds; increasing breathlessness, deep cyanosis, cardiac failure and death are usual within the first month.

On auscultation there may be a gallop rhythm and a systolic murmur.

The chest radiograph may show little abnormality at birth, but within a few days the heart becomes enlarged and the vascularity of the lung fields increased. The ECG shows little more than the right ventricular preponderance normal for this age group.

Echocardiography, especially the cross-sectional technique, is an invaluable diagnostic tool. It permits observation of the aorta, arising from the right ventricle and lying anterior to the pulmonary artery, and also allows detection of other defects.

Transposition of the great arteries is the most common cardiac cause of cyanosis at birth and of overt heart failure in cyanotic congenital heart disease within the first few weeks of life. Accurate diagnosis at this stage is urgent; it is usually fatal to await the effects of medical treatment. Investigation should be undertaken within a matter of hours. Echocardiography is of diagnostic value in showing the abnormal connections of the great arteries. If it supports the diagnosis, it is usually then necessary to proceed to cardiac catheterization which not only enables the precise nature of the anomalies to be determined but is an essential preliminary to therapy.

In the acutely ill infant, great improvement can be achieved by producing a large defect in the atrial septum to allow mixing of the blood between systemic and pulmonary circulations (Rashkind procedure). This is done by introducing a catheter with a deflated

Fig. 12.11 Transposition of the great arteries. The aorta arises from the right ventricle and the pulmonary artery from the left. Life can be sustained only if communications exist between systemic and pulmonary circulations.

balloon at its tip into the femoral vein and advancing it via the right atrium and foramen ovale into the left atrium. The balloon is then inflated and withdrawn abruptly so as to tear the atrial septum. This procedure is usually effective in the neonatal period and allows the child to live until the latter part of the first year of life when the venous return to the two ventricles is rerouted by the insertion of an intra-atrial baffle (Mustard's or Senning's operation). This operation can be carried out with a low mortality. An alternative procedure is the 'switch' operation, in which the surgeon detaches the aorta and pulmonary artery, and connects each to its appropriate ventricle.

Ebstein's anomaly

In this disorder, the posteromedial part of the tricuspid valve ring is displaced towards the apex of the right ventricle. An atrial septal defect is usually present.

Dyspnoea, fatigue and arrhythmias are usual. Cyanosis may be present if there is an atrial septal defect. There are often scratchy tricuspid systolic, mid-diastolic and presystolic murmurs, arising from flow across the abnormal tricuspid valve. Tall P waves, a long PR interval and a low voltage right bundle branch block pattern are the usual ECG features. The chest radiograph shows a large right atrium and clear lung fields. Echocardiography demonstrates the abnormal position and movement of the tricuspid valve cusp.

Death usually results from arrhythmias in childhood or early adult life, but may occur later from cardiac failure or hypoxaemia.

Partial correction, with prosthetic replacement of the tricuspid valve and repair of the atrial septal defect is indicated for the disabled case but this neither restores normal function nor prevents arrhythmias.

Dextrocardia

Dextrocardia refers to all situations where the heart is in the right chest. The lung and abdominal situs or arrangement may be reversed or normal. When dextrocardia exists with complete right−left reversal of the lungs and viscera then the heart is usually normal. When the heart is in the right chest and the other organs are normally sited, or if the heart is in the left chest (laevocardia) and the other organs reversed, then the chance of complex congenital cardiac lesions is high.

Right-sided aorta

In this condition, the aorta turns posteriorly and runs down on the right of the trachea and the oesophagus instead of arching upwards and to the left. It may continue to descend in this direction or may cross behind the trachea and oesophagus and attain the normal left-sided course.

As an isolated anomaly it is of no clinical significance. When associated with a congenital lesion of the heart, its detection may be of diagnostic assistance for it is found in 20%–25% of patients with the tetralogy of Fallot. When associated with other arterial anomalies the trachea and oesophagus may be encircled and obstructive symptoms result.

The diagnosis and management of the infant with heart failure and cyanosis

The general paediatrician and the general practitioner have the responsibility of detecting heart disease in the newborn; an expert in neonatal cardiology should be contacted without delay if there is any evidence of cyanosis or heart failure. All too frequently, the clinical evidence of heart disease is overlooked until it is too late.

Central cyanosis is a serious finding in the newborn. If it persists after exposure to oxygen therapy, and there is no evident respiratory or cerebral cause, congenital heart disease should be suspected. If the cyanosis is indeed due to congenital heart disease, the prognosis without treatment is poor. Echocardiography should be undertaken immediately. The findings of this investigation may suggest that cardiac catheterization is required: this can be combined with therapy (e.g. the Rashkind procedure, see p. 257).

The commonest causes of cardiac failure, with or without cyanosis, in the newborn, are ventricular septal defect, persistent ductus arteriosus, hypoplastic left heart, coarctation of the aorta and transposition.

The early signs of heart failure are tachypnoea, tachycardia, gallop rhythm and enlargement of the liver. Cyanosis is often present as well. The venous pressure is a poor guide to heart failure in infants. Crepitations and rhonchi are common and should not be attributed to pulmonary disease until left ventricular failure has been excluded. Oedema, which is most likely to affect the backs of the hands and feet, is a late sign, and is common in the absence of heart failure in premature infants.

Tachycardia may be difficult to assess because the pulse rate is normally fast in infants, but it seldom exceeds 140 per minute during sleep in the healthy baby or in those with respiratory disease. If the rate is in excess of 210 per minute, there is a supraventricular tachycardia requiring urgent treatment. If the heart rate is less than 50 per minute, heart block is almost certainly present.

Thirty per cent oxygen should be given to all infants who are cyanosed or in cardiac failure. The air should be humidified. Measurement of the blood gases and the correction of acidosis is an essential part of the proper management of heart failure in infancy. Frusemide starting with an oral dose of 2 μg/kg is first choice in severe failure. Digoxin may also be of value starting with 40–60 μg/kg by mouth or 40 μg/kg intramuscularly. Good nursing, temperature and humidity control, supportive frames or suspension in the propped-up position and tube feeding are essential in the early stages of treatment. Sedation with trimeprazine or promethazine may be required.

These medical measures are quite often successful in correcting cardiac failure due to a ventricular septal defect or persistent ductus arteriosus. The cyanotic infant is in a precarious state and may be dependent on a patent ductus; deterioration takes place as the ductus closes. This can usually be prevented by the intravenous infusion of prostacyclin E_1 or E_2, starting with a dose of 0.05–0.1 μg/kg per minute and slowed to one-fifth of this after 20 minutes. This therapy, which may induce pyrexia, hypertension and apnoeic attacks, is usually only a temporization measure prior to surgery.

Further reading

Anderson, R.H., Macartney, F.J., Shinebourne, E.A. & Tynan, M. (1987) *Paediatric Cardiology*. Edinburgh: Churchill Livingstone.
Perloff, J.K. (1987) *The Clinical Recognition of Congenital Heart Disease*, 3rd edn. Philadelphia: Saunders.

Hypertension and Heart Disease

Hypertension is probably directly or indirectly responsible for 10–20% of all deaths. These deaths occur because of the deleterious effects of high blood pressure on the coronary, renal and cerebral arteries, and because of the increased work load imposed on the heart.

For reasons that will become apparent, it is impossible to define hypertension. For practical purposes, the blood pressure may be regarded as abnormally high if it persistently exceeds 140/90 mmHg in a quietly resting individual. This does not imply that individuals with raised pressure necessarily require treatment. The presence of other risk factors and evidence of adverse effects must be taken into account.

The variability of blood pressure

The level of arterial blood pressure is determined by the cardiac output and peripheral vascular resistance, two factors which vary widely from individual to individual, and within one individual at different times. The blood pressure varies to a lesser extent because the changes in cardiac output and peripheral resistance often offset each other. Persistent hypertension is nearly always due to a raised peripheral vascular resistance, the cardiac output being normal. As the peripheral resistance is determined largely by arteriolar tone, it can be concluded that hypertension is the result of arteriolar vasoconstriction or organic narrowing.

Marked variations have been observed in individuals in whom the blood pressure is continuously monitored throughout the day. The mean pressure during sleep may be 30–40 mmHg lower than it is in the waking state. Factors which transiently increase pressure include anxiety and cold. Exercise leads to a brisk rise in systolic pressure but little change in the diastolic pressure. A transient doubling of systolic pressure may occur at the climax of coitus.

Certain identifiable factors are associated with persistently high blood pressure. Thus, at least in Western societies, both diastolic and systolic pressure increase with age. The blood pressure averages about 80/60 mmHg at birth and rises slowly throughout childhood. The resting blood pressure in the adolescent is often in the region of 120/70 mmHg, whilst in middle age 140/80 mmHg is more common. The systolic pressure often continues to rise into old age as the aorta becomes increasingly rigid. However, in many individuals and throughout some societies, e.g. in some Pacific islands, hypertension is virtually non-existent and there is no rise with age. In the younger age groups, males, on average, have higher pressures than females, but this tendency is reversed after the age of 45. Obese individuals tend to have pressures higher than can be accounted for by recording errors due to increased arm circumference.

The variability of arterial pressures within one individual and between individuals makes it impossible to define normality. It has been established, however, that the higher the pressure even within the 'normal' range, whether systolic or diastolic, the more likely is the occurrence of certain disease processes such as left ventricular hypertrophy and failure ('hypertensive heart disease'), coronary artery disease, cerebrovascular disease and renal disease. The blood pressure can only be regarded as pathologically high if it has caused or is likely to lead to disordered function of the cardiovascular system, brain or kidneys.

Classification by blood pressure level

Normal adult blood pressure has been defined as a systolic blood pressure equal to or below 140 mmHg together with a diastolic (fifth Korotkoff phase) equal to or below 90 mmHg.

Hypertension in adults is defined as a systolic pressure equal to or greater than 160 mmHg and a diastolic equal to or greater than 95 mmHg.

Borderline hypertension denotes a blood pressure between the normal and hypertensive levels as defined above.

Hypertension may be regarded as 'mild' if the diastolic pressure is between 90 and 104 mmHg, 'moderate' if between 105 and 114 mmHg, and 'severe' if above this. Hypertension is said to be in the *malignant* or accelerated phase if there is widespread arterial fibrinoid necrosis. The diastolic pressure is very high (often above 130 mmHg), with retinal haemorrhages and exudates and frequently papilloedema.

Aetiological factors in hypertension

In some 5% of those with high blood pressure, an identifiable cause can be held responsible. When the hypertension can be attributed to one of these, it is 'secondary'; when no such factor can be unearthed it is described as 'essential' or 'primary'.

Hypertension can be secondary to a large number of conditions of which the most important are the following:

1 Renal disease including glomerulonephritis, pyelonephritis, polycystic disease, renal tumours and renal artery stenosis;
2 Endocrine diseases including diseases of the adrenal gland such as primary aldosteronism, Cushing's syndrome and phaeochromocytoma;
3 Coarctation of the aorta;
4 Pre-eclampsia;
5 Drugs and foods including oral contraceptives, liquorice, carbenoxolone, ACTH and corticosteroids, and vasoconstrictive nose drops;
6 Acute porphyria;
7 Certain cerebral lesions such as brain tumours and bulbar poliomyelitis.

Hypertension occurring in those under the age of 40 is usually secondary, unless there is a strong family history of this condition. The relative proportion of cases with an identifiable cause decreases with age; in the elderly, secondary hypertension is uncommon.

The cause of 'essential' hypertension remains uncertain. Indeed, if it is the result of the interplay of a large number of factors, as many believe, the search for a single cause is doomed to failure. This multifactorial or 'mosaic' concept is supported by much epidemiological evidence which shows that there is an infinite gradation between the 'normal' and hypertensive' populations. As Pickering wrote:

> What causes the rise of pressure in essential hypertension? We do not know precisely. Certainly no specific fault has been identified and I am personally doubtful if one exists. But going further back we can assign roles to inheritance, which influences pressure at any age, and environment, which influences the rate of rise with age.

The influence of heredity is unquestioned, hypertension being many times more common in the families of hypertensive patients than in those of normotensive individuals. Although some have suggested that hypertension is due to a single dominant gene, most of the evidence points to the influence of many genes.

Numerous differences have been observed between groups of individuals who are hypertensive and those who are not. The significance of these as causal factors is not established.

Dietary influences. There is an undoubted relationship between overweight and hypertension. Weight loss in the very obese substantially lowers the blood pressure; in the less overweight it has little effect. Very low salt intake appears to protect against hypertension, but there is little evidence to incriminate excessive sodium chloride intake as a cause of high blood pressure. A high potassium intake may be protective. There is some evidence that a high intake of saturated fats may raise blood pressure. High alcohol consumption has been identified as a risk factor for hypertension, as has cigarette smoking, at least in regard to the malignant phase.

Haemodynamic changes. A slight sinus tachycardia and a high cardiac output may be found in early hypertensives before there is a rise in peripheral resistance. These features may result from an excessive adrenergic influence. There is good evidence that baroreceptors are reset in hypertension, as bradycardia is not induced by the rise in pressure.

Some observers have reported increases in plasma catecholamine levels; others have noted abnormal responses of receptors.

Humoral changes. The possible roles of the renin—angiotensin system and of prostaglandins are being studied vigorously at present.

The causes of secondary hypertension

Renal disease

That renal disease can be the sole cause of hypertension has been clearly established both in animal experiments and in man. The components of the renin—angiotensin system are shown in Fig. 13.1. However, the relationship between renal disease and hypertension is complex because either may lead to the other, and it is not always easy to determine which is primary.

In *acute glomerulonephritis*, hypertension is almost invariable, but is transient and not often severe. The mechanism is not clear, but sodium and water retention may play a part. Cardiac failure occurs in about one-quarter of the cases, but the hypertension is seldom an important factor in this. The diagnosis can usually be made on the basis of the acute onset, the association with preceding streptococcal infection, and the presence of peripheral oedema and disturbed renal function.

Severe hypertension is usually a late manifestation of *chronic nephritis*, and develops only when there is evidence of advanced renal failure.

There is evidence that *chronic pyelonephritis* can cause hypertension (particularly malignant hypertension) although this has been disputed. *Reflux nephropathy* is predominantly a disorder of females, and should be particularly sought for in girls with hypertension.

Hypertension occurs in more than half of those with *congenital polycystic disease of the kidneys.*

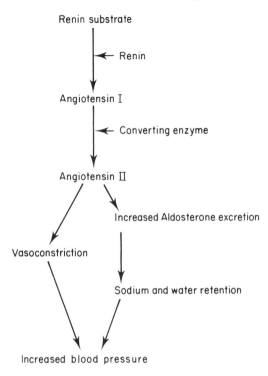

Fig. 13.1 The renin–angiotensin system.

Hypertension may also be caused by *renal artery disease*, resulting from atheromatous narrowing, fibromuscular hyperplasia or aneurysm formation. Not infrequently, only one renal artery is involved. Renal artery surgery or, if the abnormality is unilateral, nephrectomy is indicated if it can be established that the renal artery disease is responsible for the high blood pressure.

Evaluation of the patient with suspected renal disease may include intravenous pyelography, isotope renography, renal arteriography and renal biopsy.

Endocrine disease

Primary aldosteronism. Aldosterone, which is secreted by the zona glomerulosa of the adrenal cortex, promotes sodium reabsorption and potassium excretion in the distal tubules of the kidney. Normally, aldosterone secretion is largely regulated by angiotensin, but in primary aldosteronism there is an overproduction of aldosterone as a result of an adrenal cortical adenoma (Conn's syndrome) or bilateral hyperplasia; angiotensin and, therefore, plasma renin levels are abnormally low. It occurs most often in young and middle-aged females. Because of the mode of action of aldosterone, the symptoms and signs are related to sodium retention, hypokalaemia and hypertension. Frequently, the patient presents with mild to moderate hypertension, but the predominant complaints are those of muscle weakness, headache, thirst and polyuria. The hypertension is seldom severe and ma-lignant changes are rare. There is usually hypokalaemia, with a serum potassium of less than 3.0 mmol/l, and a serum sodium that is normal or high. Characteristically, there is a metabolic alkalosis and a low serum chloride. The diagnosis should be suspected in patients with hypertension and hypokalaemia, part-icularly if this is associated with hypernatraemia. However, hypokalaemia is not uncommon in other hypertensive patients, particularly if they have been treated with diuretics. Furthermore, patients with malignant hypertension develop 'secondary aldo-steronism' with low serum potassium. These patients usually do not have a high serum sodium.

The diagnosis can be confirmed by showing severe potassium loss in the urine, and by demonstrating control of the hyper-tension by large doses of the aldosterone antagonist, spironolac-tone. Adrenal tumours are probably best identified by computed tomography and should be removed surgically.

Phaeochromocytoma. Phaeochromocytomas arise in chromaffin tissue in the adrenal gland or elsewhere. Most are benign, but about 5% are malignant. The tumours usually secrete noradre-naline (norepinephrine), but adrenaline (epinephrine) may predominate.

Phaeochromocytomas may produce either paroxysmal or per-sistent hypertension. The paroxysms are associated with the sudden onset of bilateral headache, and with perspiration, palpi-tation and pallor (features often regarded as neurotic). The attacks usually last from a few minutes to an hour. If the hypertension is persistent, the clinical picture is that of severe hypertension, often of the malignant variety. Because of the hypermetabolic state induced by the phaeochromocytoma, the patients are rarely obese.

The diagnosis should be suspected in any severe case of hyper-tension. It is confirmed by the detection of high circulatory con-centrations or urinary excretion ratio of catecholamines. The tumour can usually be localized by ultrasound or computed tomography.

Phaeochromocytomas should be removed surgically. This is a potentially hazardous procedure and requires close control of the blood pressure and careful anaesthesia. Beta-adrenergic blocking drugs should not be used alone; they may induce an extreme alpha-adrenergic effect. This can be avoided by the initial use of an alpha-adrenergic blocking drug.

Cushing's syndrome. This results from cortisol excess and may be due to hyperplasia of the adrenal cortex, adrenal tumours, or to the excessive administration of glucocorticoids or ACTH. Adrenal hyperplasia is often the result of increased ACTH production by a pituitary microadenoma.

Hypertension, which occurs in more than 50% of cases, may be severe and proceed to the malignant phase. Other features of the syndrome are muscle weakness, osteoporosis, purple cutaneous striae, obesity of the trunk, a 'buffalo' hump, a 'moon' facies and diabetes mellitus. There may also be hirsutism, amenorrhoea, a liability to spontaneous bruising, and dependent oedema.

The diagnosis should be suggested by the combination of hypertension, diabetes and truncal obesity. Patients with Cushing's syndrome have an increase in urinary unconjugated cortisol excretion and the usual nocturnal fall in plasma cortisol does not occur. ACTH levels are valuable in determining the cause — being high with pituitary tumours and low if the adrenal is responsible.

Treatment depends upon the aetiology of the condition. Surgical removal of one or both adrenal glands or of the pituitary tumour may be necessary, but pituitary irradiation may be effective.

Coarctation of the aorta

See p. 248.

Pre-eclampsia

Pre-eclampsia is a condition of unknown aetiology exclusive to pregnancy, the characteristic features of which are hypertension and proteinuria. It may progress to eclampsia, in which there are convulsions.

Pre-eclampsia develops during the last 3 months of pregnancy and is most common in young primigravidae. The occurrence of oedema, hypertension and albuminuria at this time in such a patient should suggest the diagnosis, but this triad is also encountered in patients with essential hypertension, chronic glomerulonephritis and pyelonephritis.

The first abnormality is usually mild hypertension, with or without proteinuria, but oedema may be the presenting symptom. If the patient is promptly treated with rest and is carefully supervised, improvement usually takes place. However, the condition may progress until she develops headache, nausea, vomiting and drowsiness. At a later state, fits may occur, and there may be cerebral haemorrhage, renal failure and left- and right-sided cardiac failure.

There is a considerable risk of fetal death, which is roughly proportional to the severity of the hypertension.

The patient should be treated with rest and restriction of sodium intake. Methyldopa is probably the most successful drug and is freer of side-effects in this context than are, for example, beta-adrenergic blocking drugs and diuretics. In the patient with severe hypertension, especially if there are fits or pulmonary oedema, acute antihypertensive treatment is necessary. Termination of pregnancy is essential in cases not responding to treatment because this is the most effective measure for relieving 'toxaemia'.

The blood pressure of women with pre-eclampsia usually returns to normal after the end of the pregnancy. However, the affected patients seem more liable to develop hypertension subsequently than do those who have not had this condition.

Oral contraception

Oral contraceptive pills give rise to an increase in blood pressure in nearly all women. This is usually slight and falls on stopping the drug. It is wise to check the blood pressure at least during the first year of administration.

Acute porphyria and certain cerebral lesions such as brain tumours and bulbar poliomyelitis

Hypertension may occur as a feature of these conditions but is usually overshadowed by the other manifestations.

Pathophysiology of hypertension

The high blood pressure in essential hypertension is due to increased peripheral vascular resistance as a result of widespread constriction of the arterioles and small arteries. The cardiac output and the viscosity of the blood are normal. In the earlier stages, the hypertension is largely explicable on the basis of increased arteriolar muscle tone, but subsequently structural alterations take place in the arterioles. These changes may account for the fact that hypertension tends to beget further hypertension, and the removal of the cause of hypertension does not necessarily lead to a fall in the blood pressure to normal. The increased work of the heart imposed by the high resistance results in left ventricular hypertrophy and, eventually, left ventricular failure. As it progresses, the hypertrophy may outstrip the coronary blood supply, particularly if, as is so often the case, there is associated coronary artery disease.

Hypertension accelerates the development of atherosclerosis in the coronary, cerebral, renal and other arteries, perhaps because of long-standing mechanical stress. It often leads to the formation of microaneurysms of the cerebral arteries, especially those of the basal ganglia.

The clinical features of hypertensive heart disease

The development of hypertensive heart disease is usually a slow process; no symptoms or abnormal cardiac signs may occur for many years after high blood pressure has been detected.

The earliest symptom is dyspnoea, at first on exercise and later at rest. At a more advanced stage, the features of right heart failure may develop. Angina pectoris is common.

Abnormal cardiac signs include a forcible and displaced apex beat due to left ventricular hypertrophy, an accentuated aortic component of the second sound, and a systolic murmur in the right second intercostal space. Occasionally, the early diastolic murmur of aortic regurgitation is also present. As hypertrophy progresses, a fourth (or atrial) heart sound may be heard. These signs often antedate symptoms.

As failure develops, tachycardia and a third heart sound occur. At this stage, there may be pulsus alternans and the apical pansystolic murmur of functional mitral regurgitation.

Examination of the optic fundus is of great importance in the evaluation of patients with hypertension, for it is only in the retina that the state of the arterioles can be directly observed. The grading introduced by Keith, Wagener and Barker is widely used. Grades 1 and 2 include narrowing of the retinal arteries and compression of the veins at arteriovenous crossings. In grade 3 retinopathy, these features are complicated by exudates of a soft 'cotton wool' appearance and haemorrhages which are flame- or fanshaped. In grade 4 retinopathy there is papilloedema; the disc is pink with blurred edges and the optic cup is obliterated.

ECG, chest radiography and echocardiography

The ECG provides useful evidence of the severity of hypertensive heart disease. In patients with mild elevation of the blood pressure, the ECG is normal. With the development of left ventricular hypertrophy, there is an increase in the voltage of the R waves in the left chest leads and the S waves in the right chest leads. At a more advanced stage, the T waves in the left chest leads become flattened and, later, ST segment depression and T wave inversion develop. Coexistent coronary artery disease may complicate the appearances. Radiographic evidence of left ventricular hypertrophy increases with the passage of time; eventually, the features of pulmonary congestion may develop.

Echocardiography is probably the most reliable technique for evaluating the severity of ventricular hypertrophy.

Abnormalities in the blood and urine

The blood urea is often raised in patients with hypertension. In many cases, this is attributable to renal disease; in others it is secondary to the hypertension and may be corrected if the blood pressure is returned towards normal. If the blood urea exceeds 80 mg/100 ml (13 mmol/l), it is likely that renal damage is severe. The serum potassium may be reduced in essential hypertension, particularly if this is of the malignant type or if diuretics have been used. A low serum potassium in the untreated patient should lead to a search for primary aldosteronism.

Proteinuria, hyaline and granular casts may be found when there is renal disease or malignant hypertension. There is little or no protein in the urine of patients with benign essential hypertension.

Diagnosis of hypertensive heart disease: determination of cause

The diagnosis of hypertensive heart disease depends on the recognition of the high blood pressure and of left ventricular hypertrophy. However, as mentioned, coronary artery disease often coexists and may be the cause of symptoms and signs in patients with hypertension. Angina pectoris and the ECG features of myocardial ischaemia or infarction suggest the presence of coronary artery disease. Hypertension is unlikely to be the sole cause of heart failure if the diastolic pressure is constantly less than 110 mmHg.

It is of great importance to determine the aetiology of the hypertension, particularly in the younger patient in whom it is often secondary, and in whom correction of the cause is more likely to be successful. The diagnosis of acute nephritis is usually relatively easy but the differentiation of essential hypertension from chronic nephritis may be impossible unless there is a history of acute nephritis, or unless renal function is found to be worse than could be accounted for by the severity of the hypertension.

Chronic pyelonephritis may be diagnosed by the history, and by the presence of pus cells and micro-organisms in the urine. The kidneys of patients with polycystic disease are usually easy to feel; there is frequently a family history of the condition. Renal artery disease should be suspected in any younger patient with hypertension and in the older patient with an abrupt acceleration of pre-existing hypertension. A bruit over the renal arteries provides further evidence.

Primary aldosteronism (p. 265) is suggested by muscular weakness, headache and polyuria; suspicion should be aroused by hypokalaemia, particularly if there is also a high serum sodium, Cushing's syndrome (p. 267) is suggested by obesity, moon facies, purple striae, hirsutism and amenorrhoea, combined with glycosuria and an increased urinary excretion of 17-ketosteroids. Phaeochromocytoma (p. 266) is to be suspected when hypertension is paroxysmal, with severe headache, palpitation and perspiration during the attacks. In those cases in which the hypertension is not paroxysmal, there may be no clinical clues and the diagnosis depends upon the demonstration of abnormal quantities of catecholamines or their metabolites in the blood or urine.

Coarctation of the aorta (p. 248) should be sought for in all patients with hypertension. The diagnosis is usually not difficult if the femoral pulses are routinely palpated. In this condition, the femoral pulses are small and delayed and there is almost always a systolic murmur audible over the upper thoracic spine posteriorly. Confirmation is obtained by finding collateral vessels, by the radiographic evidence of rib notching and, if necessary, by aortography.

It may be difficult to diagnose pre-eclampsia (p. 267) with certainty if the patient is seen for the first time in the latter part of the pregnancy. Pre-eclampsia seldom develops until the last trimester, and is usually accompanied by a weight gain, proteinuria and oedema.

Hypertension occurs in acute intermittent porphyria, but is usually accompanied by abdominal pain, fits and various neurological lesions. These features may suggest hypertensive encephalopathy; in cases of doubt the urine should be tested for porphobilinogen.

The investigation of the hypertensive patient

A thorough search for a cause should be undertaken in all patients with severe hypertension (e.g. diastolic pressure greater than 110 mmHg) and in those under 40 years of age in whom the diastolic pressure exceeds 100 mmHg. Investigations are also required to determine what effects the high blood pressure has exerted on the heart and kidneys.

Investigations routinely necessary to determine the nature and severity of the hypertension include serum urea, creatinine, sodium, potassium and bicarbonate and urinary contents. If all these findings are normal, and there are no clinical clues to a causal disease, it is reasonable to begin treatment on the assumption that the hypertension is 'essential'. One can then reserve further investigation for those with specific indications or those in whom treatment fails.

Prognosis

Almost all patients with untreated malignant hypertension die within one year. Death is usually due to uraemia, but heart failure and cerebrovascular accidents are common.

The prognosis of benign essential hypertension is relatively good in the absence of cardiac, renal or cerebral involvement. Even in such patients, the death rate from myocardial infarction and cerebrovascular accidents is much higher than that in the normotensive population. In general, the higher the blood pressure, the greater is the risk of these complications.

Other factors related to prognosis are age, sex, cardiac status, retinopathy and renal function.

High blood pressure at any particular level is more sinister in the young patient than in the old, and in males than in females. Cardiac enlargement and the ECG abnormalities indicate a substantial risk of developing cardiac failure. Grade 3 retinal changes (haemorrhages and soft exudates) carry a prognosis only little better than grade 4 changes.

Proteinuria and urea retention are associated with advancing renal failure.

In the absence of treatment, cardiac failure and cerebrovascular accidents are the major causes of death, myocardial infarction and uraemia being less common, though not infrequent. Several studies have demonstrated the improvement in prognosis that results from antihypertensive therapy. This is most evident in those whose diastolic pressures exceed 105 mmHg, but some benefit is also achieved in individuals with diastolic pressures of 100 or even 95 mmHg. Such treatment has almost eliminated death from cardiac failure and has reduced the incidence of fatal and non-fatal strokes. There is little evidence from trials that antihypertensive treatment prevents myocardial infarction in the milder hypertensive, although it seems possible that prolonged treatment would be necessary to achieve this effect.

The treatment of hypertension

Treatment is undoubtedly indicated when hypertension has led to deleterious effects on the heart, cerebrovascular circulation or kidneys. Therefore, if there is evidence of hypertensive heart disease, or if there are advanced retinal changes with papill-oedema, haemorrhages or soft exudates, the blood pressure should be lowered. It is more difficult to determine whether antihypertensive measures are called for when the blood pressure is persistently raised in the absence of evidence of vascular or renal involvement.

Before initiating drug therapy one must ensure that no treatable cause, such as unilateral renal disease, phaeochromocytoma or coarctation is responsible for the hypertension. If surgically correctable disorders can be excluded, one should consider the most appropriate type of treatment for the individual patient. A few individuals respond well to a reduction in sodium intake or weight. However, in virtually all patients in whom there is evidence of secondary effects from the hypertension, specific antihypertensive drugs are required. Even in the absence of these complications, there is a strong case for such therapy if the diastolic pressure remains high. In the young patient, one should consider treatment if the diastolic pressure is constantly in excess of 95 mmHg. In the middle-aged or elderly patient one might raise the level for which treatment is indicated to 100 or 105 mmHg, respectively.

There are a large number of drugs in current use for the treatment of hypertension; new ones are continually being added. It is only possible to mention those which, at present, seem to be of greatest value. Every physician should be familiar with the use of four or five of these drugs as patients vary from one another in their response to therapy and no one drug can be regarded as superior in all respects to others.

Although the aim should be to make the blood pressure 'normal', too great a fall in blood pressure may impair the circulation to the heart, brain or kidneys and precipitate a myocardial infarction, a stroke or renal failure.

An important consideration is the effect of treatment on the quality of life particularly in patients with mild hypertension, only an unidentifiable minority of whom will gain benefit from antihypertensive drugs.

Drugs used in the treatment of hypertension

Drugs acting on the sympathetic nervous system

Alpha-methyldopa (Aldomet, Dopamet). This drug is metabolized to alpha-methylnoradrenaline, which replaces noradrenaline in adrenergically innervated tissues; as a consequence, there is a diminished response to nerve stimulation. Oral methyldopa begins to lower the blood pressure in about 4 hours and its effect lasts for up to 24 hours. Therapy is started with 250 mg three times a day and increased, if necessary, after a few days to 500 mg three times a day. If this dose is insufficient, a diuretic should be added. The total daily dose should not exceed 3 g. Transient sleepiness is almost invariable during the first 24 hours, but a more subtle drowsiness may persist. Other complications include fluid retention, loss of libido and a Coombs' positive haemolytic anaemia.

Labetalol. This blocks both alpha- and beta-adrenoreceptors and has proved useful both in essential hypertension (particularly in hypertensive emergencies) and phaeochromocytoma. It shares the same side-effects as other beta-blockers but in higher doses is more likely to cause postural hypotension.

Treatment may be started with oral labetalol in a dosage of 50–100 mg twice daily, and increased, if necessary, to a total of 800 mg a day.

Prazosin (Hypovase). This blocks post-synaptic alpha-adrenergic receptors. It has marked arteriolar and venous vasodilating effects and the initial dose may produce profound postural hypotension. The starting dosage is 0.5 mg thrice daily.

Beta-adrenoceptor blocking drugs (see p. 84). These are effective antihypertensive drugs whose mode of action remains uncertain. They are more effective when combined with a diuretic or other antihypertensive drugs but are often sufficient on their own and produce no marked orthostatic effects. To ensure compliance, it is best to utilize a preparation that needs to be given only once or twice a day. Provided these drugs are not prescribed for patients with obstructive airways disease or heart failure, serious complications are unusual. Minor side-effects, such as lethargy, nausea, nightmares and cold extremities are common.

Other drugs acting on the central nervous system occasionally used include clonidine, reserpine, and the adrenergic blocking drugs, guanethidine, bethanidine and debrisoquine.

Vasodilator drugs

Hydralazine. This is a potent arteriolar dilator and increases cardiac output and heart rate. It is best combined with a beta-adrenoceptor blocking agent. Initially 25 mg three times a day should be given; the dose may then be increased if necessary to a total daily dose of 200 mg. It has well-known side-effects of tachycardia, headache and a systemic lupus erythematosus-like reaction; these can largely be avoided by combining with other drugs so that only a small dosage is required.

Diazoxide. This is very effective in acute antihypertensive treatment (150 mg intravenously) but may cause diabetes in prolonged use.

Minoxidil. This is a potent vasodilator and antihypertensive. It produces a reflex tachycardia and fluid retention and should be combined with a beta-blocker and diuretic. It may cause hypertrichosis.

Nitroprusside. This is a very effective antihypertensive drug when given intravenously but should be reserved for hypertensive emergencies.

Diuretics

The mode of action of diuretics remains uncertain, but appears to have two components. Initially, there is a reduced plasma volume and cardiac output, but these are transient changes. With more prolonged treatment, the total peripheral resistance diminishes; this may be the result of changes in the sodium content of vessel walls.

Thiazide drugs. These have been used predominantly in this context and are effective, but have the disadvantage of producing hypokalaemia and occasionally hyperglycaemia and hyperuricaemia. Another side-effect is impotence.

The potassium-conserving diuretics such as spironolactone, amiloride and triamterene have only mild antihypertensive effects but can be used together with thiazide diuretics to preserve potassium equilibrium. The loop diuretics, such as frusemide, ethacrynic acid and bumetanide, may produce a considerable reduction in blood pressure when given intravenously, but they are not ideal for long-term treatment in hypertension because their effects are relatively short-lived.

Angiotensin converting enzyme (ACE) inhibitors

These drugs block the enzyme that converts angiotensin I to angiotensin II (see Fig. 13.1). They cause a fall in blood pressure by reducing systemic vascular resistance, without having any major effect on heart rate and cardiac output. This is probably mainly due to a reduction in plasma angiotensin II, but there is also a secondary fall in aldosterone.

Two drugs of this group are currently available — captopril and enalapril. Captopril exerts its maximal effect in about 2 hours. Enalapril is a pro-drug which is hydrolysed in the liver to an active metabolite, enalaprilic acid. Its peak effect is between 4 and 12 hours.

Both drugs are effective in all grades and types of hypertension, but their action is potentiated by diuretics. Profound hypotension may be induced, which may be prolonged in the case of enalapril. This should be avoided by starting with a small dose, and stopping or reducing the dosage of diuretics 2 or 3 days previously if these are being administered (Table 13.1). Renal impairment may be caused, particularly in renal artery stenosis. Hyperkalaemia may occur because of the anti-aldosterone effect; the concomitant use of aldosterone antagonists or potassium is generally unwise.

Side-effects, which are not common with low dosages, include taste disorders, nausea, diarrhoea, rashes, cough, neutropenia, proteinuria and angioneurotic oedema.

ACE inhibitors are usually well tolerated and most patients prefer them to other antihypertensive agents. They are not, however, first line treatment, partly because of their cost and partly because of their occasional severe adverse effect.

It is wise to start with a low dose, e.g. captopril 12.5 mg twice daily, or enalapril 5 mg daily (see Table 13.1).

Calcium-blocking drugs (see p. 151)

Nifedipine and nicardipine are effective antihypertensive drugs, particularly when combined with other antihypertensive therapy, such as beta-adrenoreceptor blocking drugs. Verapamil and diltiazem are also antihypertensive.

Choice of therapy for the individual patient

There is no doubt of the need for therapy when the complications of hypertension, such as cardiac failure or advanced retinal changes are encountered. However, to an increasing extent it has become clear that asymptomatic patients with hypertension benefit from antihypertensive treatment insofar as it protects them from stroke,

Table 13.1 Dosage of ACE inhibitors.

	Starting dose		Maintenance dose
	Hypertension *	Heart failure	
Captopril	12.5 mg twice daily	6.25 mg twice daily	25 mg twice daily (to a maximum of 150 mg daily)
Enalapril	5 mg daily	2.5 mg daily	10–20 mg daily

* Halve this dose (i) in the elderly, (ii) if diuretics are used, or (iii) with renal impairment (captopril better avoided).

cardiac failure and renal failure and, less certainly, from angina pectoris and myocardial infarction.

Randomized control studies of treatment in a number of countries have demonstrated clearly that if the diastolic pressure constantly exceeds 105 mmHg, antihypertensive treatment reduces the incidence of complications. Recent studies have suggested that there is a clear-cut benefit from antihypertensive treatment if the diastolic pressure is 100 mmHg or more; there is less certain evidence of those with a diastolic pressure exceeding 95 mmHg. In particular, the role of antihypertensive treatment in the elderly has not yet been defined. Currently, it seems reasonable to treat middle-aged patients whose diastolic pressure exceeds 100 mmHg with antihypertensive drugs, but to use such drugs only for patients with diastolic pressures exceeding 95 mmHg if they are young or there are features suggesting that hypertension may be causing secondary effects on the heart, kidney or retina.

One should start treatment with a single drug which has relatively minor side-effects. It is now customary to start either with a diuretic or a beta-blocker, the latter being favoured if there is angina. The next step is to try the one of these two drugs which has not been given initially and if this fails to combine the two. If such measures fail, an angiotensin converting enzyme inhibitor, a calcium antagonist, methyldopa, hydralazine or prazosin might be added. If the combination of such therapy still fails to control the blood pressure, careful review of the whole case needs to be undertaken ensuring that a secondary form of hypertension has not been overlooked and that the patient is complying with treatment. If such is not the case, then drugs such as minoxidil or the adrenergic blocking drugs might be considered.

The patient embarking on antihypertensive treatment must be advised that drug therapy will probably be required for the rest of his life. Regular checking of the blood pressure is essential.

Occasionally, urgent antihypertensive therapy must be undertaken for acute left ventricular failure or hypertensive fits. The
most effective drugs are intravenous sodium nitroprusside, (50
mg in 500 ml 5% glucose), labetalol (25 mg) and diazoxide (150
mg). All require the most cautious administration and careful
monitoring.

Further reading

ABC of hypertension. (1981) London: BMJ Publications.
Kaplan, N.M. (1986) *Clinical Hypertension*, 4th edn. Baltimore: Williams
and Wilkins.
World Health Organization (1985) *Management of Arterial Hypertension*
Geneva: WHO.

14

Diseases of the Aorta

The aortic wall is composed of an endothelial lining or intima, a media containing smooth muscle and elastic tissue, and a fibrous adventitia. The media is largely responsible for the elasticity of the aortic wall, and the adventitia for its strength and resistance to rupture.

Dissecting aneurysm

A dissecting aneurysm (Fig. 14.1) results from the entry of blood into the media, either as a consequence of the rupture of vasa vasorum or from a tear of the aortic intima. No histological abnormality is seen in the media of most cases although cystic changes are sometimes present. Dissecting aneurysm is an important complication of the Marfan syndrome and of pregnancy, but the majority of cases occur in middle-aged or elderly men with systemic hypertension. The dissection usually starts either in the ascending aorta a short distance above the aortic valve, or just beyond the origin of the left subclavian artery. The blood dissects a channel between the intima and the adventitia and usually advances distally. In so doing, it may occlude branches of the aortic arch and the descending aorta, including the renal and iliac arteries. If the dissection spreads proximally, the aortic valve may be involved, producing aortic regurgitation and, occasionally, occlusion of a coronary artery. The aneurysm usually ruptures externally into the pericardium, pleural cavity, mediastinum or retroperitoneal tissues, but sometimes it perforates the intima and the dissection 're-enters' the aortic lumen. Occasionally, the dissection becomes chronic without perforation.

Dissecting aneurysms usually present with the sudden onset of a 'tearing' pain of extreme severity. The site of the pain depends upon the location of the dissection and moves as the dissection progresses. The pain may start in the anterior or posterior chest or in the abdomen, but nearly always affects the upper back at some stage. Intervals of freedom from pain may occur; with recurrences, the pain may involve the neck, arms, chest, trunk or legs. Occasionally, the pain is slight; breathlessness or syncope may then be the presenting symptom.

Fig. 14.1 Dissecting aneurysm of the aorta. This usually starts either a short distance above the aortic valve (left) or just below the origin of the left subclavian artery (right).

On examination, the patient appears pale and sweaty and has a tachycardia; although he may have the appearance of shock, the blood pressure is usually within normal limits, having fallen from hypertensive levels. Other signs depend on which branches of the aorta are occluded. Thus, one or more of the arteries to the limbs may become impalpable. Other complications include aortic regurgitation, tamponade, hemiplegia, mental disturbances, haematuria, bloody diarrhoea and haemothorax.

The ECG is of little diagnostic value, but pre-existing hypertension may have caused left ventricular hypertrophy. The appearances of myocardial ischaemia or myocardial infarction may be present if there has been encroachment on a coronary artery. The chest radiograph shows an increase in the width of the mediastinum. Computed tomography is probably the best technique for diagnosing dissection and defining its site (Fig. 14.2). Cross-sectional echocardiography and digital subtraction angiography may also be useful. The diagnosis can be further confirmed by injecting radio-opaque material into the aorta.

The diagnosis may not be difficult when there is a severe but shifting pain associated with the occlusion of vessels. Differentiation from myocardial infarction may be almost impossible clinically. Dissection is suggested by the following: the distribution and progression of the pain, the relatively high blood pressure,

Fig. 14.2 Computed tomogram of an aortic dissection. Arrow points to detached flap in aorta.

the development of differences in the peripheral pulses, the occurrence of an aortic diastolic murmur, the broadened mediastinum and the absence of the ECG and enzyme changes of acute myocardial infarction.

Although death may be sudden and unexpected, the symptoms often progress over a period of hours or days before rupture occurs. Few patients survive more than a week and even fewer more than 3 weeks. Occasionally, a dissecting aneurysm becomes chronic and the patient may then survive for months or years.

Medical treatment is advisable during the initial phase: the fragile aortic wall makes surgery at this time hazardous. The blood pressure should be lowered to reduce the strain on the aorta; beta-adrenoceptor blocking drugs are preferred for this purpose.

When the situation has stabilized (perhaps after 2 or 3 days), surgery should be considered. As a rule, aortic replacement or repair should be undertaken if the ascending aorta is involved; surgery is only required for dissection of the descending aorta if there are continuing symptoms or major vessels are obstructed.

Saccular and fusiform aortic aneurysms

These are localized distensions of the wall of the aorta, being fusiform if the whole circumference of the vessel is involved and saccular if only part of it is affected.

Atherosclerotic aneurysms, which are usually situated in the descending aorta, result from atrophy of the media and adventitia with fibrous replacement. Syphilis, formerly the major cause of aortic aneurysm, has become uncommon. Syphilitic aneurysms usually affect the ascending aorta and the aortic arch, as a result of inflammatory changes in the aortic wall and subsequent fibrosis and calcification (see p. 300). Aortic aneurysms are also seen in association with the Marfan syndrome and coarctation of the aorta. They can also result from trauma, particularly car accidents, in which the aortic wall is partially or completely transected. A distinctive type of aneurysm is that of the sinus of Valsalva, which will be considered separately.

The clinical features resulting from an aneurysm of the thoracic aorta depend upon its size and site. When the aneurysm is in the ascending aorta, there is often associated aortic regurgitation which leads to cardiac failure. As the aneurysm enlarges and encroaches upon neighbouring structures, there may be pain as a result of erosion of ribs and sternum. A pulsating mass may be seen in the front of the chest and obstruction of the superior vena cava may occur. When the aneurysm is situated in the aortic arch, wheezing, cough and hoarseness may arise from compression of the trachea, bronchus or recurrent laryngeal nerves. Aneurysms of the descending aorta are most likely to produce symptoms as a result of encroachment on the vertebrae, ribs or spinal nerves. Often, however, an aneurysm of the thoracic aorta is first diagnosed in an asymptomatic patient by the radiographic demonstration of a localized dilatation of the aorta. The diagnosis can be confirmed by the injection of radio-opaque medium into the aorta.

Asymptomatic patients with relatively small aneurysms may survive for many years. However, the prognosis is generally poor and the patient with symptoms is unlikely to survive more than 1 or 2 years.

Most patients with aneurysms of the aorta have severe associated disorders such as hypertension, ischaemic heart disease or cerebrovascular disease, and death more often results from one of these than from the aneurysm. Perhaps only one-third of the patients die from aortic rupture; before surgery is undertaken, the cardiovascular and cerebral circulations must be carefully evaluated. Surgery should be considered for those aneurysms which are large or producing symptoms. Saccular aneurysms, which usually have a narrow neck, can be treated by transection of the neck with repair of the underlying aorta. If much of the aortic wall is involved, resection must be undertaken with replacement by a graft.

Aneurysm of the sinus of Valsalva

This is most commonly caused by a congenital localized absence of the aortic media, but can result from syphilitic aortitis or infective endocarditis. The aneurysm forms a thin-walled sac which in most instances protrudes into the right ventricle or right atrium (Fig. 14.3). No symptoms or signs are produced until the aneurysm ruptures. When it does so a fistula is formed between the aorta and the relevant chamber. Congenital aneurysms of the sinus of Valsalva are often associated with other congenital lesions, particularly a ventricular septal defect.

Sudden death sometimes occurs; more often rupture causes the abrupt onset of chest pain and breathlessness. These symptoms subside over a period of days or weeks. Cardiac failure develops subsequently, but is very variable in its rate of progression.

On examination the patient may have a collapsing pulse due to the aortic diastolic leak, and there is usually a continuous systolic and diastolic murmur, resembling that of a persistent ductus arteriosus, but loudest over the sternum at the level of the third or fourth interspace.

The ECG may be normal initially, but the signs of right ventricular hypertrophy or right bundle branch block may develop later. The chest radiograph shows cardiac enlargement with pulmonary plethora. The aneurysm may be demonstrated by echocardiography, and the shunt by Doppler ultrasound. The definitive diagnosis is made by showing the leak by aortography, and by the demonstration of a left-to-right shunt on cardiac catheterization.

The ruptured sinus of Valsalva should be treated by repair of the aortic wall.

Fig. 14.3 Aneurysm of sinus of Valsalva rupturing into right atrium.

Further reading

Dalen, J.E., Pape, L.A., Cohn, L.H., Lester, J.K. (Jr) & Collins, J.J.J. (1980) Dissection of the aorta. *Progress in Cardiovascular Diseases* 23: 237.
Liddicoat, J.E., Bekassy, S.M., Rubio, P.A., Noon, G.P. & DeBakey, M.E. (1975) Ascending aortic aneurysms. *Circulation 52 (Supplement I):* 202.

Disorders of the Lungs and Pulmonary Circulation

Pulmonary embolism, thrombosis and infarction

Pulmonary thrombo-embolism can cause or aggravate heart disease, and is a common and serious complication of cardiac disorders.

Pulmonary embolism results from the obstruction of the pulmonary arterial vessels by thrombus or by material, such as fat or air, originating in some other site. *Pulmonary thrombosis* implies the formation of clot in situ. *Pulmonary infarction* is the necrosis of a wedge of lung tissue resulting from pulmonary arterial occlusion.

Pulmonary embolism is usually a consequence of thrombophlebitis or phlebothrombosis in the leg veins but may also follow thrombosis of the pelvic veins, or clot formation in the right atrium in patients with right-sided cardiac failure, particularly if there is atrial fibrillation. Deep vein thrombosis is often asymptomatic, but the leg may be warm, tender, slightly dusky and swollen by oedema. Thrombosis is most likely to occur when there has been stasis in the veins, especially in association with childbirth, abdominal surgery, acute myocardial infarction and right-sided cardiac failure. There is a slightly increased risk in women taking oral contraceptives. Pulmonary thrombosis is uncommon except as a complication of pre-existing disease of the pulmonary arteries.

Pulmonary embolism can be prevented by measures which prevent the development or progression of venous thrombosis. Simple measures to encourage venous flow such as the use of leg exercises and elastic stockings in those confined to bed are important and effective ways of doing so. Once thrombosis has been diagnosed treatment should be initiated with heparin, unless there are contraindications. A bolus of 5000 units may be given, followed by a continuous infusion of the drug. The dosage should be controlled by the activated partial thromboplastin time (APTT) (see p. 170). Oral warfarin should be started at the same time, as described on p. 171. The INR (BCR) should be maintained between 2.0 and 3.0, unless there is recurrent thrombo-embolism when between 3.0 and 4.5 would be appropriate. Heparin may be stopped after 5–7 days. Warfarin should be continued for 3 months for calf thrombosis and 6 months for iliofemoral thrombosis.

There are three symptoms of pulmonary thrombo-embolism which may occur at different times in the same patient. They are massive pulmonary embolism, pulmonary infarction and thrombo-embolic pulmonary hypertension.

Massive pulmonary embolism

A large embolus may block the main pulmonary artery or one of its major branches, or multiple emboli may occlude many smaller branches. If two-thirds of the pulmonary arterial bed is occluded, acute right-sided cardiac failure occurs with a low cardiac output and a rise in venous pressure. Sometimes the onset of massive thrombosis is more insidious, with symptoms and signs increasing progressively over 2 weeks or more.

When massive embolism occurs, the patient may drop dead suddenly. In other cases there may be syncope, chest pain and dyspnoea. The syncope is probably attributable to a sudden fall in blood pressure, the chest pain to inadequate coronary blood flow, and the dyspnoea to impaired pulmonary ventilation and reflex factors. On examination, the patient is pale, cyanosed and breathless, with cold extremities. There is tachypnoea and sinus tachycardia. The jugular venous pressure is often raised and there may be right ventricular third and fourth heart sounds. Occasionally, there are pulmonary systolic or diastolic murmurs.

The ECG often shows the effects of acute dilatation of the right ventricle and atrium. One or more of a number of features may be observed (Fig. 15.1): a narrow Q wave and inverted T wave in lead III, accompanied by an S wave in lead I as a result of a change in the position of the heart produced by dilatation of the right ventricle and atrium; P pulmonale, or an atrial arrhythmia; partial or complete right bundle branch block; T wave inversion from V1 to V4 ('right ventricular strain') and clockwise rotation of the heart (with large S waves being seen in V3 and V4).

The chest radiograph is seldom helpful, although it may show enlarged proximal pulmonary arteries and small peripheral ones. Pulmonary angiography is probably the most specific and sensitive test for pulmonary embolism, but it is expensive, invasive and has a morbidity and mortality.

Pulmonary scintigraphy, using radioactive technetium labelled macro-aggregated albumin, is a sensitive technique for detecting perfusion abnormalities, but is not specific. A normal ventilation

Fig. 15.1 ECG appearances in pulmonary embolism. Note tall, peaked P waves, partial right bundle branch block (rSr in V1), S in lead I, Q and negative T in III, and inverted T waves in V1 to V3.

scan (with radioactive xenon) helps to confirm the diagnosis in the presence of a perfusion defect.

Massive pulmonary embolism should be suspected in any patient who suddenly develops the features of shock, syncope, acute dyspnoea or chest pain, particularly if the subject has evidence of a venous thrombosis or has been confined to bed during the preceding days. The differential diagnosis from acute myocardial infarction may be extremely difficult. The ECG is of considerable value, but the patterns associated with massive pulmonary embolism are often misinterpreted as being those of a combination of inferior and anteroseptal infarction. The appearance of Q waves and negative T waves in lead III (but not in lead II) in association with inverted T waves from V1 to V4 strongly suggests pulmonary embolism. The definitive diagnosis can be made by pulmonary angiography, but this is potentially hazardous; radio-isotope scanning is safer though less specific.

The prognosis of massive pulmonary embolism is poor; some 10% die almost immediately of a ventricular arrhythmia or circulatory failure, a further 20% die within the next few hours or days. In those who survive, complete recovery is usual, but there is a risk of further pulmonary embolism.

The patient should be treated with oxygen and digoxin. Anticoagulation should be started with intravenous heparin and continued with an oral preparation such as warfarin for 3–6 months. Fibrinolytic therapy with drugs such as streptokinase or urokinase accelerates recovery from massive pulmonary embolism and is indicated for the critically ill patient. If an appropriately skilled surgeon and cardiopulmonary bypass techniques are immediately available, the embolus can sometimes be successfully removed.

Pulmonary infarction

Pulmonary infarction follows the occlusion of smaller pulmonary arteries (and, rarely, veins). A necrotic area develops which is usually haemorrhagic because of the exudation of blood from still patent bronchial arteries. The infarction may reach the surface of the lung and produce pleurisy with an effusion which is usually blood-stained. Typically, there is a pleuritic pain accompanied by low pyrexia and, in about 50% of cases, the expectoration of bright red blood. Pulmonary infarction may, however, be silent, or cause only a low-grade pyrexia.

Often there are no abnormal physical signs, but tachycardia, tachypnoea, the signs of pulmonary consolidation and a pleural rub may occur. Right-sided failure may develop or be aggravated in those with pre-existing heart disease. The ECG is often normal but may show changes similar to those of massive pulmonary embolism. The chest radiograph often reveals small and sometimes wedge-shaped opacities. It may also show an effusion or elevation of the diaphragm on the affected side. A radio-isotope scan is abnormal, usually revealing several scattered areas of reduced perfusion.

It is frequently difficult to differentiate pulmonary infarction from pneumonia if there has been no evidence of deep venous thrombosis. Pulmonary infarction is commoner than pneumonia in hospitalized patients; it differs in that the sputum is seldom infected but is often frankly bloody, and the fever does not respond to antibiotics.

Pulmonary infarction should be treated by heparin and oral anticoagulants, the main purpose of which is to prevent further embolization.

Recurrent pulmonary emboli and thrombo-embolic pulmonary hypertension

Recurrent pulmonary embolization, which is usually associated with chronic or recurrent venous thrombosis, may appear as massive emboli, as pulmonary infarction or be silent. Eventually, the vascular obstruction may become so widespread as to cause a substantial increase in the resistance of the pulmonary arteries and lead to pulmonary arterial hypertension. Once this has become established, the prognosis is poor and most patients die within a period of 5 years. The process may sometimes be reversed or prevented from progression by permanent anticoagulant therapy. If anticoagulant therapy fails, inferior vena caval ligation or plication sometimes prevents further embolism, but is not always effective and may lead to severe oedema of the legs.

Pulmonary hypertension

The pulmonary arterial pressure is determined by the pressure in the pulmonary capillaries, the pulmonary blood flow and the resistance of the pulmonary arteries (especially the arterioles).

The small pulmonary arteries of the fetus have a thick muscular media and the pulmonary vascular resistance of the non-aerated lung is high. This muscular layer regresses over the first 2–3 months of life. As a consequence the pulmonary vascular resistance and arterial pressure start to fall shortly after birth and within a few weeks have declined to normal adult levels.

The pulmonary arteries in the adult are relatively thin-walled, the smaller vessels having considerably less muscle in their walls than corresponding systemic arterioles. The resistance to flow is much lower and the pressure in the pulmonary artery (about 20/10 mmHg) is approximately one-seventh that in the aorta. It is believed that many of the capillaries in the lung are closed at rest, particularly those of the upper parts of the lungs. When the cardiac output increases, as on exercise, the vascular resistance falls as capillaries open and small arteries dilate. As a consequence, blood flow through the lungs can increase threefold before any rise in pressure occurs.

Pulmonary arterial hypertension (greater than 30/15 mmHg) may result from:

1 an increase in pulmonary capillary pressure;
2 an increase in pulmonary blood flow;
3 an increase in pulmonary vascular resistance;

1 Passive pulmonary hypertension due to a raised pulmonary capillary pressure occurs in all conditions in which the left atrial pressure rises, such as mitral stenosis and left ventricular failure. The pulmonary artery pressure rises in proportion to the pulmonary capillary pressure and the pulmonary hypertension is not severe.

2 Pulmonary hypertension due to increased flow develops in disorders in which there are left-to-right shunts. These include septal defects and persistent ductus arteriosus. In atrial septal defect, a large pulmonary blood flow of 10–15 litres per minute may be unassociated with pulmonary hypertension because there is a compensatory vasodilatation with a fall in vascular resistance. In many cases of ventricular septal defect and persistent ductus arteriosus, there is no vasodilatation, and the resistance remains normal. The pulmonary arterial pressure may therefore rise even with comparatively small shunts. With large shunts, pulmonary arterial pressure may reach systemic levels.

3   Pulmonary vascular resistance may be increased by several mechanisms:

a   Pulmonary vasoconstriction. This may be a reaction to an elevated pulmonary capillary pressure and to hypoxia. It is particularly common in mitral stenosis, much less so in mitral regurgitation, and seldom develops unless the mean pulmonary capillary pressure is constantly in excess of 20 mmHg.
   Hypoxia is a potent pulmonary vasocontrictor and is a factor in the pulmonary hypertension that occurs in respiratory disease.

b   Disease of the small pulmonary arteries. In infants with large ventricular septal defects, there may be delay in the regression of the muscular media of the small pulmonary arteries (see above). As a consequence, the pulmonary vascular resistance may stay high, thereby limiting the left-to-right shunt. Hyaline and fibrotic changes may take place and thickening of the arteries may progress and lead to severe pulmonary hypertension (the Eisenmenger syndrome).
   Arterial muscular hyperplasia and fibrosis may take place in older patients in response to long-standing pulmonary hypertension.

c   Obliteration of the pulmonary arteries by thrombosis and embolism, of the arterioles in schistosomiasis, and of the pulmonary capillaries by emphysema.

Combinations of the three mechanisms are common. In mitral stenosis, for example, the initial phase of passive pulmonary hypertension is often complicated by vasoconstriction and by the obliterative changes of pulmonary embolism. In many cases of ventricular septal defect, both high blood flow and pulmonary vascular disease contribute to pulmonary hypertension. In emphysema, obliteration of the vascular bed and hypoxia are contributory factors.

Independent of causation, certain clinical features are characteristic of severe pulmonary hypertension. The symptoms include dyspnoea, fatigue, syncope, anginal pain and haemoptysis. Hoarseness may occur as a result of stretching of the left recurrent laryngeal nerve. Eventually, the symptoms of right-sided cardiac failure develop.

The arterial pulse is normal or small; the venous pulse is often abnormal due to a prominent 'a' wave. There is a forceful right ventricular thrust along the left sternal edge and there may be a shock in the second left interspace due to pulmonary valve closure. There is a loud pulmonary second sound, which may be followed by the early diastolic murmur of pulmonary regurgitation, and there may also be a fourth heart sound at the lower left sternal edge. Both right atrial and right ventricular hypertrophy may be seen on the ECG, and the radiograph shows prominent main pulmonary arteries with normal or unusually clear peripheral lung fields.

The prognosis of pulmonary arterial hypertension depends upon its aetiology and on its severity. Passive pulmonary hypertension responds well if the underlying disorder can be corrected. Pulmonary hypertension due to high pulmonary arterial flow can usually be reversed by the correction of the underlying congenital abnormality. Increased pulmonary arterial resistance due to vasoconstriction can often be diminished by relieving hypoxia or by the successful treatment of mitral valve disease. When pulmonary hypertension is due to severe pulmonary vascular disease, as in the Eisenmenger syndrome, the prognosis is poor and life is usually sustained for only a few years. In these cases, cardiac failure is progressive in spite of treatment and the only hope may lie in heart–lung transplantation.

Primary ('unexplained') pulmonary hypertension

Pulmonary hypertension is said to be primary when the aetiology cannot be determined. It is possible that small pulmonary emboli are responsible for some cases. The condition, which is rare, is most apt to affect young women; the first symptoms are usually fatigue and exertional dyspnoea. The diagnosis is made by exclusion in patients found to have the clinical features of pulmonary hypertension. The prognosis is poor; death is likely to occur within 5 years. Thrombosis may contribute to the progression of hypertension and anticoagulants are recommended; oral contraceptives and pregnancy must be avoided. Some improvement may be achieved by the use of vasodilators such as hydralazine, diazoxide, nitrates and nifedipine.

Pulmonary heart disease

The understanding of pulmonary heart disease (cor pulmonale) has been made difficult by problems of nomenclature. Here it is defined as heart disease secondary to disorders of ventilation and respiratory function. Right-sided heart failure due to pulmonary arterial disease or secondary to left-sided heart failure is not included in this definition, and is considered in the section on pulmonary hypertension (above).

The prevalence of pulmonary heart disease varies greatly between one geographical area and another. There is abundant evidence that heavy cigarette smoking and air pollution are major factors in the production of chronic bronchitis; cor pulmonale is commonest in those exposed to these influences. It is predominantly a disease of middle-aged and elderly men, and is uncommon in young men or in women of any age.

Pathogenesis of heart failure in lung disease

Lung disease causes heart disease mainly because of its effects on the pulmonary vessels. Due to a number of different mechanisms, there is an increase in pulmonary vascular resistance, leading to pulmonary hypertension, right ventricular hypertrophy and right heart failure.
These mechanisms include:

1 pulmonary arteriolar constriction due to low alveolar oxygen tension in areas of underventilated lung;
2 anatomical reduction of the pulmonary vascular bed from rupture of alveolar walls and from fibrotic or thrombotic obliteration of capillaries;
3 compression of pulmonary capillaries by high intra-alveolar pressures when there is air trapping.

Pulmonary hypertension is seldom severe in pulmonary disease except when there is superadded respiratory infection.

Abnormalities in the blood gases nearly always precede the appearance of heart failure due to lung disease. Hypoxaemia is almost invariable. Even if the arterial oxygen tension is normal at rest, it is reduced on exercise. The hypoxaemia results either from disturbances in the ventilation–perfusion relationship or from interference with the diffusion of oxygen through the alveolar wall.

The carbon dioxide tension is raised when the heart failure is secondary to chronic obstructive airways disease and alveolar hypoventilation. If there is a rapid rise in carbon dioxide tension, the pH is low, but in the chronic stage of the disease the renal retention of bicarbonate maintains a normal or near normal acid–base balance.

These blood gas abnormalities are responsible for many of the characteristics of pulmonary heart disease.

1 Polycythaemia and increased blood volume due to hypoxaemia.

2 Peripheral vasodilatation, due to high carbon dioxide tension, producing a large pulse and warm extremities.
3 Cerebral vasodilatation, due to high carbon dioxide tension, which leads to a raised cerebrospinal fluid pressure, with tremor, confusion and papilloedema. The more advanced symptoms of carbon dioxide retention occur mainly, if not exclusively, in patients receiving oxygen in high concentration. Such treatment is dangerous if there is carbon dioxide retention because it abolishes the hypoxaemia which is a major stimulus to respiration.
4 Impaired myocardial function due to hypoxaemia.

Diseases causing pulmonary heart disease

Diseases primarily affecting air passages of the lung and the alveoli

1 Chronic bronchitis with generalized airways obstruction with or without emphysema. In chronic bronchitis there is hyperplasia of the mucus-secreting glands of the tracheobronchial tree, with chronic infection and bronchial obstruction. In emphysema, the air spaces distal to the terminal bronchioles are abnormally enlarged, and the alveolar walls are, to a greater or lesser extent, destroyed.
2 Bronchial asthma.
3 Emphysema without bronchitis or asthma.
  In all these three conditions, airways obstruction is an important factor. This is transient in asthma and usually disappears between attacks; pulmonary heart disease is uncommon. In chronic bronchitis and emphysema there is uneven matching between ventilation and perfusion. Some alveoli are well perfused with blood but poorly ventilated, whilst others are well ventilated but inadequately perfused. Pulmonary hypertension results from a combination of hypoxia, destruction of pulmonary capillaries and the effects of high alveolar pressure on the pulmonary vessels. Often, pulmonary hypertension is experienced only during episodes of infection which aggravate bronchial obstruction.
4 Pulmonary fibrosis due to tuberculosis, pneumoconiosis, bronchiectasis, other pulmonary infections, radiation and mucoviscidosis.
  Pulmonary hypertension due to these causes is relatively uncommon, unless there is associated emphysema.
5 Pulmonary granulomata and infiltrations due to sarcoidosis, fibrosing alveolitis, berylliosis, eosinophilic granuloma, histiocytosis, malignant infiltration, scleroderma, systemic lupus

erythematosus, dermatomyositis and alveolar microlithiasis.

In these conditions there is a diffusion defect in the lung due to thickening of the alveolar membrane. Because oxygen diffuses much less quickly than carbon dioxide, this disturbance leads to hypoxaemia but not carbon dioxide retention. The hypoxaemia causes hyperventilation and eventually leads to pulmonary hypertension and cardiac failure. The early diagnosis may be difficult as the chest radiograph may show no abnormality.

6 Pulmonary resection.
7 Congenital cystic disease of the lungs.

Diseases primarily affecting the movements of the thoracic cage and respiratory muscles

1 Kyphoscoliosis and other thoracic deformities;
2 Thoracoplasty;
3 Pleural fibrosis;
4 Chronic neuromuscular weakness, e.g. poliomyelitis;
5 Obesity with alveolar hypoventilation (Pickwickian syndrome see p. 305);
6 Idiopathic alveolar hypoventilation.

In these conditions, there is inadequate pulmonary ventilation, due either to a deformity of the thoracic cage, or to interference with the function of the respiratory muscles. Alveolar hypoventilation leads to hypoxaemia and carbon dioxide retention.

Sleep apnoea. Apnoea during sleep contributes to alveolar hypoxia, carbon dioxide retention and pulmonary hypertension in such conditions as idiopathic hypoventilation, the Pickwickian syndrome, and obstruction of the upper airways by enlarged tonsils. Most affected patients have been heavy snorers for many years, and the apnoeic attacks are more often due to pharyngeal obstruction than to primary cessation of activity by the ventilatory muscles.

Clinical features of pulmonary heart disease

The patient is usually a cigarette-smoking middle-aged man with a long history of morning cough and sputum. There may have been recurrent attacks of winter bronchitis. These symptoms are slowly progressive until breathlessness becomes disabling. Overt cyanosis and peripheral oedema are usually late features but are sometimes the first clear manifestation of pulmonary disease. Recent worsening of cough and the production of purulent sputum is common.

The subject is usually breathless and wheezing even at rest. Cyanosis varies from the scarcely detectable to the gross. When carbon dioxide retention is present, there may be clouding of consciousness or confusion, accompanied by tremor of the hands. The hands are usually warm and the pulse large due to peripheral vasodilatation.

The jugular venous pressure may be raised due either to cardiac failure or increased blood volume, or because venous return is hindered by high intrapleural pressure. Cardiac failure produces oedema and hepatic enlargement. The chest moves poorly and may be barrel-shaped and hyper-resonant. Expiratory rhonchi are usual and there may be crepitations. The breath sounds are often difficult to hear.

Emphysema may make the apex beat impalpable and prevent right ventricular hypertrophy from being detected at the left sternal edge, although it may be palpable in the epigastrium. The first and second heart sounds are soft; when cardiac failure ensues there may be a right ventricular third heart sound and a systolic murmur over the lower sternum due to tricuspid regurgitation.

Electrocardiogram and chest radiograph. The ECG is often normal but may show P pulmonale, right axis deviation, right ventricular hypertrophy, right bundle branch block, or an rS pattern across the chest. In emphysema the QRS complexes are often small.

The radiological appearances depend upon the nature of the lung disease. When there is emphysema with an increased total lung volume, one may see a low diaphragm and a narrow heart. Enlargement of the main pulmonary artery and its major branches occurs when there is pulmonary hypertension. The radiograph is, however, often normal.

Pulmonary function tests. Spirometry. In chronic bronchitis and emphysema, and in bronchial asthma during the paroxysms, the forced vital capacity (FVC) is reduced, but to a smaller extent than forced expiratory volume in one second (FEV_1). Normally, the FEV_1/FVC is 75% or more; in obstructive airways disease it is considerably less. In restrictive lung disease due to pulmonary fibrosis there is no obstruction and FEV_1/FVC is often greater than 75%.

Blood gas estimations. In virtually all cases of pulmonary heart disease there is hypoxaemia. Carbon dioxide retention is usual in obstructive airways disease and in those disorders in which the movement of the thoracic cage and respiratory muscles are impaired. Carbon dioxide tension is normal or even reduced when there is a diffusion defect.

Diagnosis

Two types of diagnostic problem arise:

1   Is there cardiovascular involvement complicating known pulmonary disease?
2   Is right heart failure due to pulmonary disease or to some other factor?

Cardiac involvement in pulmonary disease is suggested by clinical, ECG or radiological evidence of pulmonary hypertension or right ventricular enlargement, by the presence of a right ventricular third heart sound and by signs of right-sided cardiac failure.

The pulmonary origin of cardiac failure is often overlooked, particularly when it coexists with known ischaemic, rheumatic or hypertensive heart disease. This is particularly the case with hypertension; mild hypertension is often blamed for heart failure which is secondary to chronic bronchitis and emphysema. The history of chronic cough with sputum and wheezing should suggest the possibility, as should poor chest movement and the presence of rhonchi. The diagnosis is usually best made by studies of ventilation and blood gases; carbon dioxide retention makes it almost certain that there is a pulmonary component in heart failure.

Prognosis

The prognosis is poor once cardiac failure has complicated pulmonary heart disease. Treatment may overcome individual attacks, but the subject is liable to further episodes with recurrent infection, and is unlikely to survive more than two or three such attacks over a period of a few years.

Treatment

When a patient is seen in cardiac failure due to pulmonary heart disease, the major objects of treatment should be to combat respiratory infection, correct hypoxaemia and carbon dioxide retention, and relieve airways obstruction.

Infection is most commonly due to *Haemophilus influenzae* and pneumococcus. The antibiotics of choice are either ampicillin or oxytetracycline in a dose of 250 mg 6-hourly for 10 days.

Oxygen therapy is essential, but oxygen in too high a concentration may lead to carbon dioxide retention and coma. The oxygen should therefore be administered using one of the special types of mask which deliver 25−29% oxygen. If oxygenation remains inadequate in spite of this type of oxygen therapy, it may be best to employ intermittent positive pressure ventilation, if necessary with tracheostomy. Bronchodilators such as salbutamol or orciprenaline by inhalation or intravenous aminophylline are helpful. Corticosteroids may be necessary in severe attacks of asthma. Digitalis and diuretics may be used, but are relatively ineffective until infection has been controlled and hypoxaemia corrected.

Once the patient has recovered from the attack of cardiac failure, efforts must be made to ensure that he does not recommence smoking, that he avoids dusty atmospheres, that obesity is corrected and that respiratory infections are promptly treated.

Further reading

Flenley, D. (1981) *Respiratory Disease*. London: Baillière Tindall.

Fuster, V., Steele, P.M., Edwards, W.D., Gersh, B.J., McGoon, M.D. & Frye, R.L. (1984) Primary pulmonary hypertension. *Circulation 70:* 580.

Harris, P. & Heath, D. (1986) *The Human Pulmonary Circulation*, 3rd edn. Edinburgh: Churchill Livingstone.

Hirsch, J., Hull, R.D. & Raskob, G.E. (1986) Clinical features and diagnosis of venous thrombosis. *Journal of American College of Cardiology 8:* 114B.

Hirsch, J., Hull, R.D. & Raskob, G.E. (1986) Diagnosis of pulmonary embolism. *Journal of American College of Cardiology 8:* 128B.

Systemic Disorders and the Heart

Infections and the heart

Infections can affect the circulation in a variety of ways:

1 direct invasion of endocardium, myocardium and pericardium;
2 toxic myocarditis;
3 acute circulatory failure due to toxic effects on the vasomotor centre or peripheral vessels, or to dehydration.

Pericarditis and infective endocarditis are considered in Chapter 9 and will not be discussed in detail here.

Diphtheria

Diphtheria causes an acute myocarditis in approximately 20% of subjects. The myocarditis is due to an exotoxin of the diphtheria bacillus rather than to local infection with the organism. Acute circulatory failure may occur in the first few days but the major cardiovascular effects are more common at the end of the first and during the second week. Tachycardia may be present in the absence of myocardial involvement and may be replaced by a bradycardia due to heart block. Gallop rhythm is common and there may be cardiac enlargement. The myocarditis may lead to cardiogenic shock, sometimes accompanied by cardiac failure.

ECG abnormalities often precede the clinical signs of myocarditis, the commonest change being flattening or inversion of the T waves. All grades of heart block may occur.

The presence of acute myocarditis is suggested by gallop rhythm, cardiomegaly, ECG abnormalities, heart block or cardiogenic shock.

Nearly all infants with acute diphtheritic myocarditis die; the mortality in adults is less than 25%. In those who recover from the acute attack, residual cardiac damage is almost unknown.

Diphtheria should be prevented by immunization; if it occurs the patient requires treatment with antitoxin and penicillin. Electrical pacing may be required for heart block; conduction disorders are seldom, if ever, permanent.

Tuberculosis

Tuberculosis may cause pericarditis, with or without subsequent constriction. It may also be responsible for heart disease secondary to pulmonary fibrosis. Tuberculous myocarditis is very rare.

Virus infections

Viruses cause both pericarditis and myocarditis. Coxsackie viruses of group B are probably the commonest organisms affecting the heart; most infections are subclinical. The clinical picture is usually one of fever, malaise and muscular pains, accompanied by evidence of pericarditis and, if there is myocarditis, tachycardia, gallop rhythm, cardiomegaly and cardiac failure. The ECG usually shows non-specific abnormalities, but there may be ST and T wave changes suggesting pericarditis or myocardial infarction. Blood levels of myocardial enzymes (such as creatine kinase) may be raised transiently. The diagnosis can be made by isolating the organism from the stool or by demonstrating a rise or fall in serum antibodies. Rest is desirable during the acute phase, and return to vigorous activity should be progressive. The patient nearly always recovers completely, but there may be residual myocardial damage and recurrences are not unusual. A myocarditis may also be associated with infectious mononucleosis, acute anterior poliomyelitis and many other virus infections.

Trypanosomiasis (Chagas' disease)

Myocarditis due to infection by *Trypanosoma cruzi* is common in South America. It is transmitted by the bite of infected reduviid bugs. There are two major forms, acute and chronic. Acute Chagas' disease, which occurs predominantly in childhood, may be asymptomatic but can produce tachycardia, cardiomegaly and cardiac failure. Much more important is the chronic form which leads to cardiac failure of insidious onset. It particularly affects men between the ages of 20 and 40. The left ventricle is enlarged, and there may be dyspnoea, chest pain and palpitation. Eventually, right-sided heart failure develops frequently complicated by thrombo-embolic events. Arrhythmias are almost invariable and complete heart block common. The ECG usually shows right bundle branch block. Death is often sudden due to ventricular fibrillation or asystole. Echocardiography shows the features of a dilated cardiomyopathy. Chagas' myocarditis should be suspected when patients who have lived in the tropical or subtropical areas of America develop arrhythmias, cardiac failure and right bundle branch block. A complement fixation test is useful in diagnosis. Treatment is essentially directed at the complications — heart failure, arrhythmias and heart block.

Toxoplasmosis

Toxoplasma gondii can give rise to a myocarditis which may complicate either the disseminated form of the disease, in which there is hepatitis, pneumonia and meningo-encephalitis, or the less acute form which resembles infectious mononucleosis with lymphadenopathy the most obvious abnormality. The myocarditis usually gives rise to tachycardia and may cause heart failure, pericarditis and arrhythmias. Complete recovery is unusual.

Syphilis

Cardiovascular syphilis used to be an important cause of death, but is now uncommon. It seldom affects the myocardium, although gummata can occur. The organism localizes in the aorta soon after the primary infection, but a latent period of 10 to 25 years elapses before clinical evidence of aortitis develops.

The initial lesion involves the vasa vasorum of the aorta which become obliterated. The muscle and elastic tissues of the media necrose and are replaced by scar tissue which becomes calcified. Atherosclerotic changes are frequently superimposed. The lesions are usually most severe immediately above the sinuses of Valsalva, and predominantly affect the ascending aorta. The inner aspect of the aorta appears wrinkled, with radial or parallel grooves. The process may involve the mouths of the coronary arteries producing stenosis and, occasionally, occlusion of the coronary ostia. Damage to the aortic valve ring produces dilatation with aortic regurgitation. Aortic stenosis does not occur. Aneurysms of either saccular or fusiform type may be formed.

The symptoms and signs of syphilitic disease depend mainly on whether there is coronary artery involvement, aortic valve disease or aneurysm formation. Coronary artery stenosis leads to angina pectoris and, rarely, myocardial infarction. Syphilitic aortic regurgitation may cause the clinical features of left-sided cardiac failure. Because syphilitic aortic aneurysms affect predominantly the ascending aorta and arch, the major symptoms are those of chest pain due to erosion of bone, cough and dyspnoea due to pressure on the trachea and bronchi, and hoarseness from paralysis of the left recurrent laryngeal nerve. The aneurysm may be visible in the second or third right intercostal spaces, and a systolic thrill may be palpable in this area. Occasionally, a tracheal tug pulls down the thyroid cartilage with each heart beat. There is often a loud systolic murmur over the aneurysm and the second heart sound may be accentuated.

The ECG appearances depend on the nature of the complications and are not specific. A chest radiograph shows a dilated aorta, often with linear calcification. Aneurysms can be difficult to differentiate from uncoiling of the aorta, which is common in the elderly. The aorta and aortic valve can be assessed by echocardiography but angiography may be needed to delineate coronary ostial stenosis.

Syphilitic aortitis should be suspected if the aorta is conspicuously dilated or aneurysmal, or if there is aortic regurgitation unassociated with stenosis. The diagnosis is confirmed by serological tests specifically directed against the treponemal antigen.

The prognosis is quite good in asymptomatic syphilitic aortitis, survival for 10 or 20 years being probable. The patient is unlikely to live more than 2 or 3 years if there is angina due to coronary stenosis or left ventricular failure due to aortic regurgitation.

Syphilitic cardiovascular disease does not develop if early syphilis is adequately treated. It is uncertain whether treatment of established cardiovascular syphilis is effective in preventing progression. It is customary to give 6 to 12 million units of penicillin over a period of 10 days in an attempt to control the infection. Surgery may be necessary for relief of coronary ostial stenosis, for the correction of aortic regurgitation, or for the repair of an aneurysm.

Endocrine and metabolic diseases

Hyperthyroidism

Hyperthyroidism (thyrotoxicosis) is a syndrome due to an excess of the circulating thyroid hormones T4 and/or T3. This may result from diffuse hyperplasia of the thyroid gland (Graves' disease) or single or multiple hyperactive nodules. Thyroid overactivity is associated with increased oxygen consumption and heat production. The augmentation in cardiac output which occurs in response to these demands, and to the direct effect of thyroid hormone on the heart, is achieved mainly by tachycardia and increased myocardial contractility rather than by an enlarged stroke volume.

The heart has to support the burden of a greatly enhanced cardiac output when its own metabolic requirements are increased. The normal heart may, in these circumstances, be unable to supply an adequate circulation; a diseased heart is likely to fail.

Clear manifestations of cardiac abnormality, such as cardiomegaly or heart failure usually imply that the hyperthyroidism has aggravated underlying heart disease. This is most commonly ischaemic but it may be hypertensive or rheumatic. Occasionally, hyperthyroidism is the sole cause of heart failure.

Most of the cardiovascular features of hyperthyroidism can be accounted for by the hypermetabolic state, but it is difficult to attribute the common complication of atrial fibrillation to this cause. This arrhythmia may be due to a direct toxic effect of the thyroid hormone on the myocardium.

Cardiac symptoms are common in hyperthyroid patients, even in the absence of cardiac disease. Palpitation is particularly frequent, and is usually attributable to the combination of sinus tachycardia and a vigorous cardiac action. Atrial flutter or fibrillation may be responsible for regular or irregular palpitation.

Breathlessness is also common, and can be due to hyperventilation, anxiety or left ventricular failure. Hyperthyroidism may aggravate angina pectoris in those with coronary artery disease. Sinus tachycardia is almost invariable if there is not atrial fibrillation or flutter, and persists during sleep. The pulse is of large volume and may have a collapsing character. The systolic blood pressure is frequently high, whilst the diastolic is normal or low.

The apical impulse is vigorous, but is usually not displaced. The heart sounds are loud, and there is often a pulmonary midsystolic murmur, due to high flow.

Cardiac enlargement and the signs of left- or right-sided heart failure may develop if the thyroid disease is of long standing or if there is coexistent cardiac disease.

The classical features of hyperthyroidism such as weight loss, moist warm extremities, tremor, lid retraction, exophthalmos and goitre are usually present, but these signs may be slight or absent in the older patient. There are no distinctive features on the ECG or chest radiograph.

Hyperthyroidism can be recognized easily if the characteristic features are present, but the diagnosis can be difficult if the abnormalities are largely confined to the cardiovascular system. It should be suspected whenever sinus tachycardia, atrial flutter, atrial fibrillation or cardiac failure are unexplained.

The diagnosis of hyperthyroidism is established by finding abnormally high blood levels of T4 and/or T3 (after allowance has been made for their binding proteins).

Hyperthyroidism may be treated by antithyroid drugs (such as carbimazole, methimazole and propylthiouracil), radio-iodine or partial thyroidectomy. Radio-iodine is the most suitable therapy for most patients with thyrotoxic heart disease (except for women of child-bearing age), but surgery may be indicated if the gland is large or if there is a danger of tracheal compression.

When the rapid control of the tachycardia of hyperthyroidism is necessary, a beta-adrenoceptor blocking drug should be given.

The atrial fibrillation of thyrotoxicosis is difficult to slow adequately with digitalis alone; a beta-blocker should be added if not contraindicated. When thyroid overactivity is controlled, dc shock is usually effective in restoring sinus rhythm.

Heart disease in hyperthyroidism usually responds well to therapy unless it has been untreated for several years.

Hypothyroidism

Hypothyroidism affects the cardiovascular system in several ways.

1 The reduced level of body metabolism is associated with a low cardiac output, a diminished peripheral blood flow, a reduction in venous return, and sinus bradycardia;
2 The deficiency of thyroid hormone seems to be responsible for interstitial oedema and mucoid infiltration of the myocardium, and for a pericardial effusion;
3 The hypercholesterolaemia characteristically present may be responsible for premature coronary atherosclerosis and ischaemic heart disease; the evidence for this is inconclusive;
4 'Myxoedema coma' is associated with hypotension and bradycardia.

The patient with hypothyroidism seldom has cardiac symptoms, except for angina pectoris due to coexistent coronary disease. The symptoms and signs of cardiac failure rarely, if ever, occur in the absence of some additional form of heart disease.

The pulse rate is usually between 50 and 60 per minute. The sluggish apex beat is difficult to feel and the heart sounds are soft.

The ECG is abnormal in showing low voltage of all components of the PQRST complexes; the T waves are flattened or inverted. The chest radiograph reveals a large cardiac shadow, often accompanied by a pericardial effusion; on fluoroscopy, cardiac movement is seen to be diminished.

Hypothyroidism is usually suspected because of the general sluggishness, the cold and thickened skin, the husky voice, the coarse but scanty hair and the slow pulse, but minor forms of the disorder may easily escape detection. Blood levels of T4 and T3 are low. The most sensitive test for primary hyperthyroidism is the high serum level of thyroid-stimulating hormone (TSH) but this is not raised if hypopituitarism is responsible.

Treatment with thyroid substances is effective but may provoke angina pectoris. For this reason, in those suspected of having coronary disease, small doses (e.g. thyroxine 0.0125 mg) should be used initially and the dose should be increased very cautiously, if necessary, but not beyond 0.15 mg. The serum TSH level can be useful as a marker of the adequacy of replacement therapy. The addition of a beta-adrenoceptor blocking drug may protect the patient from angina but often fails, in which case coronary artery bypass surgery may be required.

Carcinoid syndrome

Malignant carcinoid tumours with metastases in the liver may be associated with pulmonary stenosis and regurgitation, and with tricuspid stenosis or regurgitation, the valve cusps being fixed by fibrosis. The cardiac lesions are probably due to the actions of kinins or of 5-hydroxytryptamine (5HT, serotonin) secreted by the tumour. These substances are also responsible for the flushing attacks, telangiectasia, diarrhoea and bronchospasm characteristic of this syndrome.

The cardiac findings in the carcinoid syndrome are those of the particular valve lesion and of right-sided heart failure. The diagnosis is established either by identification of the tumour at laparotomy or by the detection in the urine of large quantities of 5-hydroxy-indole acetic acid (5-HIAA), a breakdown product of 5-HT.

Treatment is unsatisfactory, the diarrhoea may be controlled by codeine, and the flushing by ketanserin (a 5-HT blocker): cardiac failure is treated on conventional lines, valve replacement occasionally being necessary.

Haemochromatosis

In this disorder, which is mainly encountered in older males, there is excessive iron storage associated with cirrhosis of the liver, diabetes and pigmentation of the skin, and a substantial proportion of patients die from a cardiomyopathy, which may be restrictive, but is usually of the dilated congestive type. Treatment of the failure may be temporarily effective as may repeated venesection, but the prognosis is poor.

Gout

There is a statistical association between hyperuricaemia and coronary artery disease, but there is no definite evidence of an increased incidence of coronary disease in those with clinical gout. Gout may be provoked by diuretics; it may occur in severe cyanotic congenital heart disease in association with secondary polycythaemia. It occasionally causes an acute pericarditis.

Glycogen storage disease

In this autosomal recessive disorder, excessive glycogen is deposited in skeletal and cardiac muscle. Breathlessness, feeding difficulties and muscular weakness usually develop about the third month of life and the progression of cardiac failure is relentless. The ECG and the chest radiograph demonstrate biventricular enlargement. Death occurs before the age of 3 years — usually within the first year of life.

Obesity

This is associated with heart disease in a number of ways. In the first place, obese patients often appear to be hypertensive. This is to some extent, but not exclusively, due to falsely high blood pressure recordings in those with fat arms.

A specific Pickwickian syndrome of hypoventilation with carbon dioxide retention, hypoxia, somnolence, polycythaemia and right-sided heart failure is sometimes caused by obesity. The obesity is directly responsible for the hypoventilation because it restricts respiratory movement; improvement can be achieved by weight loss.

Obesity is important in patients with cardiac disease of any type because the demands on the heart are increased. Weight reduction is an essential component in the prevention and treatment of angina pectoris, hypertension, and cardiac failure.

Beri-beri

This disease is due to thiamine deficiency, which is usually the result of a diet with a high proportion of polished rice in eastern countries but is associated with alcoholism in North America and Europe. The deficiency leads to a lack of co-carboxylase which is necessary for the oxidation of pyruvic acid to acetyl coenzyme A. The citric acid cycle is inhibited and the accumulation of lactate and pyruvate may lead to peripheral vasodilatation and impaired cardiac function. The characteristic haemodynamic features are those of a low peripheral vascular resistance and a high cardiac output. Cardiac failure eventually occurs and in the later stages the cardiac output may fall.

The clinical features of beri-beri heart disease include palpitation, fatigue, breathlessness and peripheral oedema. In some cases there may be acute circulatory failure with hypotension and syncope. There is usually sinus tachycardia with a large pulse and right-sided cardiac failure. The heart is enlarged and there may be a gallop rhythm and systolic murmurs.

The neurological features are those of an ascending peripheral neuritis, commonly accompanied by mental confusion. Paraesthesiae occur in the hands and feet and there is weakness of the legs. The calf muscles are tender and areas of anaesthesia occur.

Neither the ECG, which usually shows non-specific T wave changes, nor the chest radiograph, which reveals cardiomegaly, are helpful in diagnosis. This is usually achieved by obtaining a history of nutritional deficiency or of alcoholism, and by finding evidence of both peripheral neuritis and cardiac failure.

Most cases respond quickly to thiamine chloride, 50 mg intramuscularly per day. Subsequently, thiamine should be given orally in dose of 10–20 mg.

Alcoholic cardiomyopathy

There is increasing evidence that a large intake of alcohol, even in the absence of nutritional deficiency, can lead to cardiomyopathy. The patients are often middle-aged men who are excessively fond of both food and alcohol. The initial symptom is either breathlessness or palpitation, due to ectopic beats or atrial fibrillation. The ECG may show low, dimpled T waves. In the early stages, abstinence may reverse the picture, but otherwise there is progression with increasing cardiac failure to death.

Treatment consists of complete abstinence from alcohol and the use of conventional measures for controlling atrial fibrillation and cardiac failure.

Miscellaneous disorders

Rheumatoid arthritis and the connective tissue disorders

Rheumatoid arthritis. This is accompanied by valve disease rather more often than would be expected by chance, although by no means as frequently as is rheumatic fever. Acute pericarditis and pericardial effusion are quite common; pericardial constriction is rare.

Ankylosing spondylitis (rheumatoid spondylitis). This is associated with aortic regurgitation due to focal destruction of the elastica and media of the aorta.

Reiter's disease. This is characterized by urethritis, seronegative arthritis and conjunctivitis. It is sometimes complicated by pericarditis, myocarditis and aortic regurgitation.

Systemic lupus erythematosus. This often affects the heart, although cardiac symptoms and signs seldom dominate the clinical picture. Acute or chronic pericarditis, with or without effusion, is usually the most obvious evidence of cardiac involvement. Myocarditis sometimes develops, and may be due to disease of the small coronary vessels. Endocarditis also occurs, with large warty excrescences which may involve any of the four heart valves. These lesions seldom give rise to clinical heart disease, but may act as a focus for infective endocarditis.

Polyarteritis. This may result in myocardial infarction, or in cardiac failure without evidence of infarction. The heart failure may be, in part, the result of hypertension which is common in this disorder. Pericardial effusions occasionally occur.

Scleroderma. This may lead to cardiac failure either by producing a cardiomyopathy, usually of the constrictive type, or as a result of pulmonary heart disease secondary to diffuse pulmonary fibrosis.

Pseudoxanthoma elasticum. This is a familial disease affecting connective tissue associated with calcification and proliferation of the media of the coronary and peripheral arteries which may give rise to ischaemic heart disease and vascular insufficiency. The skin, particularly in certain areas such as the elbow creases and back of the neck, takes on a crêpe-like appearance with much redundant tissue. Characteristic dark 'angioid' streaks occur in the fundi; there is a liability to hypertension, gastrointestinal haemorrhage and blindness.

The Marfan syndrome

This familial disorder of connective tissue may result in many skeletal, cardiovascular and other abnormalities. These include great height, long limbs with spidery fingers (arachnodactyly), a high arched palate and dislocation of the lens.

A weakness of the aortic media is common and leads to dilatation, aneurysm formation, and dissection. Aortic regurgitation may follow dilatation of the valve ring. Mitral valve disease may result in cusp prolapse and regurgitation.

These abnormalities can be evident in childhood but may not develop until the fifth decade.

There is no specific treatment. Surgery may be required for the valve disorders and aortic disease.

Cardiac tumours

Cardiac tumours are rare. The commonest is the *myxoma* which occurs most frequently in the left atrium, but occasionally in the other chambers. It varies from 1 to 8 cm in diameter, and is usually attached by a pedicle to the atrial septum. Because its position may vary with posture, transient or complete obstruction of the mitral valve may result. The tumour may prolapse into the left ventricle and cause mitral regurgitation. The haemodynamic effects of left atrial myxoma usually resemble those of mitral stenosis. The tumour may also be responsible for embolic phenomena, and can produce constitutional effects such as fever, weight loss, anaemia, finger clubbing, raised sedimentation rate and abnormal serum proteins. The obstruction of the mitral valve may lead to dyspnoea and, rarely, syncope or vertigo related to posture. Variable mitral systolic and diastolic murmurs may be heard, and there may be a loud first sound and opening snap. The diagnosis should be suspected in patients with signs of mitral stenosis, who have a history of syncope, or variable murmurs, or unexplained fever with a high ESR. The diagnosis can be most readily established by echocardiography which demonstrates a mass within the left atrium (Figs. 16.1A and B). The tumour should be removed under cardiopulmonary bypass.

Trauma

Traumatic lesions of the heart may be due to penetrating chest injuries as, for example, from gunshot wounds or stabbing, or from non-penetrating injuries produced by blows to the chest such as steering wheel accidents.

Penetrating injuries may cause lacerations of any of the heart chambers or great vessels, and death may ensue from haemorrhage or cardiac tamponade. If the victim does not die within a few hours, late complications may occur due to infective pericarditis, valve damage or intracardiac shunts. The diagnosis is usually not difficult and can be deduced from the site of the injury, the evidence of blood loss or cardiac tamponade, or ECG abnormalities.

The chest radiograph may be valuable in locating foreign bodies in or around the heart; echocardiography is useful in detecting pericardial fluid. Pericardial aspiration may relieve tamponade, but for the other serious complications, immediate surgery is usually necessary.

Fig. 16.1A Parasternal M-mode echocardiogram of a left atrial myxoma. Multiple echoes are seen behind the anterior mitral valve leaflet in diastole as the tumour prolapses downwards towards the left ventricle. IVS = interventricular septum. T = tumour.

Fig. 16.1B Cross-sectional echocardiogram of myxoma. There is a large tumour (T) situated in the mitral valve orifice.

A substantial proportion of blunt chest injuries seen in hospital have some cardiac damage. This may take the form of myocardial 'concussion' in which there is functional impairment but no structural damage, or 'contusion' in which there is myocardial necrosis. Myocardial infarction may occur from direct trauma to the muscle, or as a consequence of injury to a coronary artery. In either case, any of the complications of infarction may be seen, including arrhythmias, rupture, and aneurysm formation. In addition, valves and chordae tendineae may be ruptured, and haemopericardium and tamponade may occur. Aortic transection is relatively common, particularly in acceleration accidents.

Unless tamponade or murmurs develop, cardiac damage may not be suspected. Chest radiography, ECG and cross-sectional echocardiography should be undertaken in all cases of severe blunt chest trauma. Aortic damage is probably best located by computed tomography. The patient may require surgical treatment for tamponade, aortic rupture or valve regurgitation.

Anaemia and the heart

Anaemia imposes increased demands upon the heart and, at the same time, impairs its function. It aggravates the symptoms of the patient with heart disease and has important circulatory effects even in the individual with a normal heart.

The haemodynamic effects of anaemia probably result mainly from a decrease in blood viscosity and from tissue hypoxia, which is responsible for peripheral vasodilatation. As a consequence, the peripheral arterial resistance is diminished, the diastolic pressure falls and the pulse pressure widens. Ventricular afterload is decreased. The stroke volume and cardiac output are increased when the haemoglobin falls below 7 g/100 ml blood, and both respond to exercise to a greater degree than normal. The hypoxia produces coronary vasodilatation when this is possible, but in the patient with coronary artery disease the ability to dilate is restricted. If anaemia is both severe and prolonged, fatty degeneration of the myocardium takes place.

For the reasons described, anaemia may precipitate or aggravate cardiac failure in the patient with pre-existing heart disease, and it may induce or exacerbate angina in those wth coronary artery disease.

It is rare for either heart failure or angina to develop in anaemic patients with normal hearts, but signs and symptoms may occur in such patients which mimic those of heart disease. Dyspnoea, tachycardia and peripheral oedema are common in patients with chronic and severe anaemia.

Anaemia produces the warm skin and bounding arterial pulse of the high output state. A venous hum in the neck is common. Cardiac enlargement may be seen in the advanced case. The murmur most commonly found in anaemia is systolic and situated in the second or third left intercostal space close to the sternum. It is probably due to turbulence resulting from increased flow and reduced blood viscosity. There is often a loud third heart sound and, in very severe cases, there may be a short mitral mid-diastolic murmur, due to increased flow.

The ECG is usually normal, but non-specific ST and T wave changes may occur and the ST depression of myocardial ischaemia may develop.

The clinical features of anaemia are usually readily corrected either by appropriate drug therapy, or by blood transfusion. Rapid transfusion is dangerous, particularly if there is heart failure; in this situation, it is advisable to use packed cells. If whole blood only is available, a diuretic such as frusemide 40 mg should also be given.

Pregnancy and the heart

Pregnancy imposes a substantial load on the heart and circulation. The cardiac output and blood volume increase from the second month onwards, until, about the 30th week, they are some 30−50% above normal levels at which they remain during the rest of pregnancy. During the last 8 weeks, the inferior vena cava may be obstructed by the uterus when the subject is supine; as a consequence, the cardiac output may fall when this position is assumed. Other factors affecting the cardiovascular system are an increased metabolic rate, a corresponding rise in oxygen consumption, the arteriovenous shunt in the uterus and an elevation in the venous pressure due to the increased blood volume.

These circulatory changes produce characteristic physical signs in the normal pregnant woman. The hands are warm and the pulse is large. A tachycardia is present and the venous pressure slightly raised. The apex beat is vigorous and may be displaced outwards, partly as a consequence of cardiomegaly and partly by the high diaphragm. The high flow almost always produces a soft pulmonary midsystolic murmur and a third heart sound. These are often mistaken for cardiac disease. The chest radiograph shows an increase in cardiac diameter.

The circulatory burden of pregnancy frequently reveals pre-existing heart disease for the first time. Symptoms may start at about week 12 and tend to progress until they may become severe from week 24 onwards. A period of particular danger occurs after delivery, when the sudden reabsorption of blood from the uterus into the circulation may precipitate pulmonary oedema.

Heart disease in pregnancy is frequently rheumatic; mitral stenosis is the most serious lesion encountered. Patients wih tight mitral stenosis may become breathless in early pregnancy and progress to pulmonary oedema or right-sided cardiac failure. Even those with less severe lesions may develop symptoms during the last months or shortly after delivery. Patients with mild mitral stenosis, mitral regurgitation and aortic regurgitation usually tolerate pregnancy well, but may become increasingly breathless.

The management of rheumatic heart disease in the pregnant woman depends upon a number of factors including her age, parity and religious beliefs, the stage of the pregnancy, the nature of the lesion, and the response to treatment. In the patient with severe mitral stenosis, pregnancy should be avoided or deferred until mitral valvotomy has been performed. If such a patient becomes pregnant, a decision should be made before week 16 as to whether valvotomy should be undertaken or the pregnancy terminated. As pregnancy progresses beyond this time, both termination and valvotomy become more hazardous. If the patient is seen for the first time at a later stage of pregnancy, she should be managed medically, for with adequate bed-rest, digitalis and diuretics, the maternal mortality is low.

Patients with rheumatic valve lesions other than mitral stenosis should be managed medically or have the pregnancy terminated.

Prosthetic valves pose a special problem in pregnancy. Warfarin, particularly in the first trimester, may induce congenital abnormalities, but the discontinuation of anticoagulants exposes the patient to an increased risk of thrombo-embolism. Heparin may be preferable for this early phase as well as for the last few weeks of pregnancy. The British Society for Haematology has recommended 10 000 units subcutaneously 12-hourly or 7000 units 8-hourly up to 16 weeks and from 36 weeks to delivery, with warfarin as an alternative from 16 to 36 weeks. If possible, prosthetic valves should not be inserted in women who are likely to become pregnant.

Patients who were born with congenital heart disease are being seen with increasing frequency in pregnancy, but the cardiac abnormality is usually mild or has been corrected by surgery prior to conception. Pregnancy is tolerated well if there is an uncomplicated septal defect or persistent ductus arteriosus. Severe pulmonary hypertension of whatever aetiology is extremely hazardous, with a 25–50% risk of maternal death during the pregnancy or in the puerperium; termination in early pregnancy is to be strongly recommended.

Toxaemia of pregnancy is discussed in Chapter 13.

Cardiomyopathy ('peripartal') of unknown aetiology some-times develops during later pregnancy or the puerperium. Although about one-third of patients recover permanently, there is a risk of progression and of recurrence during subsequent pregnancies.

Termination of pregnancy

With good medical preparation and skilled anaesthesia there is little risk in terminating a pregnancy in the presence of cardiac disease. This procedure is indicated in women with advanced heart disease and severe symptoms in early pregnancy, if they are not suitable candidates for mitral valvotomy. Termination should also be considered for those with less severe disease who would find the care of an additional child burdensome.

Sterilization

This should be considered in patients with heart disease who have completed their families or in whom further pregnancies would be harmful. It should not be undertaken lightly. The religious beliefs of the patient must be respected, the risk of psychological disturbance considered, and the possibility of surgical correction of the cardiac lesion borne in mind.

Contraception

Patients with cardiac disease may wish or need to practise contraception. Advice should be proffered to those for whom pregnancy is temporarily inadvisable.

Oral methods of contraception have the major advantage of reliability. The combined oestrogen and progestogen pill increases the risk of arterial and venous thrombosis, and exacerbates systemic hypertension and pulmonary hypertension. It should, therefore, be avoided in women known to have or be at high risk of these conditions. Women over 35 who smoke should not take the combined oral contraceptive because of the greatly increased risk of cardiovascular disease. Less information is available on the progestogen-only pill, but the risks seem to be substantially less.

Intra-uterine devices are better avoided in congenital and valvar heart disease because of the risk, albeit small, of infective endocarditis.

Further reading

Acromegaly Mather, H.M., Boyd, M.J. & Jenkins, J.S. (1979) Heart size and function in acromegaly. *British Heart Journal 41:* 697.

Alcohol Regan T.J. (1984) Alcoholic cardiomyopathy. *Progress in Cardiovascular Diseases 27:* 141.

Anaemia Varat, M.A., Adolph, R.J. & Fowler, N.O. (1972) Cardiovascular effects of anemia. *American Heart Journal 83:* 415.

Carcinoid syndrome Clarke, B. & Hodgson, H.J.F. (1986) Carcinoid syndrome. *British Journal of Hospital Medicine 35:* 746.

Coxsackie infection Smith, W.G. (1970) Coxsackie B myocarditis in adults. *American Heart Journal 80:* 34.

Friedreich's ataxia Child, J.S., Perloff, J.K. et al. (1986) Cardiac involvement in Friedreich's ataxia. *Journal of the American College of Cardiology 7:* 1370.

Giant cell (cranial) arteritis Huston, K.A. & Hunder, G.G. (1980) Giant cell (cranial) arteritis. *American Heart Journal 100:* 99.

Hypothyroidism Aber, C.P. & Thompson, G.S. (1964) The heart in hypothyroidism. *American Heart Journal 68:* 428.

Marfan syndrome Roberts, W.C. & Honig, H.S. (1982). The spectrum of cardiovascular disease in the Marfan syndrome. *American Heart Journal 104:* 115.

Pregnancy Szekely, P & Snaith, L (1974) *Heart Disease in Pregnancy.* Edinburgh: Churchill.

Sarcoidosis Fleming, H.A. (1986) Sarcoid heart disease. *British Medical Journal 292:* 1095.

Scleroderma Goldman, A.P. & Kotler M.N (1985) Heart disease in scleroderma. *American Heart Journal 110:* 1043.

Syphilis Webster, B., Rich, C., Dense, P.M., Moore, J.E., Nicol., C.S & Padget, P. (1953) Studies in cardiovascular syphilis. *American Heart Journal 46:* 117.

Systemic lupus erythematosus Doherty, N.D. & Siegel, R.J.: (1985) Cardiovascular manifestations of systemic lupus erythematosus. *American Heart Journal 110:* 1257.

Thyrotoxicosis Sandler G. & Wilson, G.M. (1959) Nature and prognosis of heart disease in thyrotoxicosis. *Quarterly Journal of Medicine 28:* 347.

Toxoplasmosis Harvey, H.P.B., McLeod, J.C. & Twitter, J.R. (1966) Myocarditis associated with toxoplasmosis. *Australian Annals of Medicine 15:* 169.

Trauma Taggart, D.P. & Reece, I.J. (1987) Penetrating cardiac injuries. *British Medical Journal 294:* 1630.

Psychological Aspects of Heart Disease

The relationship between psychological factors and heart disease is complex. Many anxious individuals believe, erroneously, that they have heart disease; anxiety and depression often complicate and aggravate organic heart disease.

Psychological factors in the genesis of hypertension and coronary disease

The blood pressure rises acutely on emotion; it is therefore reasonable to speculate that there is a relationship between chronic emotional stress and sustained hypertension. This would be very difficult to establish and, as yet, the evidence is equivocal. Nonetheless, hypertensives and their normotensive children appear to have exaggerated responses to emotional stimuli, and relaxation techniques are antihypertensive in some individuals.

There has been much interest in psychological factors in coronary heart disease. Rosenman and Friedman described a 'specific overt behaviour pattern' which they designated type A, characterized by aggression, ambition, impatience and preoccupation with deadlines. They reported a high incidence of coronary disease in such individuals and have also claimed that they could be trained out of these habits after myocardial infarction, with beneficial results. Some have confirmed their observations; others have not. If what they say is true, it is surprising that coronary disease is now commonest amongst manual workers. Other psychological characteristics have been related to coronary disease — perhaps the most persuasive evidence points to hostility as a risk factor. There is certainly little to suggest the view that stressful occupations (traditionally doctors and lawyers) lead to coronary disease.

On the other hand, there can be no doubt of the importance of emotional stress in precipitating episodes of angina pectoris. Rarely, there is strong circumstantial evidence that emotional stress has been a contributory factor in causing myocardial infarction or fatal arrhythmias.

Anxiety state and the heart

Individuals with an anxiety state often have complaints suggestive of heart disease. A large number of labels have been applied to the complex of symptoms of such patients, including 'effort syndrome', 'cardiac neurosis' and 'neurocirculatory asthenia'. It is particularly common in the armed services during war-time, and has therefore been called 'soldier's heart', but it also occurs frequently in civilians.

Breathlessness, palpitation and fatigue are almost invariable, and are usually accompanied by feelings of faintness and dizziness. Chest pain is less common, but is often the reason for referral to a physician.

The breathlessness may be related to exertion, but also occurs at rest. Frequent complaints are that 'I can't take a deep breath' or 'I can't get enough air'. The palpitation is usually the awareness of a sinus tachycardia, but can be due to ectopic beats which cause the patient to think that his heart is about to stop.

The chest pain of anxiety state is usually situated in the left sub-mammary region but may be elsewhere in the left chest and may radiate to the left arm. It is sometimes provoked by effort, but tends to come on after exercise rather than during it; it can develop at rest and at night time. It often takes the form of a persistent ache lasting for hours or days; sharp momentary stabs of pain are also frequent. The patient will often say that the pain is 'in his heart'. The muscles in the area may be tender, and in some cases the pain can be abolished by infiltration with local anaesthetics.

Whilst recounting his history, the patient gives an impression of distress, and is tense or rather withdrawn in manner. Sighing respiration is common and there may be hyperventilation. Sinus tachycardia is usual, and palpation reveals a hyperdynamic heart. The hands are often sweaty but cool; there may be a coarse tremor.

The ECG confirms sinus tachycardia and may show non-specific flattening or slight inversion of T waves.

The diagnosis can usually be made from the characteristic symptoms and from observing the patient. The poor relationship of the breathlessness and pain to exertion, and the site, character and duration of the chest discomfort differentiate the syndrome from angina pectoris. The palpitation can be distinguished from that of paroxysmal tachycardia by the lack of sudden onset and by the relationship to emotion.

The prognosis with regard to the relief of symptoms is poor if it is a chronic condition or if there is a serious personality derangement. If the complaints have occurred in response to an obvious emotional stress, the outlook is relatively good. When anxiety about the heart has been induced by the thoughtless or ill-informed comments of physicians, it is particularly difficult to eradicate.

Psychiatric treatment is necessary for the more severe cases, but strong reassurance by the physician may be effective in those patients in whom cardiac symptoms predominate, particularly when an unfounded fear of organic heart disease has provoked them. The patient should be instructed to embark upon a pro- gramme of gradually increasing physical activity. Sometimes, it may be necessary to give tranquillizers such as diazepam (Valium) 2−5 mg three times a day. Propranolol in a dose of 10 or 20 mg four times a day is helpful if the palpitation of sinus tachycardia is distressing.

Psychological disturbances in patients with heart disease

Many individuals equate heart disease with total disability and death. Patients with cardiac disorders may regard themselves and be considered by others as 'invalids', even though their lesion may be of little importance or be correctable.

Fear of sudden death is common in those who experience angina and palpitation. Anxiety and depression are important causes of symptoms and disability in patients who have sustained a myocardial infarction or have undergone coronary surgery (see Chapter 8). Headache in hypertensive patients is usually due to tension and only rarely to the high blood pressure.

Excessive anxiety can be prevented by thoughtful management of the patient and his relatives. Frankness should be combined with optimism. One must be careful in one's choice of words; if such terms as angina, murmur or heart failure are to be used, they must be explained in such a way that they do not cause alarm.

Advanced heart disease can cause confusion and delirium as a result of hypoxia or hypotension or, when associated with pulmonary disease, carbon dioxide retention. Similar symptoms may arise from lignocaine overdosage, or following cardiac sur- gery. Depression may result from a number of cardiac drugs including methyldopa. Fatigue is common in patients on beta- blocking drugs. These psychological disturbances, which are sec- ondary to medical disorders, should be treated by correcting the underlying cause.

Surgery and the Heart

Anaesthesia and general surgery in patients with heart disease

Anaesthesia is potentially hazardous in the patient with heart disease because it may cause hypoxaemia, hypercapnia, hypotension and cardiac arrhythmias; these complications can be almost completely avoided by skilful management. The choice of anaesthetic technique is dependent on the type and severity of the cardiac lesion and the nature of the operation being undertaken.

The period of induction is particularly dangerous, as hypotension may result from the intravenous barbiturates commonly used, and endotracheal intubation may stimulate vagal reflexes with resultant bradycardia, heart block or asystole. The dose of barbiturates should be small; muscle relaxants facilitate quick intubation. Halothane may be employed for maintenance of anaesthesia but should be avoided if a fall in blood pressure is undesirable; it causes direct myocardial depression. Spinal, epidural and regional anaesthesia cause little myocardial depression, but may produce hypotension, especially in the hypovolaemic patient.

Patients with heart disease often tolerate major operations without serious complication but the necessity for surgery must always be balanced against the cardiac risks. The greatest problems usually arise in those with ischaemic heart disease because hypotension may provoke serious arrhythmias or result in myocardial infarction. These risks diminish as time passes after a coronary occlusion, being high during the first 3 months, and reaching a relatively low level by the end of a year. Only surgery which cannot safely be deferred should be undertaken in those who have had a myocardial infarction within the preceding 6 months. On the other hand, when a patient has survived a year or more after a myocardial infarction without major disability, it is reasonable to consider cholecystectomy, prostatectomy and other major, but relatively elective, procedures. Nonetheless the patient should be carefully monitored over the succeeding 2—3 days.

Hypertensive patients usually tolerate surgery well, provided no sharp fall in blood pressure is permitted. It is generally wiser to continue the antihypertensive therapy, with close observation of the blood pressure during and after the procedure.

Major surgery should, if possible, be avoided in those with severe heart valve disease; it is better to defer this until the valve lesion has been corrected. However, if prosthetic valve surgery is contemplated, it may be preferable to carry out general surgery first in order to avoid operating on a patient receiving anticoagulants.

Particular care is required in the presence of pulmonary heart disease. Affected patients tolerate surgery poorly, and are susceptible to respiratory infection, pulmonary collapse and bronchitis postoperatively. It is important that these individuals stop smoking some weeks prior to surgery and are free of pulmonary infection.

Cardiac failure and arrhythmias should always be brought under control as far as possible prior to surgery. Complete heart block should be managed by temporary or permanent insertion of an endocardial pacemaking electrode. Special care is needed when electro-cautery is used in the presence of an implanted pacemaker; advice from the cardiologist responsible for the patient is necessary.

Fluid and electrolyte balance is of great importance in these patients. Large volumes of fluid are required during major surgery. Patients are usually fluid depleted before they come to the operating theatre and lose substantial amounts (from the wound and the respiratory tract) during this procedure. Particular attention should be paid to avoiding or correcting hypovolaemia.

Surgery for heart disease

Indications and contraindications

Most types of congenital and rheumatic heart disease are amenable to surgical treatment (for discussion of individual lesions see Chapters 11 and 12). Surgery also has a major part to play in the management of ischaemic heart disease, infective endocarditis, pericardial constriction and in diseases of the aorta. In deciding whether surgery is necessary in an individual case, one must weigh up the prognosis of the patient without surgery and the risks of morbidity and mortality imposed by surgery. For example, most patients with atrial septal defects or persistent ductus arteriosus are asymptomatic, but have a life expectancy reduced to about 40 years. Surgery in childhood is justified in these cases because the mortality is very low. At the other end of the scale, severe aortic stenosis carries a very poor prognosis and surgery should be undertaken in spite of a mortality which commonly exceeds 5%. Contraindications to surgery include poor left ventricular function, extreme pulmonary hypertension and advanced disease of other organs such as the brain, liver and lungs.

Types of cardiac surgery

Cardiac surgery may be 'closed' or 'open'. In closed-heart surgery, the circulation continues through the patient's heart throughout the operation, and the interior of the heart is not inspected. The operations are relatively simple and safe but are limited in scope to such procedures as mitral and pulmonary valvotomy, pericardiectomy for pericardial constriction, division of persistent ductus arteriosus, resection of coarctation and shunt operations for tetralogy of Fallot. In experienced hands, the mortality of these operations is low, but postoperative complications include systemic embolism (after mitral valvotomy), arrhythmias, pulmonary collapse and infection, pulmonary embolism and the postcardiotomy syndrome.

In total cardiopulmonary bypass, the heart and lungs are completely excluded from the circulation. Venous blood is drained by gravity into an oxygenator through cannulae inserted into the inferior and superior venae cavae. A pump is used to recirculate the blood through a cannula positioned in the aorta (Fig. 18.1). When operations are undertaken on the mitral valve, the aortic valve prevents regurgitation into the left ventricle of the blood pumped into the aorta by the artificial heart—lung apparatus. When operations are being carried out on the aortic valve, the aorta must be clamped below the origin of the innominate artery to permit a dry surgical field. The coronary arteries may be supplied with blood through special coronary cannulae. Hypothermia is often employed, either through the use of a heat exchanger or by directly cooling the surface of the heart.

With total cardiopulmonary bypass, the cerebral circulation is maintained, and operations on the open heart lasting up to 5 hours can be performed. The potential risks are considerable; the major hazards are cerebral air embolism, trauma to blood by the pump-oxygenator, and electrolyte and acid—base disturbances. The lungs often become abnormally stiff in the postoperative phase, and the pulmonary atelectasis and infection are common. If perfusion has been inadequate, renal failure may occur. In the first few days after operation, arrhythmias are frequent, because of the trauma to the heart and because perfusion may lead to hypokalaemia and unmask digitalis toxicity.

Open-heart surgery with total bypass is suitable for all surgically treatable lesions. Because of the risks involved, it should be undertaken only by an experienced team of surgeons, anaesthe-

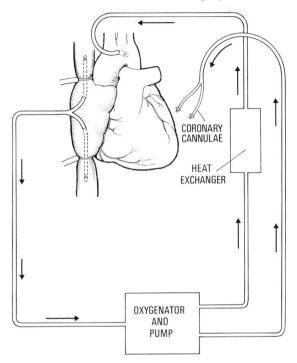

CORONARY
CANNULAE

HEAT
EXCHANGER

OXYGENATOR
AND
PUMP

Fig. 18.1 Cardiopulmonary bypass. Venous blood drains from cannulae in the venae cavae into an oxygenator, and is then returned to the femoral artery or aorta by a pump. The temperature of the perfusing blood can be controlled with a heat pump. The coronary arteries can be selectively perfused.

tists and ancillary staff. In the best hands, the mortality of the bypass technique itself is less than 1%.

The postoperative management of the patient subjected to open-heart surgery is more difficult than that of closed-heart surgery, the risks of haemorrhage, pulmonary complications and arrhythmias being increased.

The replacement of heart valves (see also Chapter 11)

Heart valves may be replaced by prostheses, homografts or heterografts. In appropriately selected cases, valve replacement leads to the amelioration or abolition of symptoms and striking haemodynamic improvement.

There is a large variety of prosthetic valves available, of which the Starr—Edwards ball valve has been the most widely used

(Fig. 18.2). With all artificial valves, there is a risk of thrombosis and of infection in relation to the prosthesis, and of haemolysis. Long-term anticoagulant therapy is necessary to prevent embolism; it is particularly important that good control is maintained. The INR should be kept between 3.0 and 4.5. If homograft or heterograft valves are used, haemolysis is rare and anticoagulants are unnecessary unless there is some other indication, such as atrial fibrillation.

Prosthetic valves produce characteristic clicks, a mitral prosthesis causing a 'first sound' and 'opening snap', and an aortic prosthesis an 'ejection click' and 'aortic second sound'. The mechanical prostheses now available seem likely to maintain their function for many years, but are liable to be the source of emboli and of infection. Bioprostheses are not prone to thrombosis. They are liable to deteriorate after a period of 7−10 years, especially in the young. For this reason, heterografts should be avoided in children and young adults; homografts are more satisfactory in the young.

Intra-aortic balloon pumping (counterpulsation)

Mechanical support may be given to the circulation by a balloon introduced via a femoral artery into the descending thoracic aorta which is inflated in diastole and deflated in systole by an external pump. This reduces afterload and increases coronary and peripheral diastolic blood flow. It greatly improves the patient with poor cardiac performance, particularly immediately after bypass surgery. It is of value in cardiogenic shock, as after myocardial

Fig. 18.2 Starr−Edwards caged ball prosthesis in the aortic valve position.

infarction, only if it allows the patient to survive until some corrective surgical procedure can be undertaken.

Cardiac transplantation

Cardiac transplantation is now an established treatment for patients in advanced cardiac failure whose expectation of life is not thought to exceed 6–12 months. The results have progressively improved, particularly since the introduction of cyclosporin. The upper age limit for the procedure is 50–60, depending on the centre. Many transplant recipients return to nearly normal lives. Survival averages some 80% at 1 year and 65% at 2 years. Immunosuppressant therapy has to be carefully monitored. One as yet unresolved problem is the rapid development of coronary disease in many of the transplanted hearts.

Combined heart and lung transplantation has had some measure of success, but long-term results at present are not so good as heart transplants.

Artificial (mechanical) heart replacements are still in the experimental phase.

Further reading

Bonchek, L.J. (1981) Current status of cardiac valve replacement. *American Heart Journal 101:* 96.
Goodwin, J.F. (1986) Cardiac transplantation. *Circulation 74:* 913.
Schroeder, J.S. & Hunt, S.A. (1986) Cardiac transplantation: where are we? *New England Journal of Medicine 315:* 961.

Index

Mexiletine, 83
Micturation syncope, 94
Minoxidil, 275
Mitral atresia, 250
Mitral regurgitation, 217−221
  pregnancy, 312
  with,
    mitral stenosis, 214
    tricuspid regurgitation, 236
Mitral replacement, 216
Mitral stenosis, 205−216
  pregnancy, 312
  with,
    mitral regurgitation, 214
    tricuspid stenosis, 234
Mitral valve, 7, 8, 204
  disorders,
    atresia, 250
    pregnancy and, 312
    prolapse, 217
    regurgitation, 214,
      217−221, 236
    stenosis, 205−216
  replacement, 216
  valvotomy, 215−216
Mitral valve prolapse, 217
Mitral valvotomy, 215−216
Mortality, 1
  diphtheria, 298
  myocardial infarction,
    167−168
  surgery, 319−320
Murmurs, heart, 110−112
  classification of intensity,
    112
  continuous, 116
  diastolic,
    early, 115, 231
    mid-, 115−116
    presystolic, 116
  misinterpretation, 214
  systolic, 114−115
    benign, 114
    mid-, 112−113
    pan-, 113
Musculoskeletal pain,
  147−148

Mustard's operation, 258
Myocardial infarction, 154−155
  complications,
    early, 156−160
    late, 174
  defined, 137
  diagnosis, 166−167
  ECG, 160−164
  echoradiography, 166
  pericarditis comparison, 180
  physical signs, 155−156
  prognosis, 167−168
  pulmonary embolism
    comparison, 287
  radionuclide studies,
    165−166
  rehabilitation and secondary
    prevention, 174−175
  serum enzymes, 164−165
  treatment, 77, 168−174
Myocardial ischaemia, 90−91
Myocarditis, 186−187, 298, 307
Myocardium
  contractility, 5−6
    impaired, 12
    increased, 19
  normal functioning, 2−9
  perfusion studies, 128−129
  see also Cardiomyopathy;
    Myocardial infarction;
    Myocarditis
Myosin filaments, 2−3
Myxoma, 308

Nephritis, chronic, 264
Neurocirculatory asthenia,
  316−317
Neuroendocrine system,
  heart failure response, 13−14
New York Heart Association,
  patient classification, 95−96
Nicotinic acid, 142
Nifedipine, 152
Nitrate treatment, 149−150
Nitroglycerin, 150
Nitroprusside, 275
Nodal ectopic beats, 56

Nodal rhythm, 57
Nodules,
in finger and toe tips, 192
subcutaneous, 199

Obesity, 142, 305
Oedema, 27, 92
Opiate treatment, 168
Optic fundus,
examination, 269
Oral contraception, 268, 313
Orthopnoea, 88
Oxygen therapy,
pulmonary heart disease,
296–297

P wave, 38
Pacemakers
artificial, 76–78
natural, 32–33, 53
Palpation,
abdomen, 106
chest, 103–106
Palpitation, 91–92
Pancarditis, 198
Papillary muscle,
rupture and malfunction,
160, 217
Paracentesis,
pericardial, 186
Paroxysmal nocturnal
dyspnoea, 88–89
Partial thromboplastin time
(PTT), 170
Percussion,
heart, 106
Pericardial effusion, 121,
181–182, 306
Pericardial friction (rub), 117
Pericardial tamponade,
182–183
Pericarditis,
acute, 178–181
constrictive, 183–185
Pericardium, 178
calcification, 121
friction (rub), 117
effusion, 121, 181–182, 306

paracentesis, 186
tamponade, 182–183
see also Pericarditis
Peritoneum,
ascites, 92
Phaeochromocytoma, 266–267
Phonocardiogram, 106
Phosphodiesterase inhibitors,
19
Pleurisy, 180
Pneumonia,
pulmonary infarction
comparison, 288
Pneumothorax, spontaneous,
180
Polyarteritis, 307
Polyarthritis, 198–199
Porphyria, acute, 268
Post-cardiotomy syndrome, 216
Post-myocardial infarction
syndrome, 174
Postural syncope, 95
Potassium ions,
depletion, 21
PR interval, 39, 70
Prazosin, 274
Pre-eclampsia, 267, 271
Pre-excitation, *see*
Wolff–Parkinson–White
syndrome
Pre-hospital care,
of myocardial infarction
patients, 170
Pregnancy, 116, 311–313
congenital heart disease and,
239–240
pre-eclampsia, 267, 271
Preload, 4, 10
Prinzmetal's angina, 138
Procainamide, 82
Propafenone, 83
Prothrombin ratios, 171,
285–286
Pseudoxanthoma elasticum,
307
Psychological disturbances,
anxiety state, 316–317